The Surgery of Master Jehan Yperman

(1260?—1330?)

BOOKS I and II
Translated in French From Old Flemish From Manuscripts At Cambridge And Brussells, With An introduction By

Doctor A. De Mets

Paris
Editions Hippocrate
7 Rue des Grandes-Degrés
MCMXXXVI

and

BOOKS III THROUGH VII
Translated In Italian, From The Same Mss And The Ghent Codex
As "Jehan Yperman, Padre della Chirurgia Fiamminga" With Introduction and Notes By Mario Tabanelli

Firenze
Leo S. Olschki Editore
MCMLXIX

ENGLISH TRANSLATION
By Leonard D. Rosenman, M.D
San Francisco
1996-2002

To order additional copies of this book, contact:
Xlibris Corporation
1-888-795-4274
www.Xlibris.com
Orders@Xlibris.com
16654-ROSE

THE SURGERY OF MASTER JEAN YPERMAN

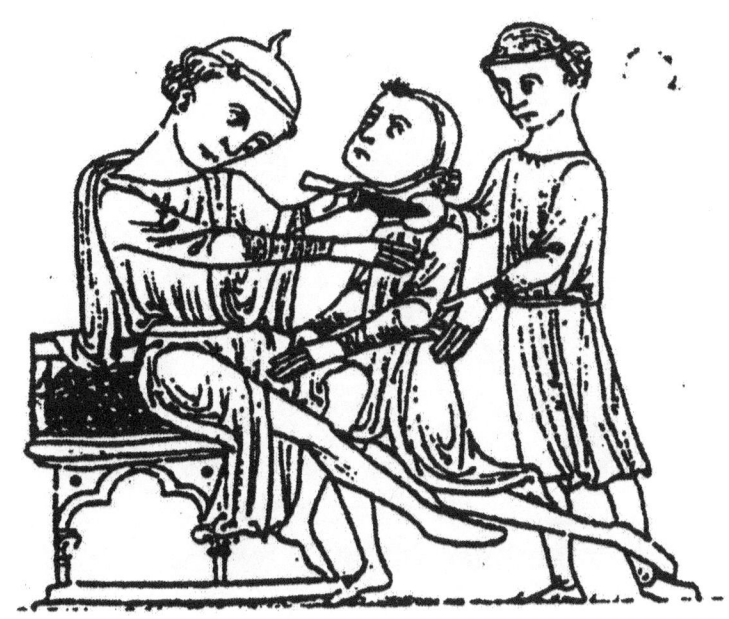

Frontispiece

SURGEON CUTTING FOR GOITER

Plate 46 from
THE MEDIEVAL SURGERY
By Tony Hunt
(see Bibliography, page 21)

For Susan, David, John and Amy

Contents

THE SURGERY OF JEHAN YPERMAN BOOK I
THE HEAD

BOOK II: THE EYE AND THE TREATMENT OF OCULAR DISEASES, ACCORDING TO THE INSTRUCTION OF MASTER JEHAN YPERMAN.

BOOK THREE: THE NOSE

BOOK IV THE MOUTH AND ITS CONTENTS

BOOK V THE EAR

BOOK VI THE NECK AND THE THROAT

BOOK VII THE BODY BELOW THE NECK: THREE PARTS

PART I
FORTY CHAPTERS FROM THE BRUSSELLS CODEX

PART II FIFTY-ONE CHAPTERS FROM THE CAMBRIDGE CODEX

PART III ELEVEN CHAPTERS TAKEN FROM THE GHENT CODEX

ENGLISH TRANSLATOR'S NOTE AND BIBLIOGRAPHY

During the one hundred fifty years preceding Yperman's activity as a surgeon, the profession was reborn in Europe, growing from seeds brought from the orient and from scraps discovered in Byzantine monasteries. The seeds and the scraps had Greek and Roman sources. During those one hundred fifty years only a few names remain marked large for us to remember as founding fathers: they are Roger Frugard, Roland of Parma, Bruno of Longoburgo, William of Saliceto, Lanfranchi of Milan, the unnamed Four Salernitan Masters, Hugh of Lucca, Theodoric of Bologna, Jean Pitard, Henri de Mondeville, Jean Yperman. I draw a line to separate the epochs of Yperman and his contemporary Henry of Mondeville from their more famous follower, Guy de Chauliac. The last named was different from the others before him and he may be considered more as a forerunner of the great renaissance in surgery that came with the famous men of the 16th C; our earlier surgeons were the links to the past, whose discoveries reawakened Europe to the possibilities of surgical treatments.

All the earlier group were Italians with three exceptions, Henri de Mondeville, Pitard and Yperman. However, all of them had Italian teachers, among them Lanfranchi who, in mid-career, left Milan and became a Parisian. Yperman alone from the north was Flemish. Like today's mid-western American students who attend Ivy-League universities or who attain to Rhodes scholarships at Oxford in England, and who return to their homes with adopted mannerisms and habits of dress and with altered accents of speech, so did Yperman return to Ypres to flaunt the Frenchness of his Parisian years

Of the less than a dozen remembered names we have original writings of only eight, not counting the glosses of the Four Salernitan Masters. They are Roger, Roland (who reproduced Roger's book with some additions), Bruno, Theodoric, William, Lanfranchi, Henri and Yperman. Now we have modern English translations of all of their surgical books, and four, including this volume, are in print: Roger, Roland, Bruno and Yperman.[1] The French translation (1936) by Dr. DeMets and the Italian translation by Tabanelli (1969) are the sources for the English edition of Yperman which follows here. It will provide easier access for English-speaking students who are interested in our surgical antecedents, easier than the French and Italian—and in part Flemish—versions provided by Dr. DeMets and Tabanelli. Furthermore, this translation is rendered from the viewpoint of and with the comments and notations of an experienced modern surgeon.

One may ask why do we save Yperman's curiously confused book for posterity? It lacks the orderliness of some of his predecessors and it does not have the greater detail and more complete resources of his coeval's. One finds seemingly careless repetitions which suggest that the author wrote it piecemeal between frequent and often-long interruptions when he was called to serve in his primary role as a military surgeon. His phrases often are tortured, a sign that in spite of his better-than-ordinary education, he remained a home grown Flemish soldier who was not expected to be literary and capable of writing elegant Latin. Perhaps that was one reason that he wrote in the familiar tongue, by necessity rather than only by choice.

What can we discover in his book? We see in it the dispersion into the northern Flemish hinterlands of the conflicts among the medical professionals that began when Louis IX of France granted Jean Pitard the privileges of academic status for surgeons, and which led to the flowering of the College of St. Comé which came after the arrival at Paris of Lanfranchi, the Milanese. Yperman's book is prideful and

---

1See my Bibliography, below. Short sections of Roger Frugard's, Lanfranchi's and Henri de Mondeville's books were Englished by Prof. Michael McVaugh in *A Source Book in Medieval Science*, E. Grant, Editor, Cambridge, Harvard Univ. Press, 1974. Drs. LM Zimmerman and I Veith translated a short piece from Yperman and another from Mondeville in their *Great Ideas in the History of Surgery*, Baltimore, Williams and Wilkins, 1961. CG Cumston translated parts of Mondeville, mostly from the Antidotary. in Buffalo Medical Journal, Vol 58, 1903, pp486-504; 549-565; 642-656 (LDR).

disdainful of the practices of the unlettered practitioners, many of whom were outright charlatans who deserved his disdain. Yperman sheds light on those early turf battles and shows us how far back in the centuries go the same sort of arguments that beset us today. However, if one wishes to see the town-gown conflict in its first great scenes he should read Henry of Mondeville's book. Yperman expressed similar attitudes but he was less wordy than the Frenchman.

Next, Yperman is of interest because he was the first medieval surgeon who wrote in a language that could be read by those who knew only a mother tongue. He wrote in his local Flemish (Thiois) with occasional bits in Picardese-French and Latin.

Third, we find expression of a defensive attitude that we do not find so strongly stated by the Italians of that era. Yperman offers us a 13thC version of what we in the last decade of the 20th C call "outcome credentialing". Yperman more than once warns the surgeon not to undertake to treat a certain patient or to use a certain treatment lest he expose himself, as the surgeon, to criticism from his competitors or to defamation by an unhappy patient or by the survivors. His warnings oppose such actions not so much because they may destroy a patient or because they may fail in a desperate situation when there is only a small hope for a successful outcome; rather he says don't do it because it will reflect badly on you, and that may impair your career as a Master Surgeon!

Fourth, Yperman gives us some good advices about techniques that are not far from what we consider good surgery today. For example, observe his instructions about the placement of incisions for cosmetic benefit and for small scars. Although it is not nearly as complete as those found in Henry's or Guy's books, the list of his medications has its own charm for those who are curious. The Compendium Surgical Pharmacopeia in Appendix I, is added by this translator; it contains all of the items mentioned in the translations of De Mets and Tabanelli.

Yperman's Treatise had seven Books; the numbering of them is confused among the various codices, and I shall ignore that confusion here. Dr. De Mets translated only portions of the few manuscripts of *Chirurgia* which had been discovered in the nineteenth century and Tabanelli has accepted the invitation in the final paragraphs of De Mets' edition and has offered a more complete work.[2] This English translation contains the two Books in De Mets' edition and the last five in Tabanelli's.

While all translators, including the great ones in all languages, seem apologetic or at least a little embarrassed, they all seem to agree that the original can only be diluted in translation, as if a great wine has been watered. Yet most scholars agree that new translations are necessary for new generations of readers, leaving unanswered the question why the originals maintain through the centuries their untarnished qualities for the readers who can see the authors' own words. And we all agree that translations of translations are suspicious items.

Yet consider Yperman who read Bruno's and Theodoric's medieval Italianate Latin—they who cited Constantine's African Latin—who in turn had translated the Greeks and the Arabs, who got theirs from the Greek of Galen and of others who wrote in Rome and Byzantium and Alexandria. Yperman wrote in his district-Flemish (Thiois) which De Mets took into French, and Tabanelli took – with some of it from Latin copies—into Italian. And here I offer both of the last two moderns in English. The text is translated with an intent to conserve meaning rather than to make literal transformations. I have changed the arrangements in many sentences and paragraphs and I have altered punctuation marks for the sake of a clear English text.

This offering is not meant to ring true the sounds of medieval Flemish, yet I hope that the reader will get the 'feel' of a medieval surgeon's problems, his skills and his attitudes. The reader may evince wonderment how he managed to cure anyone, lacking the tools that we today find in our hospitals and clinics. To that end I insert the insights and an overview of an experienced surgeon. "But to clarify what was ambiguous in the original is not translation but explication"[3]. So be it; the many parentheses and footnotes are explicative. The translator, as usual, apologizes, yet only half-way.

2. Tabanelli, p.7: "Here for the first time the complete Chirurgia of Jehan Yperman is presented in a modern language, translated from the ancient Flemish." (T)

3. Sidney Alexander, translator of F. Guicciardini, *The History of Italy*, (1561), MacMillan Company, New York, 1960, p xxix.

The Pharmacopeia in Appendix I is taken from my *Medieval Surgical Pharnacopeia and Formulary* (see Bibliography). In that compendium, all the medications mentioned in De Met's and Tabanelli's books are explained and their use by Yperman is marked by a **Y.** Most of the medicines will be numbered in parentheses only when they are first mentioned in the text, to identify them in the Pharmacopeia. Those with common names (celery, carrot. etc.) do not require additional indicators

The Names and Places that are cited in the Glossaries of De Mets and Tabanelli are combined in Appendix II. The works of authors cited in the text and in the footnotes are annotated in the several bibliographies as well as in Appendix II.

Acknowledgments

I thank the patient librarians at the Mount Zion Hospital of UCSF for assistance whenever needed, Mme. O. LePendu for assistance with obscure French phrases, and Mr. William Wright for his careful and meticulous proof-reading.

This English translation is a product of the Department of Surgery at The Mount Zion Hospital of the University of California at San Francisco, encouraged and supported by the Chairman, Professor Orlo H. Clark. Also, I am deeply indebted to the Mount Zion Health Fund for assistance in publishing this book.

The De Mets edition of 1936 is long out-of-print, and to the best of my knowledge its Publisher is no longer in existence. However, Sig. Alessandro Olschki, the proprietor of Casa Editrice Leo S. Olschki at Florence, Italy, has kindly permitted me to use Professor Tabanelli's Italian edition of Yperman's *Chirurgia*. The color-plate of the Zodiacal Man is reproduced with the kind permission of Mr.G.Miller of the George Braziller Company. The Frontispiece is taken with permission from Tony Hunt's edition of The Trinity College Ms.of Roger's Chirurgia.

TYPOGRAPHICAL NOTES

Comments by me inserted pari passu in the text are in parentheses that begin with (ie). The few footnotes inserted by DeMets all end with (DM), those by Tabanelli with (T). The many footnotes inserted by me all end with (LDR).[4]

BIBLIOGRAPHY

Albucasis. *On Surgery and Instruments.* transl. by MS Spink and GL Lewis. Univ. of California Press, Berkeley. 1973. The Surgery is the last of Albucasis' grand medical compendium of thirty treatises published just before or after 1000.

Baas, JH. *Outlines of the History of Medicine,* Transl. and supplemented by HE Henderson. reprinted by Krieger Publishing Co., Inc. Huntington, NY, 1971. from the original German edition of 1889

Bruno of Longoburgo. see Tabanelli (Bruno)

Daremberg, Charles. *Introduction To The Glosses Of The Four Salernitan Masters.* in S. De Renzi's Collectio Salernitana, Vol. III, pp. 205-254. English transl.by LD Rosenman in *The Surgery of Roland of Parma.* see below, Tabanelli (Roland)

Four Salernitan Masters. See Daremberg and Roland

Guy de Chauliac. See Nicaise.

Henri de Mondeville. See Nicaise

Hunt, Tony. *Popular Medicine in Thirteenth-Century England.* Woodbridge, Suffolk, The Boydell Press, 1990

Hunt, Tony. *The Medieval Surgery.* Woodbridge, Suffolk, The Boydell Press, 1992.

Lanfranchi of Milan. *The Science of Surgery* (1295). From a Middle-English Ms. of 1380. Edited by Robert von Fleischhacker. Early English Text Society. London, 1894. Engl. transl. by LD Rosenman. 1999. Awaiting publ.

---

4 The authors cited in the text are in the Biographical Appendix II (LDR).

Nicaise, E. Guy de Chauliac's *Grand Chirurgie*, 1363; edited and translated by EN. Germer, Balliere et Cie, Paris, 1890

Nicaise, E. Henri de Mondeville's *Chirurgie*,1306-1320; edited and French transl. by EN. Germer, Balliere et Cie, Paris, 1893. Engl. transl. by LD Rosenman, 1998, awaiting publication.

Roger Frugard see Stroppiana and Spallone

Roland of Parma. See Tabanelli

Rosenman, LD. *A Medieval Surgical Pharmacopeia and Formulary*, 1999. Awaiting publication

Sarton, George. *Introduction to the History of Science.* Williams and Wilkins Company, Baltimore. Three Vol. 1927-1948

Stroppiana,L. and D. Spallone, *The Chirurgia Of Roger Frugard.* Rome. Istituto di Storia Della Medicina Della Universita Di Roma, 1957. English transl. by LD Rosenman, Philadelphia, Xlibris Co., 2002

Tabanelli, Mario. An Italian Surgeon of the Thirteenth Century, Bruno of Longoburgo. Leo. S Olschki, Florence. 1970. Engl. transl. by LD Rosenman, Pittsburgh, Dorrance Publishing Co. 2002.

Tabanelli, Mario. *La Chirurgia Italiana Nell'Alto Medioevo. Ruggiero (pp.x-105)-Rolando-Theodorico.* Leo S Olschki, Firenze. 1965. An English transl. of *The Surgery of Roland of Parma*, with *An Introduction To The Glosses Of The Four Salernitan Masters*, by LD Rosenman. Philadelphia, Xlibris Company, 2002

Theodoric Of Bologna. The Surgery. edited and English transl. by E.Cambbell and J. Colton. Appleton-Century-Crofts, Inc. Two vol. 1955 and 1960

William of Saliceto. Chirurgie. edited and French Transl. by P. Pifteau. Imprimerie Saint—Cyprien, Toulouse.1898. Engl. transl. by LD Rosenman, 1997. awaiting publ.

Both Dr. De Mats and Professor Tabanelli wrote extensive and detailed Introductions for their books, dealing mostly with the same materials. I have used De Mets' Introduction as the basis for the following section—it antedated Tabanelli's by thirty years – and have supplemented it with Tabanelli's carefully wrought additions placed in footnotes.

The Surgery
of Master Jehan Yperman

BOOKS I and II

BOOKS III THROUGH VII

INTRODUCTION

Little more than one century has elapsed since first were revealed to the general public the works and the name of a Flemish surgeon who had lived during the 13th and 14th centuries; he was Jehan Yperman. A veil of oblivion weighted by 5 centuries had hidden him. That veil was lifted on the occasion of the sale of the collection of a famous bibliophile, van Hulthem, the scion of an ancient patrician family of Ghent. Van Hulthem had devoted his life to the arts and the sciences and during the ruinous times of the reign of terror of the French occupation of the Belgian provinces, he earned great credit for saving from wanton destruction quantities of objects of art and of books belonging to the then-detested churches and convents. He succeeded in depositing them all in the church of St. Peter belonging to the ancient Benedictine Abbey. He was, at that time, a Deputy in the "Five Hundred"[5] and together with the other Belgian deputies he bravely denounced the vicious destruction by the Commissars of the Republic.

Among the large number of manuscripts listed in the sixth volume of the catalog of van Hulthem's library[6] was a group of items which he had purchased at London at the sale of the library of Richard Beer and which had special interest for him. Van Hulthem asked one of his friends, J.-F. Willems, an expert bibliophile and antiquarian to prepare a detailed description. I append that at the conclusion of this introduction.

J.-F. Willems gave the title: *Trés ancienne histoire naturelle physique belge de l'homme aux XIIIe et XIVe siecles. (A very old Belgian medical text by a man of the thirteenth and fourteenth centuries.).* The collected items are at present (ie 1936) in the Royal Library at Brussells, listed as 156.24-156.41.

Archeologists and bibliophiles were at once greatly excited by the discovery of those documents. At that time, M. Diegerick, the archivist for the city of Ypres was the first to establish the source. Thanks to

---

5 The Five Hundred was a provisional governing body early in the French revolution. (LDR).

6 The catalogs of van Hulthem's library exceeded 6 volumes. After his death the whole collection was purchased by the Belgian government for about 300,000 francs (DM).

him and to his source-materials at Ypres—which, sad to say, were destroyed by fires during the war of 1914-1918—we learned that Jehan Yperman, whose name appears frequently in the manuscripts, was a contemporary of our very great Flemish poets, van Maerlandt and van Boendaele and that he was the author (ie of the manuscripts), both as a surgeon and a physician.

Some have stated that Yperman was born in 1280 or thereabout. That is incorrect. M. de Saegher, archivist for Ypres, with proof in hand, showed that he came well before that date. He published the marriage contract of Yperman, signed in the presence of the magistrates of Ypres in 1285.

"Know all ye here present that Johannes Yperman, citizen of Ypres, has given his consent and his oath as a bridegroom, to hold and to maintain every responsibility as set forth in this year of Our Lord 1285, in the month of August, on the Saturday following the Saint's day of Our Lady"

He was born around 1260.[7] Some authors have it that he studied medicine at Paris, where the university attracted large numbers of Belgian students who sought that knowledge. All agree that in 1297 the municipal authorities of Ypres granted him a quarterly stipend of 50 paris sous. That fact is cited in the "Miscellaneous persons accounts" of the municipal rolls.

We are led to believe that Yperman must have had an academic background that allowed him to take the courses at the University of Paris, and that he knew both Latin and French. That was not unusual for those times in Flanders, because large numbers of Latin schools, the so-called papal schools, were there.[8]

Yperman himself stated that he attended the professional lectures of Lanfranchi of Milan, who was a refugee from Milan at Paris (ie after 1295) fleeing the political disturbances in his own country. The teachings of Lanfranchi, condensed in his book of surgery, were treasured. The leading physicians (ie of Paris), including the Dean of Passevant and the bachelors (ie those with degrees from the Univer-

---

7 We again cite Snellaert (see DM and T's *Cited Authors*) who believed that Yperman was born at Poperingen, a town near Ypres (T p.13).

8 There is no evidence that Yperman ever was a clerical student, although Carolus believed it so, and Diegerick strongly disagreed. Furthermore, Yperman was married and had at least one son. And, every time a sectarian person was

sity) pleaded for him to give his highly recommended lectures on operative surgery and that he write a book that would set forth the principles and all related matters, with his own commentary.

Yperman's material existence at Paris was that of the countless 'scholars', the impoverished residents of the colleges, where they found their bed and board.[9] At that time the Parisan School enjoyed great fame. The University, controlled by clerics, dominated the affairs of the city. It was a light that shone over France. Paris was a brilliant salon and it attracted from all the neighboring countries the young students who were eager to learn.

Is it true that Yperman really attended Lanfranchi's lectures where the exercises attracted a crowded audience? One passage in Yperman's *Surgery* is testimony to that and allows us to accept it almost without question.When he discussed injuries to the cranium Yperman wrote "about that, I advise what Lanfranchi taught me."

That phrase is what brought Dr. Tricot-Royer with good reason to contradict von Leersum, to whom we are indebted for his fine complete edition of Yperman's *Chirurgia* (Flemish,1912).

Yperman succeeded in his efforts as a student and thereafter maintained the aura of a scholar who had been well trained in the liberal arts. He succeeded in making a deep and lasting reputation. Furthermore, he did not conceive of practicing surgery without a suitable medical preparation and, proud of his 'clerical culture', he showed a haughty disdain for the ignorant lay surgeons.

The archives indicate his presence at Ypres in 1303. The city records of 1304 inform us that "To Master Jehan Yperman for his year of service at the Hospital del Belle, four pounds." [10]

The Hospital Del Belle was one of the principal hospitals established in populous Ypre, which at that time contained at least 200,000 inhabitants. He practiced there during almost 30 years. While there, especially in his home near the hospital, a part of which was rented out by him to the city fathers, he wrote his two works, the *Surgery* and

---

named as a master he was called a Presbyter rather than a Master, the title given to a lay person. including Yperman. Those are sufficient evidence that Yperman did not belong to any religious order (T. p 25).

9 A document cited by Ghelforf, Diegerick and DeMets could be offered, perhaps as evidence, that he lived at Paris and received, thrice-yearly, a stipend of 50 Parisian soldi during the year 1297 (T).

the *Medicine*, using the local language of the surgeons who knew no Latin and to serve for his own son who could not deal with the complexities of Latin grammar. Yperman's mother served as a nurse at the Hospital of Notre Dame on the Marchiet. That service is noted in the account book for single entries as follows, "To Kateline Yperman's (the s is the Saxon genitive, customary in Flanders, meaning a woman of the Yperman family) for her service at the hospital." Later, in the records for 1306, one may read, "To Kateline Yperman's, for her service, item, 6 livres."[11]

In the early years of practice, Yperman had a house outside the city walls in the suburbs where lived a large population of weaving-mill workers in pinched circumstances. Although Yperman had already purchased his house there, the city magistrates insisted that Yperman's presence was needed in the city itself, and that he should live within the walls which were locked shut at night. They were determined to set up the Master in town and to grant him a subsidy of 7 livres and 10 sous for his lodging. Even better, after Yperman had moved into the city the city council requested that he rent to them a room in which they would hold their meetings. That was alongside the hospital on the Rue de Lille. The archives state "To Master John Yperman, for a room on South Street where, the magistrates meet. They apply for the rental of that room from now until the middle of March."

The city's archival texts are a mixture of picardese-french dialect and flemish (Thiois). "Master John Yperman has earned a salary for military service: 10 livres that is for service in the army during the expedition of the Yprois against the Count of Flanders, Louis de Crecy".

In 1312, the Yprois held forth in battle at the Castle of Wynendaele.

---

10 T. claims it was only 3 pounds, and cites Diegerick that the account ledger of Ypres was the first time that Yperman was titled "Master", sometime after 1297. The 'paybooks' are fragmentary. They exist for 1297 and from 1298 to 1304 they are lacking. However, after 1304, that is, in 1305, we find the salary (ie 3 pounds). In 1308 he was paid 3 Parisian lbs. and 8 soldi for services at the Hospital del Belle, and during 1309, 1311, 1315 he was paid 4 lbs per annum. In 1317 he was paid 6 lbs (T p.18,19).

11 De Mets is not correct. The entry in the account book for 1304 cites two persons named Yperman. One was Kateline Ypermans and another Kateline who was her daughter (T p.21)

A small item in a local document states that the Yproise militia while fighting at Groningen, near Courtrai, had Yperman leading their surgical corps. It was bloody affair and the surgeons and their assistants had a busy time of it.[12]

The records for 1327 contain the following: "To Yperman 10 Livres for a year of services to the local poor and 8 livres for rental of the meeting room."[13]

After 1332, Yperman's name is gone from the account book, replaced by Master Henry le Bril, "7 livres for supervision and treatment of the sick." The Doctors of Medicine (ie in contrast with the surgeons) were treated more royally. As examples, "To Master Servais Lecupre, physician, 80 Livre; to Master John de Lille, 35 Livres; to Master John Leclers, 13 Livres."

The two large Flemish cities of that very turbulent era, the thirteenth century, were easily pushed into battles against each other or each against the ruling prince. Each sought to dominate the economy of Flanders, belligerently to excess. The Lion of Bruges versus the Lion of Ghent, a contest that led both of them to succumb under the domination of Burgundian princes and, centuries later, under Charles V (ie Holy Roman Emperor).

White banners, green banners, troops of mercenaries and militias of the local working folk who had been placed under arms all were accompanied into battles by surgeons with their movable equipment and personnel as was customary for the time. The Annals of Bruges reveal details of that activity. The Bruges militia was present at the battles of Zeeland, Lessines, Cassel, Gravelines, Audernaerde, Courtrai and Lille. The surgeons were there with them. Here are some details of the account books:

1302–7 livres to Lippine the arsâtre[14] and his squad.

1302–25 livres to Master Gilles the arsâtre, the doctor and his horse.

---

12 The date of Yperman's death on De Mets' Title Page disagrees with the dates of battles given in this section. Probably he lived until 1330 or soon after; see below and nb the date in Bk.VI., Ch.5 (LDR).

13 The last stipend noted in the account books was paid to Yperman in 1329 for surgical services at the Hospital del Belle. That leads us to conclude that Yperman's career ended around 1330 or 1331. Daremberg's or perhaps even Carolus' guesses that 1310 was his date of death ceratainly are wrong. Snellaert's guess, 1350, is possible but probably much too late (T. pp 24-25).

1303–6 livres and 3 sous to Master Janne the arsâtre and his
doctors and for his service at Lessine.

1304–20 livres to Lippine the arsâtre for the activities at
Gravelines, Cassel and Courtrai.

1306–43 livres to Master William, the surgeon at Zieriksee.

1312–4 livres to Master Jan Raefe for his cart and horse at
Wynendaele.

1378-79–139 livres and 16 sous to Master Peter Pature, the
surgeon, and to Master Janne the arsâtre and their horses
at Audenaerde.

1498–4 livres and 12 sous to Master Diderich, the surgeon, for
the happy outcome in the case of the poor valet who had to
undergo an amputation and who recovered with the help
of the Lord.

We had stated above that ancient cities in their customary activities, awarded stipends to young men to allow them to continue as
students. The following is a delightful item that was culled from the
archives at Bruges by Dr. De Meyer:

"Every town had two categories of educated clerics in its service.
Some of them were well-versed in both natural and codified law, and
were able to clarify knotty issues and to give advice in cases that were
brought before the judicial courts. The other group were learned in
the sciences and were on hand to assist the citizens when they were
ill, available to every one in need who could turn to them for help.
Therefore, the benevolent magistrates of Bruges, being aware of the
talents of Master Janne van Moorbeke, son of Master Benoit, who is 27
years of age and a bachelor of medicine, and already known to be
zealous in his professional activity, the above-named magistrates, after
mature reflection and after due consultation with the leading citizens of the above-named City of Bruges, have decided to send the
above-named Master Janne van Moorbeke to the Schools (ie The
Studium of Paris), where to study Medicine for an additional 3 years.
For that purpose he will be paid a stipend of 60 parisian sous, payable
in two moieties, the first at mid-winter and the other on Saint John's

---

14 Arsâtre probably was the cauterizer or the handyman for setting up the
cauteries. From Ars - burn, and Âtre -furnace. (LDR)

Day. It is our purpose that the above-named Master Janne de Moorbeke will be able to be well-advanced in the art of medicine at the end of 3 years and that he will return to offer his services to the good people of the magistracy of this city and to situate himself to serve them and other people as well.

As a loyal and honest man, Master Janne van Moorbeke has agreed to these terms. Enacted on the sixth day of November, 1418.

Signed: Auebs, Vos, Jacob, Hildeballe, Zarre, Volkaerst, Greine, Aertricke, Leffin and others.

We may agree that the case of Yperman was the same as that of Van Moorbeke. No doubt, Van Moorbecke was sent to the Paris Studium and that he would have arrived at an enraged Paris just at the time of the civil insurrection that was instigated by the assassination of Jean Sans Peur (ie Sept. 10, 1419).

THE TREATISE

Yperman's Treatise (*The Surgery*) is a precious testament; it was written in a mother-tongue two hundred years before Ambroise Paré. The latter was the first in France (ie but not the first in Europe) to free Medicine from Latin (which he himself did not know) and whose work was published in the French language of the streets.

Yperman himself explained why he wrote in Flemish.[15] The prologue of his work follows (in Latin):

"This is the theory and practice of Jehan Yperman, being in the prime of his life, written in Flemish for the use of his sons (ie who do not understand Latin). He willingly transmits what he himself has learned from works of many teachers: Lanfranchi, The Four Masters of Salerno, Galen, Roland, Roger, Bruno, Rhazes, Hugh of Lucca and Albucasis."

Therefore, Yperman knew Latin. Although some have said that

---

15 (*Tabanelli's comment*) What may we infer from the following brief statements? Some are written in Latin, the common language of the scholars of that epoch; others are written in 'thiois' the language of western Flanders. Some important questions appear: 1. Why did Yperman write in Flemish instead of Latin? 2. Was it only to render it understandable by his son? 3. If so, can we thereby plausibly date the book as well the as the time of Yperman's death? Let us try answer the questions?

his original work was drafted in Latin, there is no basis for that conjecture. We can go back farther, to those times (ie to dispute that). In Yperman's time we find that the civil documents were written as much in Flemish as in French (picardian dialect).

The manuscript in the Library of Brussels (The Burgundian) is on parchment, folded in quarto, 147 leaves forming 294 pages without a cover. It was bound in 1351, according to this note by the copyists at the end (the 14th section,"on Urine"), "Thank the Lord. By Johann of Aeltre." It contains many interesting drawings of instruments. Dr. Carolus had the commendable initiative to translate the first two books. He published a valuable commentary which had the added credit of calling attention to the great work (Bulletin de la Societé De Médecine de Gand, 1854, XXXII).

Dr. Snellaert wrote a note about a second copy which he owned and which ended up at the Library of the University of Ghent. That copy also is illustrated. The circumstances of Snellaert's disturbed life and premature death prevented him from completing the work that he had planned. He had the foresight to have made a copy of the manuscript at Cambridge, which copy came finally to the Library at Brussels (No. 21833).

Later on another manuscript was discovered at London and another, a fragment, at Leiden.

The handwriting of the 14th century is neat and graceful, the abbreviations are clearly marked. The language is Flemish coming from West Flanders, and probably was the spoken tongue of that region.

Yperman was a contemporary of our first great writers in Flemish argot, so-called 'Thiois', van Maerlant and van Boendaele. He rightly deserves the title Father of Flemish Surgery (ie having written in the native tongue). He knew those authors and he owned works by them. He was especially attracted to the teachings of Lanfranchi whom he often cited. He looked back into the works of the Arabs and the Arabists (ie Bruno) and he bypassed the scholastics who dominated Montpellier. Fifty years after Yperman, Guy de Chauliac as well was able to distract himself from them. Yperman practiced ligature of arteries and also he investigated the maneuver of torsion of arteries (ie to establish hemostasis without ligature) which was a method used by the ancient surgeons. Yet, 200 years later the use of ligatures on arteries was accredited to Ambroise Paré. And, even into the 19th century, Amusat credited Paré with the invention of the technique of torsion!

The Regulations of the Hospital of Notre Dame on the Marchiet at Ypres (1218), recently published in the (Journal) Hippocrate, were written in picardese French.[16]

In the epoch in which Yperman practiced (it is clear that he was successful), the activity of dispensing pharmaceuticals was regulated by the magistracy of Ypres, set down as follows in a manuscript of 1309, The Book of All The Hours of Ypres, including articles relating to the pharmaceutical establishments which were often the shops of the spice-grocers:[17]

---

16. Some historians hold to the belief that Yperman wrote first in Latin, denying Carolus' statement that he was the first to have written a surgical treatise in his 'mother tongue'. Haeser (p. 769) said that the initial Latin version came when the son was very young. Neuburger (p. 519) agreed, and Pagel (p.738) also speaks of a Latin text that was not saved. Van Leersum (1.c) said that the first part of the Proem was put into Latin by some copyist much later, noting the 'classical tone' of the writing. That will explain why the Codex at Cambridge has a double opening, Latin and then Flemish. 2. We read the following in the opening statements: In the Cambridge Codex," quam ipse compilavit et redegit in teutonico filo suo." In the Brussels Codex, "quam ipse tractavit in flammingo ad utilitatem filii sui." followed in Flemish for the rest. "He composed this work in the thiois idiom to favor his son who was too young to be able to understand his father's books (written in Latin) (ie belonging to but not necessarily written by him). He would understand them better by reading them himself than by listening to them being read aloud by someone. That is why he writes this book in Flemish; he wants his son to profit from it; to retain the knowledge that has brought his father so much praise." Therefore, we conclude that the opening Latin phrases were written by a copyist rather than by Yperman, although we cannot really prove it so. We have no knowledge of the son other than what appears here. Yet there may be another reason for Yperman's writing in Flemish, as suggested by De Mets. The local western Flemish dialect was used so the apprentice-surgeons and the barbers who lacked Latin could profit from his treatise. That second hypothesis has merit especially if we consider what happened to Guy de Chauliac's book later in the century. The original Latin soon was translated into common French to expose it to a wider readership than simply the academic surgeons, rather more to the barbers. 3. Now we consider the continuing uncertainties about the dates of the writing and the publication of Yperman's book. I do not doubt that it was written during the years when he was called 'Master' and when he was at work at the Hospital del Belle at

Ypres. Therefore, it was not before 1305; that was the year of publication of Bernard of Gordon's *Lilium* which Yperman cited. More likely, the *Chirurgia* was written after 1328. That is consistent with what Yperman himself wrote in Book VI, Chapter VI: " having treated a young beguine at Ypres in 1328" (Brussels Codex). The London and the Cambridge Codices give the year 1321 (ie *I think Tabanelli has slipped. See Fig.1 taken from the Cambridge Codex which clearly shows 1328*). Furthermore, the frontispiece of the Ghent Codex shows the date 1328. I cannot really understand or explain away the date, 1310, that appears in the London Codex, except to attribute it to a copyist's error. Van Leersum provides an elegant examination of the materials dealing with the end of Yperman's life as they appear in the Codices at Cambridge and London. In the first we find, "in the city of Ypres where we prcticed his profession, he died in 1330. He had written this treatise in the Flemish thiois dialect for the favor of his son." The fiigure ?used to designated 30, was interpreted by Carolus to mean the Roman numeral 10. And he is right in having examined other Mss of the era in which the 15thC Cambridge Codex was written.. For example, an account-ledger in the Medicean Library at Florence writes the date 1420 as MCCC and ? ?. Those figures are the same as that in the Cambridge Codex. The London Codex uses the same symbol. However, the date is in conflict with the date given in the text itself and is further invalidated by the word *then*. "He practiced his profession until he died; in the year MCC e ? (ie ? a misprint for MCCC) , and *then* he edited this book in the thiois language."

Aside from the date 1310 there is nothing to question the date of his death before the date 1328 given in his book for the treatment of the beguine, and the date 1329 in the account-ledgers of Ypres that mention payment for his work at the hospital. It remains for us to determine the date of publication. We have demonstrated the conflict between the dates 1310 in the Codex and the date 1328 in the book itself. It is not easy to set an exact date today. The available data are scarce and they favor a date near the end of Yperman's work at the hospital, that is, not later than 1328 to 1330. That period corresponmds to a time when our Author could have honed the literature and had the experience to enable him to produce a work of such importance as his. Also, that date agrees with the 1328 found in the Ghent Codex, although that was written by someone other than the copyist, evidently at a more recent date.

We really do not know how widely disseminated was his book among the flemish surgeons of his epoch. We can be doubtful of a wide extent because so few mss have come down to us and the fact of no early printed editions. Van Leersum insists that the book was read long after the Author's death, and was studied in a large part of the region. I cannot find how VL arrived at his optimistic estimate and find agreement with later statements (ie by VL), " we find no influence of Yperman on his contemporaries; and we do not know if he taught or if he had any students." And at the end, "I cannot find any references to Yperman in the various surgical codices collected by Thomas Schelink, the Fleming , up to the years 1343."

And how can we expect to find certain written evidence after the great convulsions, the near and far destruction of precious materials, artistic, literary, and scientific in the endless warfare that overran Flanders in the centuries that followed (T p.30).

"Article 5. All grocer-apothecaries must agree to own the book called the Antidotary of Nicholas, a complete true copy.[18] and[19]

Article 6. (Item) He must possess weights ranging from one ounce up to a noir tournois (ie a local term) which are standard and match those of other good cities.

Article 7. (Item) He must not substitute one medicine for another nor give other than the specified amounts (ie in the prescription).

I must add to Tabanelli's remarks: The Great Plague in the decade that follwed Yperman did more to disrupt the progress of Surgery than any other cataclysm of the era. The break between the epoch of the surgeons of 1170 - 1330 and that of Guy de Chauliac who appeared after the Plague, is clearly marked (LDR). This statement about the place of Yperman's mother's employment adds evidence for the use of the local argots in official documents, rather than the usual "Law-Court" verbiage which was Latin. (LDR)

17 The term Antidotary meant more than a prescription against poison. It was a book of prescriptions, as is a modern Pharmacopeia. Also, it could have been an herbal, such as a Book of Hours. It could designate the shop where an apothecary dispensed his wares. It could be the name for an apothecary himself. (LDR)

18 We must give full credit to the erudite bibliophile, M.O. Van Schoor for his precise definitions of 'The Antidotary of Nicholas':
1. A work, Περι Φυτων (Concerning Plants), is ascribed to a Syrian at the time of Christ, known as Nicholas Damascenus. The work was published for the first time in the 14th century as translated from Greek into Arabic by Chase Ben Honain, and then translated back into Greek, as published.
2. Nicolas Myrepsos, also known as Alexandrinus after the city of his birth, lived in the court of Emperor John Vatatzes in Asia Minor from 1222 to 1255 (ie the Byzantine Emperor John III Batazes). He wrote an antidotary containing 2656 formulas arranged in 46 categories.
3. Nicholas Praepositus Salernitatis was the director of the School at Salerno around 1100. He was called Ialeusius. The details of his life are not known. Following the tradition of Saledino d'Ascolo he wrote 2 antidotaries: "The Antidotary Magnum" which was too large for general use and "The Antidotary Parvum - Containing Everything in Common Use".
The A. Parvum was the official text for apothecaries all through the middle ages, along with the works of Nicholas Myrepsos, Mesûe and the Luminaro Magnum of Manlius de Bosco. The A. Parvum was first printed at Venice in 1594. The A. Magnum, seldom used, has not come down to our time.
We are indebted to Van Schoor for his fine descriptive edition of the frontispieces of all the extant pharmacopeias of which he is the proud owner. The series begins with the Receptaires of Florence (first edition, 1498 (DM).

19 Here and in many places to follow, I obtain my data from G. Sarton's magnificent *Introduction to the History of Science (see Bibliog.)* De Mets' needs some emendation. 1. Chase Ben Honain was Hunain Ibn Ishaq, a Nestorian who lived in in India and then in Bagdad around 850. 2. Saledino d'Ascolo was Saladin of Ascoli who lived at Naples around 1440. 3. Mesûe was Mesûe the

Article 12. (Item) He must agree to list the contents and the date they were compounded and to discard them when they are spoiled.

Article 15. (Item) No apothecary will give or sell any medicines that can be used to produce an abortion. If he should do so by order of a physician he will suffer his own conscience.

Did Yperman conduct a school? No one has identified a disciple. His own son did not follow him, the very son for whom he wrote his 'Surgery' (see fn 11).

Fifty years after the Master's death his great name had dimmed. The great plague of 1349 and the siege of 1383 together had reduced the population to 20,000. One can search in vain for the site of the old hospital that was Yperman's base for 30 years. The old city of Ypres did not arise from its ashes. Its eternal glory now rests on its fame for having set itself as the unbreachable wall against an invader (ie Germany in two World Wars and breached in both!).

The banner of Yperman waves only in his fatherland. He did not have the same fortune as Ambroise Paré whose works came 250 years after his and which remain objects of study by doctors and book collectors.

We hope that the injustice of the historical denial of Yperman one day will be repaired. We hope that a doctor of medicine and a historian familiar with the old-country dialects will combine their efforts and will produce a definitive edition of his works, complete with a French translation and a set of well-researched notes. That will contribute to the relighting of the flame of a glorious past now lying dormant. It will give Yperman's life-work the great and the public exposure that it deserves.[20]

Let my essay (*with Tabanelli's additions*), derived from the beautiful collection of Prof. Laignel-Lavastine, be added to the admirable studies that already have already been published about

---

Younger, also known as Masawaih al Maridini who wrote the Grabadin at Bagdad around 1000. 4. J.J.Manlius de Bosco wrote his Luminaro Major in 1525 (LDR).

20 See fn. 2 in the English Tranlator's Preface (LDR).

Yperman and be a contribution to that body of international research.

DE METS' AND TABANELLI'S BIBLIOGRAPHIES COMBINED

L.-J. Willems—Note on a manuscript collection: 'The very ancient Belgian natural history by a man of the 13th and 14th centuries' inserted in the catalog of the van Hulthem's collection, 6th volume, at present at the Royal Belgian Library, the Burgundian Collection, No.s 15624-15641.

This manuscript, on parchment, folded in quarto, consists of 147 leaves in 294 pages without cover sheets. The calligraphy is of the 14th century, and, as we will see later, it was rebound in 1351. We conclude that it was a product of a Belgian hand because it is in the Flemish language, a very rare occurrence in those times, which merits attention. That this book was copied from even older versions can be demonstrated by spaces and absent lines which the copyist probably had intended to fill. The writing is readable, the style and the orthography are generally consistent and the abbreviations seldom are equivocal. The double i is written ii and not y. Every page has three columns for lines of verse and two columns for prose. Each page contains about 50 lines. The only ornamentation is red color for initial letters.

The manuscript formerly was owned by Godfrey Leonys, a pharmacist and notary at Malines, as shown by a note on a separate sheet at the end.

As to content, it is a fairly complete collection of short pieces and of longer articles that deal with natural history (ie science) and human medicine, beginning with the influences of the stars and the planets and ending with anatomy and surgery.

Part 1. A sheet 1 to 6 recto containing a poem about the history of the universe which, rightly or not, is attributed to a certain Fra Gheraert. It has 1,610 lines.

Part 2. From folio 6 verso to 8 verso. It contains recipes for waters and medicinal oils followed by a short chapter on the signs of impending death.

Part 3. From folio 9 recto to 22 verso containing the Antidotary of Nicholas (ie obligatory at Ypres, cf footnote 6), composed of pharmaceutical compounds listed alphabetically. At the end we find the date expressed in Roman Numerals (ie MCCCLI):

> Finito libro sit laus gloria Christo
>
> Dexteram scribentis benedicat lingua legentis

Part 4. From folio 22 to 27 verso, presenting a 'Treatise on Urine' according to Gilles of Salerno who copied Isaac.[21] It is in two parts and at the conclusion of the second we read' "Deo Gratias. Per Johannem de Aeltre, probably the name of the copyist.

Part 5. From folio 28 verso to 45: 'The Medicine of Avicenna (the major work of Avicenna)', preceded by a table of contents of the 48 chapters in the treatise.Therein are cited many authors including the name of a Flemish doctor, Jean Braemblat. Included are the Flemish names of many of the herbs.

Part 6. From folio 46 to 47: 'On the complexions or temperaments' according to Hippocrates and Galen.

Part 7. From folio 47 to 48 recto: 'On Human Physiognomy', after Hippocrates.

Part 8. From folio 48 to 50 verso; 'On Knowlege of Urine' after Gilles of Salerno, Isaac and Théophile. (See footnote 16).

Part 9. Folio 51 recto and verso: Some pharmaceutical and medical definitions.

Part 10. From folio 54 recto to 75: "Treatise on Medicine by Master Jean Ypermans divided into 42 chapters and a table of contents at the end. It begins with

Ephemeral Fevers and ends with a chapter on gonorrhea which the author thought was a loss of semen. In the chapter on epilepsy he mentions the Flemish language. The treatise concludes with an

---

21 The Treatise on Urine, here ascribed to Gilles (again in Part 8, below) probably can be traced to Galen. Gilles was Giles of Corbeil who flourished at Salerno, then Montpellier and Paris around 1200. He wrote a metrical reduction of a text composed by a contemporary of Paul of Aegina, Theophilus Protospatharios around 650 in Constantinople. His source was Galen. But Theophilus was translated by Isaac Judaeus the Elder about 900 at Tunis. Isaac, in turn was brought into Europe by Maurus of Salerno about 1200. Maurus' text was widely accepted in medieval times (LDR).

afterword in Latin : Master Jehan, called Yperman expounds on Medicine. Thank you, Lord. Amen.[22]

Part 11. From folio 74 recto to 75 recto: a metrical exposition of 484 verses stating the the principles of hygiene. I think that it is taken from the *Heimelycheid der Heimelycheden* [23], especially that part which deals with hygeine.

Part 12. Folios 75-77 recto: Extracts from the poem Natures Flowers by van Maerlant, that part which relates to medicine.

Part 13. From folio 77 verso to 85 verso: A poem on the 'secret parts' of men and women, as indicated at the beginning, whereas at the end one reads, in Latin, an explanation of the secrets of women.

Part 14. Folios 85-88: On Magic (Chiromancy) divided in 17 chapters.

Part 15. Folio 89: A poem about ascetic love which has nothing to do with medicine but is quite unusual in its rhythms and rhymes.

Part 16. From folio 91 to 107 recto: *The Herbal of Dioscorides and of Circumstance*. This herbal, or rather, this pharmacopeia is presented in alphabetic order and describes the 202 plants and their special virtues. The article on mandragora is notable for the strange properties that he ascribes to it.

Part 17. From folio 108 to 147 verso. Here is the *Surgery* of Master Jean Yperman who began with this introduction (partly in Latin followed by Flemish): "Here begins the *Surgery Of Master Jehan, Called Yperman*, which is written in germanic (ie there being no other Latin word for Flemish!) for the benefit of his son. I have wished that by diligent study he will profit from what I teach and from what I have learned from the very great masters and have taken from the very great authors of the past."

---

22 This second Treatise in Flemish is in the Brussells Library. Broeckx says that it is not a complete text, not enough to present a full picture of Medicine during Yperman's epoch. Broeckx published it in Antwerp in 1863. Buschmann. (T)

23 Those Flemish terms refer to another work dealing with a woman's 'private parts', a sort of gynecology of the times. See Part 13 (LDR).

PRINTED WORKS

Blommaert. Old Flemish Poets

Broeckx, C. The Surgery of Jean Yperman. The original text from the Cambridge Codex. Annales de la Academie d' Archeologie of Belgium, Antwerp,1863.

Broeckx, C. The Medicine of Yperman. Commentaries and the original flemish text, from Brussells Codex. Buschmann, Antwerp, 1867.[24]

Carolus, J . A French translation of the first three books of **The Surgery**, published in The Annals of the Society of Medicine of Ghent, Glyselysch. Vol. 32, 1854.

Carolus, J. The Surgery of Jehan Yperman, Father of Flemish Surgery. Idem. Vol 32, 1854.

Chereau, A. Jehan Chereau. Chirurgien flammand des XIII et XIV siecle. Union Medicale, (I(I series) Vol. 26, 1865

De Flov and Gailliard, Copies of Flemish Mss in England. Royal Flemish Academy. 1897

De Marez, G and de Sagher, F. The Account Records of the City of Ypres, Librairie Kiessling et C. Hayez. Brussells, 1909

De Sagher, F. A Note Concerning The Death of Yperman. Janus: 19, 33, 1914.

De ten Brink, Jan. The History of Netherlandish Literature, 1897.

De Wachter, P.F. On the Surgery of Jehan Yperman. Annals Of Soc. of Med. of Antwerp, Vol. 24, fasc. 521. 1863.

Diegerick. Bibliography of all references bearing on the Ms of Yperman, father of Flemish Surgery. Annals of Soc. Of Emulation of Western Flanders. Vol 61.1857

Elaut, Jehan Yperman, West Vaanderen. Vol 12, p 201. 1965

Gerrits. The History of The Netherlands in French Literature in Flanders 1855

Guislain, H, (also Glyselynk). Notes on the manuscript by Yperman. Ibid, 1854. Idem.1854

Guislain, H. A Discussion on the Birthplace and the Work of Yperman. Bull. Soc. Medicine of Ghent. Vol XXII, 1855

Gurtl, E.J. Jehan Yperman. Geschichte der Chirurgie, II, 1898

24 See fn 16 (LDR).

Haeser, H. Übersicht der Geschichte der Chirurgie. Stuttgart, Verlag Enke, 1879

Jonckeere, Jehan Yperman. Le Scalpel. 10:326, 1957

Lafaut. Jan Yperman. Annals of the Society for History, Ypres, 1908.

Lonneville, Georges . Belgian Journal of Stomatology, 1932. Diseases of the mouth and teeth. Le Scalpel, XXXV: 44, 1932 Diseases of the Ear, 1932. Idem, XXXVI, 31. 1933 Diseases of the neck and throat 1933.

Neuberger, O. Jehan Yperman. Geschichte derf Medizin, II:430 and 519. 1911

Pagel, H. Handbuch der Geschichte der Medisin. Berlin. Karger. 1915

Samel and Schamelhaut. Flemish Medical Practice. A Bibliography before the 19thC. Nu en Straks (a periodical) 1897-1901

Dr. Snellaert. Comments about **The Surgery of Yperman** and about the translation by Carolus. Bull. of the Society of Medicine of Ghent, Vol. XXVIII, fasc. IX 1854. **te Winckel, I.** On The Development of Netherlandish Literature, 2 vols. 2nd ed. 1927.

Tricot-Royer, P. Jehan Yperman, Father of Flemish Surgery. Medieval Leaves, Vol. 2 pp.58-62, 1931, pp 66-94, 1931-1932.

Van Leersum, E.C. The Surgery of Master Jan Yperman, Leiden, Sijthoffs uitg.1912. (from the Brussells, Ghent and Cambridge Codices).

Van Leersum, E.C .. Did Yperman die inm 1310? Janus, Vol 14, fasc. 393, 1909

Van Leersum, E.C. Notes Concerning the Life of Yperman. Janus;, Vol.18, pp, 1-15, 1913

Van den Peereboom, A. Notices, etc. re Ypres. Ypriana, I, IV. 1878-1880.

Verdam. Library of the Middle-Netherlandish Literature (Catalogue), Leyden, 1912.

Willems, J.-F. Note on the Manuscript Collection: Notes. 15624-15641 See above, Item 1.

DE METS' AND TABANELLI'S NOTES ON THEIR SOURCES CONDENSED AND ADAPTED FOR THE ENGLISH VERSION

For the translation of Book I (The Head) both De Mets and Tabanelli used the manuscript at Cambridge, illustrated by pen drawings, which were edited and published at Antwerp in 1863 by Dr. Broeck, at the request of the Belgian government. The perfect copy was made by Verachter, archivist of the city of Antwerp. Tabanelli's Edition includes ten black-and-white plates taken from the Codex; I have inserted them in my translation of De Mets' Book I, which I use for this English version. However, the Frontispiece is from the Brussells Codex and appears in De Mets. The color-plate of the Zodiacal Man in Book I, Ch.16 has an extraneous source.(see Acknowledgements)

The Cambridge Codex completely lacks the Book On the Eyes. Therefore, for the translation of Book II (The Eyes) both Authors used the manuscripts of The Royal Library of Brussels (the Van Hulthem collection, 15624 to 15641). That manuscript is considered to be the oldest and the most beautiful. It is on vellum whereas the other manuscripts of The Surgery are on paper. However, it is not illustrated. As I did for Book I have used De Met's edition for Book II; it is complete, and as in Book I, the Two Sources are alike in content and meaning.

De Mets's Edition is limited to Books I and II. Therefore, the remainder of the English Edition comes from Tabanelli. He used several Mss (see below) as his sources, and they will be noted.

Besides the Cambridge and the Brussells manuscripts, three other manuscripts of the Surgery of Yperman and a modern edition are in existence:

1. The manuscript of Ghent (collection of Dr. Snellaert) which is illustrated, but has missing items.
2. And 3. The manuscripts at London and Leiden, which are fragments.
4. The edition put out by van Leersum, derived from four manuscripts. It is very elegant, but we criticize the copyist who took it upon himself to complete the many abbreviations and to have used a system of spelling that is too different from the old and original Flemish language.

YPERMAN'S TEXT

DEDICATION
To the Blessed Mary, Mother of God

We must dedicate our opus to God The Father, to The Son and to The Holy Ghost in three entities: The True Lord, The Father who has no beginning, The Son sired by the Father, born of the Virgin Mary who was ever a Virgin, The Holy Ghost derived from The Father and The Son, the three entities stemming from the Father, a single will and a sacred God. Here I pray to the Virgin Mary, the great supporter of the world, that she be willing to pray for the author of this work: that his own son be filled with the inspiration and the knowledge that he would discover in the surgical authorities; let this work be of use to wounded persons or to those who have been afflicted with injuries and illnesses, as they are found in the surgical texts, that they may be cured with the help of The Lord and with the assistance of those authors. By the Saints Cosmos and Damien, gloried martyrs for The Lord, and by Saint Luke the glorified attendant of Our Lady Mary, let them all pray to The Lord for him (ie this author) and for all those who work diligently according to the principles set forth in this treatise, in the manner prescribed in its good rules.

PROEM

Here begins **The Surgery** of Master Jean Yperman who writes it at Ypres and sets it down in Flemish for his son, in the hope that he will profit from his (ie the author's) skill and teachings. That instruction has been extracted from the books of many great surgeons and great writers. That debt will be acknowledged as we proceed.

CHAPTER 1.
THE STRUCTURE OF THE HEAD

First of all observe that the head is spherical, thereby enabling it to contain more in the least volume (ie surface area). Furthermore, the rounded shape is the most beautiful. As a result of its roundness it follows that blows and projectiles make less contact and are more readily deflected.

Observe that the head is the root-stock of the human body, whence come the nerves and the senses deriving from the brain and from the spinal marrow (ie the medulla oblongata and the spinal cord as a single structure) which arises from the brain and which, as is the case of the brain, is covered by two membranes. That marrow is called the *nucha* in Latin.

Three tissues compose the head: bone, fleshy tissues and brain. The last is the marrow of the head. The flesh is muscular. The skin which covers it (ie the scalp) is full of roots of hairs.

The muscular tissues (ie galeal, fibrous) is tougher than other muscle but less so than nerves or cords or tendons and bone.[25]

The hair that grows from the scalp protects the bony calvarium and the fibrous layers against the cold and other injurious agents.

The scalp contains many pores which pass completely through it as if it is a sieve to allow the brain to dispel the excesses vapors and heat that would be harmful to it. Similarly, the membranous layers beneath the skin are full of pores[26]

---

25 Although the medieval surgeons used the word *nerve* at various places in their works to mean nerves, tendons, ligaments or fascial bands, here Yperman clearly indicates nerves as we know them (LDR).

26 Here I have used *pores* where De Mets used *poils,* meaning hairs, which clearly was an editorial error (LDR).

The hair of the scalp serves two functions: the first is to protect the pores against the cold; the second is to adorn the head.

The skin of the scalp is thicker than elsewhere on the body, with two exceptions: the soles of the feet which serve us in walking and the palms of our hands which do our work.

A single hair, or occasionally two or three, traverses every pore in the scalp. The skin itself is bound to the underlying muscular tissues by small filaments of nerves that come from the brain, by some tiny venules which derive from veins which come from the liver and by tiny arterioles that are called *arteriae* in Latin which come from the heart. Nature provides this ingenious scheme of attachment of the skin over all the parts of the body.

The bones of the cranium are neatly put together of many pieces, each with an internal and external table; the internal table faces the brain, the external the muscular tissues. Between the two tables is a layer rich in small arteries and veins which provide heat, nourishment and the essentials of life into the bone. The arterioles provide warmth and vitality, the venules give warmth and nourishment.

The head has three regions: anterior, middle and posterior. The anterior, beginning at the face, is warm, dry and full of vitality, but it has little marrow. The middle region is full of marrow (ie brain) and vital spirits, being warm and moist. In the center of the middle region are the ears which lie in the two bones, called the temporal bones.[27] The posterior region is cool and dry, lacking both vitality and marrow.

It is important to be aware of the nature of those parts because the treatment you apply must follow from that knowledge. For example, warm and dry parts require the opposite, that is, cool and moist medicines. That policy will be true for all sorts of afflictions.

The anterior region contains the eyes, the nose and the mouth. Above the eyes are bony ridges that really should not be considered part of the cranium, but rather as shields for the eyes. They have a transverse position under the eyebrows.

There are many good reasons why the cranium is composed of many pieces. First, we find passages for the nerves in the interstices where the bones meet. There, too, the arteries and the veins that

---

27 De Mets uses 'rochers', a metonomy implying the rocky hard substance of the temporal bone. We use the term 'petrosal' with the same implication of hardness (LDR).

warm and nourish the brain go through the passages with the nerves. Furthermore, the interosseous commissures allow the escape of excess heat that could damage the brain. Fourthly, the dura mater, the membrane over the brain, itself is anchored at the sinus (ie the sagittal) and at the temporal and occipital sutures. Those attachments serve to suspend the brain in a membranous envelope within the bony box, called the cranium, the structure which protects the pale and soft brain.

Here the Author digresses from his topic.(ie De Mets ommitted the section).

Let us return to our discussion of the three regions of the head. The anterior division contains the parts of the brain that govern vision, taste and olfaction; that is where lie the faculties that grant us the sense of black and white, of clarity or cloudiness etc; the distinction between the flavorful (ie salted) and the unflavored etc.; the recognition of pleasant versus disagreeable odors.

In the middle region we find the cerebral centers of intelligence and audition. We can question and answer intelligently and we can understand what we hear. With that portion of the brain we create all of the ideas that are human.

In the posterior portion is the part of the brain that harbors memory, which allows us to retain the experiences of the present and of the past. Roger (ie Frugard) stated it concisely in Latin, as passed on to us in Roland's *Commentary on Roger:* "in the frontal section is Image; in the middle is Reason; at the rear is Memory."

The brain is enclosed within two membranes; one is the dura mater, the other is the pia mater. The dura is thicker and tougher and because of its proximity to the calvarium there is constant friction against it. The dura may become inflamed and be injured, yet it can heal and the damage not be necessarily lethal.

The pia mater is delicate and is the intimate covering of the brain. When it is injured or inflamed recovery is rare. However, Galen reported that he had seen a person who had suffered a wound to both membranes who had recovered. He added a comment that the wound was small and that no brain was extruded. Theodoric also reported that an armor-maker at Lucca had suffered the loss of the back part of his skull and yet had recovered. What is more, he had lost none of his faculties.

Occasionally, after a fit of anger or of fear or of intense fever, and with no other observed events, a thick deposit may form between the dura and the pia. Also, from time to time, at the sites of cranial fractures the dura may be injured and undergo suppuration, and give forth a thick drainage. Some lay surgeons (ie the uneducated ones) mistake that for brain substance. Take no heed of it: they are deceived and they teach that deception to others. When the brain itself suppurates it is beyond recovery, because it is the necessary organ whence flows the fundamental sources of human life.

So much, then, for generalities. Let us now discuss matters that relate directly to Surgery.

CHAPTER 2.
ON THE DIFFERENT WOUNDS OF THE SKULL AND THE SIGNS BY WHICH WE CAN RECOGNIZE INJURIES TO THE DURA MATER AND PIA MATER.

Wounds of the head are frequent. At times the injury does not include fractures of the cranium; at other times fractures compound major scalp wounds or a fracture will lie under a small wound. You will find that cranial fractures in the presence of large scalp wounds are more favorable (ie to treat) than those with small wounds. In the latter cases one must enlarge the wound in order to tend to the fractured bone. In addition to the assessment of the fracture, one must always examine for damage to the meninges, either to the dura mater or the pia mater.

Injuries to the dura are manifest by these symptoms: First, there is a feeling of heavy-head as a result of the separation of previously joined structures. The face is flushed and the eyes are glazed because of the surplus of vital spirits. The tongue is reddened by fever. The patient becomes delirious as his vitality and his humors are disturbed.

When the pia mater is damaged the following symptoms appear:

The patient loses his senses of taste and smell. His digestive functions cease. He becomes speechless as part of the general disturbance of the vital functions and of the vapors which provide normal motor function. In this case the nerves that supply the tongue are impaired. Similarly, the other organs fail in their natural functions.

These are the signs of impending death in cases with injured pia mater [28]:

In some cases spots appear on their faces. In some the bloody discharges from the nose and eyes are mixed with pus. Those are the signs that death is near, especially if chills and fever occur as often as three or four times every day. All of the symptomatic patients, especially if the meninges are torn, usually will die at the appearance of the next new moon, if not several days before. That is because the planetary bodies dominate certain regions of the body. The moon is the dominatrix of wetness on Earth; the wetness of the moon added to the terrestrial wetness increases the wetness (ie edema) of the brain. It becomes extraordinarily swollen and it cannot maintain its normal functions, especially since it is no longer contained within intact meninges.

So dies the wounded man. In this way we describe the risks of death after injuries to the head, and we state that much skill is necessary in their treatment.

Bruno (ie da Longoburgo) stated that in his experience with many victims of wounds of the dura mater complicating skull fractures, none of them survived who exhibited the symptoms given here. However, he wrote that he had cured some with small wounds of the pia mater in whom brain tissue had not extruded. Galen in his *Commentaries on The Aphorisms* (ie of Hippocrates) which is a medical text, also stated that he had cured many patients with small wounds of the pia. However, he expressly added that if the wounds were large enough to allow herniation of brain tissue, death was inevitable.

---

28 For a full discussion of the importance of those signs in the medieval world see F.S.Paxton, Signa Mortifera: Death and Prognostication in Early Monastic Medicine. Bull.Hist.Med., 1993, 67:631-650 (LDR).

Chapter 3.
On The Parts Of The Head And On How One Must Treat Each Part.

The diseases of the head are manifold. There are cephalalgias, monophagias, migraines and many other maladies that are not in the province of surgery and we will not deal with them here; rather, we will limit our discussion to matters in the field of surgery.

Frequently the wounds to the head are in the front part where The Authorities expressly decry the application of warm and dry medicines, because that part of the head already is hot and dry. That is despite the fact that warm medications favor the repair of tissues in many other places in the body. As a general rule, hot and moist applications favor the natural regeneration of tissues. Nevertheless, The Authorities state that one may not apply them even in cases of injuries to the middle part of the head, because, there it already is warm and moist, and by reason of the large amount of marrow (ie brain substance) in that region the risk is great that the heat will cause necrosis. On the other hand, you may use medications with those qualities at will in wounds of the posterior part of the head because there by nature it is cool and dry.

When the cranium is fractured, healing usually takes 30 to 40 days until there is complete union of the fragments. Children and persons younger than age 18 are the exceptions because they still are endowed with the vitality conferred by Their Lord (ie the ages of divine innocence), that which we call "the paternal seed". Above all, in any case, you should from the beginning base your treatment on The Lord. When He so wills in your favor you will be successful. You must invoke The Lord in all of your enterprises because He is the mainstay in all that we surgeons do. And you who aim to be surgeons must have these qualities : conscience, intelligence, divine protection and the full control over your limbs (ie the arms and hands).

CHAPTER 4.
ON THE NECESSARY QUALITIES OF A GOOD SURGEON.

The following qualities are required of a good surgeon:

1. He must be healthy in both mind and body. Rhazes commented that he who has the bearing of an ill natured or nasty person seldom is naturally a good man; his disposition is bad and his tendency is to have evil thoughts and to commit improper acts. Avicenna on the other hand offered a corollary, saying that even he who has a fine appearance may have evil habits.

2. The surgeon should have graceful hands and slender fingers and a sturdy frame that has no tremors. He should have sharp vision and be able to think clearly. He must be able to react promptly and unwaveringly. More than that, he must not be money-hungry, because avarice may lead one away from the righteous path.

3. Galen said that he must be modest and yet be courageous in his works.

4. The surgeon should be broadly educated beyond the realm of medicine. He should have studied the books of science and philosophy, including grammar, logic, rhetoric and ethics. With a background of knowledge in those four subjects he will have learned to assess rationally all that he will face.
   Logic is the art of reasoning.
   Grammar educates one in the fine points of Latin.
   The surgeon should know Rhetoric if he wishes to speak with ease and elegance about all sorts of matters. Witness the lawyers who learn that art by practice, not by reading it in books.
   The surgeon should understand Ethics which teaches one good habits.

5. He must not be a libertine. Rather he should maintain sobriety and chastity.

6. His religious faith should be beyond question.

7. He must devote himself completely to his patients, in such a manner that, with God's help, there will be nothing in his treatment nor in the attentions that he gave to them that can be reproached by his patients.

8. When he is in the patient's home he will not disclose in any details that are related to his treatment, nor dally at length with the housewife, her daughter nor her servants. He will not reveal information to others about the concerns of the sick man. It is especially important that he not give hints with frivolous glances (ie smirks, winks etc.) because they (the curious onlookers) are a malicious sort and the circumstances (ie if known) may make enemies among them.[29] Rather, in that manner, the surgeon should comport himself as everyone's friend.

9. I advise that he not make small talk with anybody because he may not know that the badinage may be offensive to the listener.

10. Do harm to none. Treat honorably all other surgeons and clergymen and express no envy of their successes.[30]

11. He should not flatter himself.

12. He should have a serious mien and seek to earn a good reputation.

13. He should not offer a cure for a serious illness when there is no hope for success. If the surgeon should yield to entreaties to go ahead, he should tell the patient's friends that he will do only as best he can.

14. He will always offer solace to the patient.

15. He will state the condition clearly and accurately when the prognosis is very bad.

16. As to fees: he will take recompense according to the patient's financial means. He will treat the poor gratis, for the sake of his love of God who endowed him with the ability to do so.

---

29 Yperman is emphatic about the surgeon's responsibility for the patient's privacy (LDR).

30 *Clergymen:* Probably the reference is to the clerical Doctors of Medicine. (LDR)

Chapter 5.
On The Primary Dressing And Suturing Of Wounds In Different Parts Of The Body

1. When you are called upon to treat fresh wounds, first examine them carefully and determine their causes: blows, missiles, falls etc. If necessary (to properly inspect it) wipe the wound clean with a sponge and lay on a wad of oakum steeped in beaten egg white. By whipping the egg white you eliminate a lot of its moisture which will cause it to run and plug the pores of the skin near the wound. If you do not have sufficient egg white at hand you may soak the oakum in the blood from the wound itself. That works very well by drying the wound as the pad hardens (ie clots). Whereas other surgeons soak the tow in water and vinegar, I always use the blood from the wound for the dressings, to my satisfaction.

If the wound is a large one, as caused by a sword blade or a similar weapon, you should suture it, beginning at the middle if the wound requires three sutures.[31] When only two sutures are needed place the needles equidistant away from the ends. Place a drain at the lower end to allow the escape of pus. The sutures should be placed deeply enough to approximate the full thickness of the wound's surfaces, thus avoiding a deep recess for accumulation of pus. That is what will happen if you bring together only the superficial edges of the wound. The resulting deep abscess will continue to drain as a fistula and will require treatment later on.

The threaded needle for suturing should be triangular (ie in cross section, having cutting edges) and the eye of the needle should be channeled (ie a trough between the eye and the end of the needle) such that the threaded end will not be too large and you can draw it through with ease. Use twisted waxed thread that will not rip the tissues, either red or white silk (ie instead of rough-edged linen or cotton even when waxed).

---

31 If the wound is stellate or if one edge of a lunate wound is much longer than the other, one needs at least three sutures (LDR).

Before you proceed with the suturing, seek and remove splinters of bone and other foreign bodies.

2. If instead of a fresh wound you are called to treat wounds with dry surfaces, you first must freshen them. Use a scraper or use a knife to cut the tissues back to bleeding surfaces before going ahead with the sutures.

If the edges of the wound are widely separated, avail yourself of a third person's hands (ie an assistant in addition to the surgeon and the patient) to approximate the wound-edges (ie before you sew them).Tie the sutures with double knots and always be certain that your knots will hold.[32] Then dust a powder, which you had prepared beforehand, over the sutures to harden the tissues along the wound-edges (ie by its astringent effects).[33] Here is the prescription as used by Roland:

Take 1 ounce each of grand mélisse and bolo d'armenie (59). Add 3 ounces each of Greek tar (colophane, 126) and 5 ounces each of mastic (122) and small white frankincense perles (188) and 2 drams each of sangdragon (408) and minium (241).[34] Grind and mix well; pass it through a fine sieve; keep it in a box, where, if kept dry, it will remain useful for over twenty years. Roland called it his Red Powder (377b). Not only was it hemostatic, it also favored the appearance of tissue (ie granulation tissue). It can be used in treating open fractures if first it is diluted with egg-white and mixed with dust of milled wheat flour (177). We will return to the last item in a chapter on fractures of the limbs. The powder also favors the regeneration of skin that has been sliced off, especially if it is used along with water cress leaves or other medicinal leaves that are applied over the defect.

Albucasis recommended another powder for use over the sutures.

32 To obtain sufficient length for a 'running' suture as well as anchoring at the ends of wounds (LDR).

33 Perhaps the coagulated skin where the sutures made their perforations would hold the sutures and not be cut through by the thread (LDR).

34 Hereafter I will place a number in brackets after the first mention of the medication in the text. That will locate it in the Pharmacopeia in Appendix I. In some cases the contents of the Compounds will be listed in the footnotes, as here I will use DeMets' French terminology for Yperman's Flemish. Grand Melisse is a cordial made from the flowers of Melissa officianalis, the Lemon Balm (LDR).

Take care to use it only over the sutures and not to dust it between the edges of the wound. Here it is: Take 3 parts of chaux vive, 2 parts of small perles of white frankincense and 1 part of dragon's blood. Pulverize and force it through a sieve and save it for use as needed. You may use your fingers to dab it directly on each suture. The same author added that if nothing else is available you may use fresh lime alone to achieve almost the same results.

CHAPTER 6.
ON WAYS TO CONTROL HEMORRHAGE IN WOUNDS.

When the surgeon encounters a wound from which blood is flowing he must find the source. Bleeding that comes in spurts and jets obviously is arterial and the blood is watery and bright. If the blood flows slowly and is of a darker color it comes from veins, which are everywhere, bringing nourishment to the body.

Arteries come from the heart and they have two coats: one is gristly and never seals because the blood is thin, hot and ever in motion.

Veins arise in the liver and they carry brownish and thick blood slowly. For that function it needs only one loose coat.

Most often the arteries and veins bleed in the same wound. Seldom is there arterial bleeding alone because the arteries lie deeper in the tissues than the veins.

Be aware that arterial hemorrhage is much more dangerous than venous; it is especially threatening when it is profuse. That is why I advise immediate control whenever possible, to avoid the grave complications and threatened death preceded by spasms, a problem which we will discuss later. At this point it is will be sufficient that you know that when spasms accompany arterial bleeding, it is a mortal sign, as are also prostration, cessation of intestinal activity and delirium. Now I will tell you how to arrest arterial and venous bleeding.

Bleeding from small veins is easily controlled with a pack of oakum that you have allowed to dry and have bandaged in place. You may have soaked it in the blood of the wound itself or in egg-white (163) (ie see above, Ch.5).

Bleeding from large veins may be treated in the same way. Sometimes that method is unsuccessful. In that case do as follows. Press down on the oakum pack with your fingers to hold it in place and to prevent a free escape of the blood. Then pour in water to cool the region, thereby to diminish the local fever and to promote coagulation (ie the blood becomes thicker). The coolness also causes the skin, the muscles and the vessels to contract and the lumens of the vessels become narrower. Be aware that you must prevent the water from entering the veins themselves thereby causing serious complications, and if you must irrigate a wound while it is bleeding the cold water entering the vein may damage the vessel's coats, because they are tendinous (ie nervous). Later, when wounds that were irrigated have to be sutured, you must rub them to make them ooze before you go ahead with the sewing.

If yet the bleeding has not stopped you should resort to the following medicines which have hemostatic properties in varying degrees, one more potent than another. I will describe them in the order of their hemostatic potency.

In all cases of venous or arterial bleeding (ie after the previously stated methods have failed) press your thumb or another finger on the open vessel so to stem the flow. The longer you hold fast the better are the chances of the blood coagulating, which coagulum becomes an excellent hemostat. Then lay on the dry oakum pad or one that you have soaked in vinegar and water or egg white or the blood from the wound, and then dust on the following powder, which Bruno approved [35]:

Take equal parts of small white frankincense, hepatic aloes, dragon's blood and bol de' armenie. Pulverize and pass through a sieve. Hold the pack in place with a bandage that is not so tight as to provoke inflammation.[36] Galen taught that the humors and spirits (ie airs) always flowed (ie preferentially) toward the injured regions, adding that nothing will impair the healing of a wound more than inflammation.

---

35 Bruno da Longoburgo. In Chapter 15 Yperman calls this powder the Theodoricon (LDR).

36 More often than for other meanings, Inflammation in the ancient surgical texts meant Infection, manifested as what we call Cellulitis. That was different from non-invasive Suppuration on the surfaces of a wound which was thought to be a natural and desirable part of the processes of healing. Here, the author repeats the warnings against too-tight wrappings which caused ischemia and favored the development of the invasive infections (LDR).

You may add to the above-mentioned powder some egg-white and poils de lievre (356), finely minced with a scissors diluted to the consistency of honey. Take several strands of oakum, about the width of almonds and fill the wound and lay over that a lot of dry oakum. If you lack sufficient oakum use a wad of lint and pile it atop the other. Bind it in place but not too tightly.

An even more powerful hemostatic powder is made as follows:

Take equal parts of chaux vive, sangdragon, the stone of which they make small lanterns and white frankincense. Mix that all with some haresfoot or cobwebs, and prepare it and use as you did the others.

Another hemostatic powder which Galen used follows here: Take 16 drams of red or yellow atrament (356), 16 drams of white frankincense, 8 drams of aloes (19), 8 drams of silex (430a), 4 drams of orpiment (327) and 20 drams of stones for lanterns.[37] Pulverize and pass through a fine sieve and apply the fine powder atop the strands (ie described above) that you had placed in the wound.

All these powders were taught by Bruno who had found them in older texts. Theodoric, who compiled and commented on Bruno, used them, too, in practice in suitable cases.

But now I want to bring you up-to-date with Lanfranchi's comments on this subject.[38] He had been summoned to treat a child who had fallen on a knife which had cut his hand and injured the radial artery—an appropriately named vessel. Before Lanfranchi's arrival the child had lost so much blood that he was taken for dead. Lanfranchi found his pulse barely perceptible and that the blood was pale, still flowing from the wound. He grasped the wound with his fingers and held on for a long time, during which the child came to and opened his eyes. Lanfrance sent to an apothecary for the following powder:

Take 2 drams of thick white frankincense and 1 dram of hepatic aloes. Pulverize to a powder and dilute with egg-white to a consistency of honey. Then mix with finely chopped haresfoot clover (356) and apply it in the wound on a pad of dry oakum. On

37 Pierres De Lanternes are not identified (LDR).

38 Yperman's bows to his great teacher remind us of Theodoric's devotion to his own mentor and father, Hugh of Lucca (LDR).

top lay dry oakum and bind in place as tightly as can be tolerated by the patient. He left it in place until the following day.

Then, when Lanfranchi returned, he found the child to be strong, having had no further hemorrhage. The boy's father requested a change of dressing which the Master refused until the fourth day. Then he took equal parts of egg-white and oil of roses and mixed in some of the powder already used, making it all quite fluid. He poured it over the powder that remained in the wound (ie after removing the wadded oakum) and left it all for an additional week. At his visit on the eighth day he found the wound had healed with sound scar. That was a source of great marvel in the father.

On another occasion the arm of an 18 year-old child (ie the stated age is questioned by De Mets) was pierced by a small knife wielded by another child. A vein was entered and a nerve nearby was injured causing severe pain. Lanfranchi saw blood pouring from the wound and reflected for a moment. He withheld his usual medicaments because the cool and sticky egg-white would have plugged the pores of the skin. Therefore, he said to flex the child's arm a bit (ie so to relax the wound) to enable him to grasp the vein and apply a ligature, and at the same time he would be able to relieve the nerve-pain by pouring rose water into the wound. The distraught mother sought a lay practitioner who advised the opposite. Lanfranchi left the scene and the laic applied his usual hemostatics and nothing happened; the bleeding continued and the child weakened. Then a physician was summoned, a friend of the mother, and he sent for Lanfranchi, who wanted no more of it. But the doctor himself went to consult Lanfranchi who repeated the advice he had given the mother. The physician insisted that the lay practitioner follow that advice, which he did. He applied a ligature and stopped the bleeding. Later on, when he was asked why the child, who had endured the hemorrhage for so long a time, had not suffered spasms, Lanfranchi casually explained it as an occasional happening with bleeding.

I wrote all the above to show how much you must know about

what to do in those circumstances. You must not be stubborn and follow your own fixed prescription.

I will reaffirm here that when you see that your hemostatic powders or other measures have failed to arrest the hemorrhage, then you will fall back on the ligature. Use a needle threaded with a waxed thread and pass it under the vessel, taking pains not to puncture the vessel with the needle. Then tie the ends of the thread.

Another way: Use a strip of metal that has a small hole bored through and place it on the wounded surface so the hole lies over the opening in the bleeding vein. Take another metal strip (ie such as a thick probe) which you have heated to redness and pass it through the hole in the metal, therewith to cauterize the hole in the vein, just where it crosses the hole. Be careful not to char the vein elsewhere and avoid contact with adjacent nerves. Arteries should be cauterized enough to form a char, the burning being somewhat more intense on arteries than on veins. However, if you are concerned that the eschar will slough away and allow a renewal of hemorrhage, use the more secure technique. Grasp the vessel, twist it and ligate it.[39]

In summary: Hemorrhage can be controlled in four ways:

1. By compression of the vessel until a clot fills the opening.
2. By cooling the region with irrigations.
3. By use of the actual or potential cautery (ie hot metal or hemostatic medicaments).[40]
4. By ligation and torsion of the vein or artery.

Some practitioners apply ashes (38) of feathers, hair and the like on the opening in the vessels. As for me, I have taught what were the most tested methods of the Old Masters and what I have found to be most successful. As for you, when you enter practice,

---

39 One of my own Masters, Robert Linton, MD, favored that technique. He grasped the vessel with a fine hemostat near the bleeding site and twisted it, thereby stopping the flow. Then he ligated the vessel or sutured the hole if the vessel was a large one. He used that method, rather than attempting at the outset to find the opening itself, wasting time with multiple attempts with the hemostat (LDR).

40 Bruno, Chirurgia Major, Part II, Chapter 18 offered Albucasis' definitions. "Cauteries are either actual or potential. The actual is heated by fire; the potential uses corrosive medicaments such as cantharides, garlic etc."(LDR).

always be careful with the hemostatic medicines that you use in open wounds and on open vessels. The medicaments which you use in great quantities and leave for a long time will come away on their own (ie as sequestered sloughs). In any case, do not change the hemostatic dressings before the third or fourth day unless there is raging inflammation. Then you must examine the wound and proceed to treat it prudently according to its severity.

CHAPTER 7.
ON WOUNDS OF THE HEAD WITHOUT FRACTURES AND ON THE FOUR SEASONS

When you encounter a scalp wound without a cranial fracture, simply apply a strip of oakum or lint soaked in egg-white (simple or beaten) and atop it a wad of a like material. But, during the winter soak the strip in egg yolk; during the spring and autumn use the whole egg; during the summer use only the egg-white. Suture the wound if you think that is necessary.

If the wound is full thickness down to the bone, or if the skin alone is divided, and you treat only the outer layers without cleaning up what is deeper, the result often is a fever that comes from the wound and it may spread beyond your ability to treat it. Therefore, I advise what Lanfranchi taught me and what I took to heart, to wit: Take warm oil of roses in which you have soaked the strip, as warm as is tolerable, and lay the strip in the wound. Continue to treat it in that way (ie at more frequent intervals) until the

---

41 Yperman does not imply that the gaping wound edges a will be united by scar. Rather the intent is to promote the coverage of the base of the wound on the surface of the calvarium. The adherence of the overlying scalp to that surface will prevent infection from entering the subgaleal space. Subsequent treatment will allow the wound to contract and to be covered with new epithelium, forming a broad scar (LDR).

42 Black Ointment. It also was called The Ointment of the Twelve Apostles for its 12 main ingredients, as well as other names by various authors. Guy de Chauliac described it as follows (Nicaise edition, p 617): white wax, resins, ammoniac, opoponax, verdigris, round aristolochium, frankincense, myrrh, galbanum, bdellium, litharge, and common oil or vinegar. When the mix is heated it turns black See the fn that follows for Yperman's own recipe for Black Ointment (LDR).

wound is united by an exuberant growth of granulation tissue.[41]
Then lay the linen lint or tow in the wound, atop which you spread
a black ointment,[42] and over that you place a pad of oakum or
linen folded to double thickness. Hold it all in place with a bandage.

CHAPTER 8.
ON THE LUMPS WHICH FOLLOW BLOWS TO THE HEAD
AND STRIKES BY PROJECTILES
ON THE WOUNDS WHICH COMPLICATE THOSE LUMPS.

Not infrequently the head suffers severe blunt injuries, whether
by clubs, fists, stone-missiles or arrows, and the cranium is not fractured. The injury may or may not wound the scalp or form soft or hard
tumors (ie edema or hematomas).

If the scalp is opened, shave the region and sew the wound. Dress
it with oakum or lint strips which have been soaked in egg-whites or
yolks according to the time of the year. If an infection appears by the
third day, apply this plaster to treat it, which Roland described as
taken from Roger. Do as follows:

Macerate saffron (395) in water until the water is colored. Add
wheat-flour and boil until properly thickened. Apply the mixture
hotter than merely tepid, all over the head. The plaster will ease the
pain of the wound.

But, if you must induce suppuration, take equal amounts of sureau
(165), some parsley juice (244), bees-wax (293), lard (206), olive oil
(312) and wine (496). Beat it all together and add wheat-flour to
thicken it to the consistency of honey (220). Then lay it on the inflamed wound. Do not use this mixture on wounds that are near
commissures or close to nerves, because fatty stuff is contraindicated
at those regions. However, use it without fear in wounds of the scalp
or soft tissues. As Roland taught, use it hot, not tepid. It is a good
remedy in the proper case.

In its stead you may prefer Lanfranchi's plaster made from 1 part
olive oil, 2 parts water and some wheat-flour (187). Boil it until it is
not quite as thick as bread dough and apply it when warm on the

wound. It will cleanse the wound. Then you sponge the wound with warm wine and apply the lint pads as described. Then add the black ointment. Before you use it, be sure that the brain has not been damaged. In those cases the brain substance is fatty enough; one should not add oil or other fats. The black ointment will be useless.

That ointment is made as follows: Take one pound each of olive oil and lard; five pounds of pine tar (379); 3 ounces of colophony; in summer take 3 ounces of wax and in winter use 2 ounces: 5 ounces each of mastic, olibanum (316), ammoniacum (23), serapinum (429), opoponax (321) and terebinth (489).[43] Combine as follows:

Put the oil, lard, tar, wax and the gum-resins that cannot be pulverized, such as the galbanum, ammoniacum, serapinum and opoponax in a metal pot and melt them over a low flame. When they are well blended add the mastic, the olibanum and the opoponax which you had ground into powder beforehand. Mix that with the oil and the others while stirring continuously with a spatula. You will know when it is ready when you drip a bit onto a polished marble slab. It will be smooth and uniform and will stick between your fingers. Then remove the pot from the fire and add the terebinth all the while mixing it with care. Then squeeze the whole through a thin hemp or linen cloth and set the filtrate aside for use when you need it. The ointment is used in all recent wounds where it favors the appearance of granulation tissue, of surface suppuration and of the scar (ie which will unite the wounds edges).

One may use Theodoric's method for treating wounds. For wounds of the head he took some properly prepared lint, free of starch, and made a pad by soaking it in warm wine. After squeezing out the wine he laid the warm pad on (ie not in) the wound. Alongside the wound he place bolsters of lint which he held in place with bandages, That effectively brought together the full thickness of the wound edges. When suppuration occurred he wiped the wound dry with warm wine and put on the plasters as we have described.

43 Yperman's Black Ointment and other recipes in Chapter VIII: Some of the ingredients vary from Guy's recipe. Ammoniacum, Goudron (naval tar, 304), Aristolochium (32); Bdellium (53); Galbanum (194) serapinum a gum resin of ferula plants; Litharge (253); Mastic, Myrrh (299), Olibanum, Opoponax, another gum resin of Commiphora family, as bdellium and myrrh; Serapinum, Terebinth, Verdigris (482), (as used in Guy's recipe for Black Oint. See fn 18) was green copper acetate; Cumin (145) (LDR).

However, if the suppuration was excessive he used the following. He had previously boiled mauve (273) leaves in water and he had saved the water for later use as an irrigant. He then chopped the leaves into tiny bits and dried them before placing them in a box to be used when needed. When he wished to use them, he moistened some with wine and added some finely milled wheat-flour and worked them to the consistency of a roux or of honey. He put the mixture right into the wound as hot as the wounded man would allow. The plaster relieved the inflammation of the wound. After that he treated the wound with the wine-soaked lint.

If only lumps appeared after blunt trauma and there were no open wounds, he laid on unbeaten egg-whites until the third day. Then he applied the following plaster as hot as possible to the previously shaven head.

Take 3 ounces each of dried laurel berries (238), washed cumin and pure anise (27). When the cumin and anise have been thoroughly dried in an oven, pulverize them (with the dried berries) in a mortar and sift them through a sieve. Then take 1 ounce each of mastic and frankincense and crumble them into a container with care that the powder not become lumpy. Boil the first three powdered with a small amount of wine and gradually add the others while mixing continuously. Then add 3 ounces of fine wheat-flour to make it all glutinous. Add some honey to make it as thick as a roux and spread it on a cloth. Apply it to the head while it is still hot. Let it remain for three days. Then you replace it with a freshly made plaster. Continue that treatment as long as the boss is puffed up or suppurates or persists as a soft mass.

In that fashion, I, Jean Yperman, have cured many patients of their tumors that other surgeons wished to incise. Macer [44] used crushed

---

44 Macer was not a person. The name was given to an herbal, The Macer Floridus, probably by the French monk Odo von Meudon, d. 1161 (LDR).

45 The Four Masters were a group of surgeons at Salerno about 1250 who composed a commentary on the text of Roland of Parma (see Daremberg in the Bibliography) (LDR).

fennel (180) in vinegar (484) in a plaster on the head-lumps and claimed to cure them.

When the hair-bearing skin alone is edematous use a method recommended by the Four Masters [45] in their gloss of Roland and Roger: Boil mallow and absinthe (1) leaves in water and lay them on the swelling. That will make the edema recede.

CHAPTER 9.
HERE WE LEARN HOW TO RECOGNIZE AND DIAGNOSE FRACTURES OF THE SKULL WITH OR WITHOUT LUMPS OR OPEN WOUNDS

When lumps on the head appear after blows that do not cause open wounds, shave the head and apply unbeaten egg-white. Then fasten a waxed string between the teeth (ie probably the semiconscious patient held the string by biting) and wind it around his thumb and index fingers. If his skull is fractured the victim will signal you to stop when you ever-so-slightly turn his head by tugging the string. Even if the distortion is merely the width of a finger nail it will be painful. [46]

Lanfranchi used another test. Insert a roof-thatch reed between the teeth of the patient. If he does not bite down on it that is a sign of a cranial fracture. The same is true for failure to crack a nut, or (ie the opposite) if the patient cannot relax his jaws to allow the admission of the end of one's thumb to the second phalanx.

A third test is done this way: Make a plaster of 1 pound of fresh beeswax, 2 pounds of labdanum (234) and 5 pounds of frankincense. Pulverize the frankincense, then mix in the labdanum and wax. Stir it over a fire and make a plaster (ie with flour, honey, olive oil, wax, cloth etc.) and keep it on the patient's head for a full day and night. The

---

46 The use of passive movements of the head for diagnosis and prognosis was well accepted in ancient surgery. Probably the most famous example was the case of Henry II of France in 1559. A jouster's lance had struck him through his eye and had unhorsed him. The surgeon of record was Paré and the consultant was Vesalius. The latter placed a handkerchief in the almost comatose patient's mouth and jerked it. When the royal victim cried out in pain, Vesalius said that the prognosis was bad. The royal patient died. (LDR).

following morning peel it off quickly in one piece. If the cranium had been fractured the plaster will have molded itself in the form of the defect. That method was taught by William of Saliceto and William Congenis.

Let me assure you that, with the exception of the infallible plaster mold, all the tests often have been false. However, I have often enough been successful with the string between the teeth.

CHAPTER 10.
ON WOUNDS CAUSED BY SHARP EDGED WEAPONS, WITH LOSS OF TISSUE, WITH OR WITHOUT FRACTURES

A stroke of a weapon can slice off a portion of the scalp and carry with it a piece of calvarium and yet not reach the brain (ie the inner table remains intact). In such a case you first must detach the fragment of bone from the soft tissues and freshen the edges (ie all around) until they ooze blood. Then suture the flap, beginning at the middle, placing the needle punctures a finger's breadth apart so to fit the flap in place. Take care not to close the lower end where you will insert a wick to allow the escape of pus. Do not keep the drain in place for too long, lest it cause necrosis of the bone. After the closure place one of the powders that we have described on the wound.

If the flap has been completely detached or if the attachment cannot provide nourishment, the flap will wither. Then you must use the ointment that Roland taught or black ointment or Agrippa's ointment as described in Nicolaus' *Antidotarium.* You can find that book at the pharmacist's shop.[47] Atop the ointment place a pad that brings

---

47 See Introduction by De Mets and Tabanedlli, fn 13 (LDR).

48 In a century when the Clerical Physicians were debating how much of either Universals and Particulars were the essence of Medicine, our Jehan forthrightly says that Surgery is the Art of the Ad Hoc. It remains so. See N. Siraisi, *Taddeo Alderotti and His Pupils,* Princeton, Princeton Univ. Press, 1981, p.124 ff. (LDR).

the scalp into contact with the calvarium. Do not press too hard because that will keep the nourishment from the wound.

Be prepared for anything that you may encounter in any circumstance.

That must be your goal to which you devote your entire self, your talent and your thoughts. Therefore, If you adhere to that principle no one can speak ill of you.[48]

Chapter 11.
Wounds With Sharp Weapons That Expose The Dura Mater

Now we come to those cutting wounds that slice off scalp and a piece of calvarium (ie both tables) and expose the dura mater, which is the membrane over the brain. It transmits the pulsations of the brain as it derives from the same tissues that form the arteries that take origin at the heart.

If the bone is still hanging from the flap, detach it. Carefully feel with your fingers to find jagged edges of the damaged remaining calvarium which you trim away before suturing the wound. Even better, slip a lead strip (under the edge of the intact skull) to separate the brain (ie the dura) from the bone, and use a small biting tool to cut away any overhanging spicules. The splinters can be removed with large and small forceps. I advise the use of the lead strip, as above, for safety whenever you must use sharp instruments in operations near the brain.

After you have evened the edges, insert the suture needle inward through the flap then out through the intact scalp. Then you proceed to dress the wound you have approximated (ie loosely with perhaps only one or two sutures, to allow insertion of the wicks (see below).

To protect the dura from the accumulations of pus, do this. Take clean pieces of red sidon[49] and cut them to the shape of but a little larger than the area of the wound in the bone. Soak the pieces in egg-white. Slip the pieces, two or three plies, over the surface of the brain

---

49 Sidon, a soft crimped cloth, similar to the modern silk crepe (LDR).
50 Bago, cotton-wool (LDR).

(ie the dura) and under the edges of the bone (ie before suturing the scalp). Why use sidon? Because it acts as a better wick than linen net and it is softer. On top lay some white bago[50] which is a good absorbent for the pus, and the sidon is not. Then cover it with oakum saturated with egg-yolk alone or, better, also with oil of roses. The former absorbs, the latter fortifies. In addition use this absorbent ointment: Take equal parts of the drippings of roasted meats (206) and oil of roses, add some saffron and grind all in a mortar. Rub it on the scalp alongside the wound, excepting on the suture punctures where you dust the red powder

When the proud flesh has regenerated between the scalp and the bony fragments, scrape it smooth (ie the granulation tissue that extrudes along the loosely sutured suture line) with a knife and remove the sutures. Then complete the treatment with warm wine and black ointment, or another like it.

When a blow has cut a flap of scalp along with some bone and the dura mater remains intact, and when there are no perforations by splintered bone, do this. Be certain of the latter and then remove the attached piece of bone and suture the scalp in place, making a careful match-up of the edges. Apply the red powder except where you have left a gap for the wick which will carry off the pus. Lay on a pad so to maintain the contact (ie between the under surface of the scalp and the outer surface of the inner table of the calvarium). Keep the wound wet with compresses of warm wine during the first four days. Then sponge it clean and dust on the red powder until full recovery.

When you are convinced that the wound-edges are united remove the sutures, one at a time according to your assessment (when union is secure). Follow with treatments as above.

Some surgeons insert drains between each pair of sutures, and in their failure to understand the rationale of the sutures, they interfere with their real purpose. The suture really is the only a way to bring the edges of a wound into contact for nice healing. Skin is its own father (ie provides the natural substance to regenerate skin) as is bone (ie for bone) and all the other tissues—including muscle, blood and fat. In this case the skin (ie of the intact portion of scalp) would not regenerate fresh new skin in the absence of a cicatrized (ie healed) suture line. The same would be true for bone without callus and for nerves and blood vessels without their own regenerative materials.

If the scalp wound spared the bone, sew it up and treat it as any uncomplicated wound, as I have taught you to do.

Many practitioners use oakum soaked in mothers' milk. That, of course, defeats Nature's own wisdom. Why do that? When Nature proves insufficient, then you should offer help in a reasonable manner: stimulate the whole patient either by invigorating or by etiolating the body with suitable regimens.

If a patient's blood is too rich, offer him beverages and foods which have weakening effects. If the blood is too weak, provide nourishment that is easily digested, such as chicken, stewed partridge, tender vegetables and fruits and diluted wine, all of which are to be used only if the patient is not feverish. Remember, chicken feeds a fever. I will expand on that in a chapter devoted to the diets that are prescribed for sick persons.

CHAPTER 12.
SPLINTERS IN HEAD WOUNDS CAUSED BY SHARP-EDGED WEAPONS

This is how to manage wounds caused by swords, axes and other sharp-edged weapons that cut the scalp and split off small splinters of bone. Carefully detach the bony fragments from the soft tissues and suture the wound. Then apply black ointment.

I must warn you, if you do not meticulously remove the splintered fragments of bone, the wound will not really heal. And even if the scalp wound heals over the retained bits of bone, they will cause a delayed abscess. What began as a single problem becomes a double malady when the fleshy tissues atop the splinters slough. In that event you will have to use a powder of colchicum (124a) which goes by the Latin name "Hermodactyl"(219), which eats away the sloughing tissue.

A second warning: If the bone fragments have been cut loose from all attachments, the subsequent exposure to air will cause their necrosis (ie as sequestra) as a complication which few wounds of that sort can escape.

If the wound penetrates only the outer table of the calvarium scrape it with a doubly curved burin deeply enough to achieve a flat surface, going, as previously stated, to the very edges of the bony defect. Then healthy granulation tissue will be generated at the exposed base of the defect where the blood vessels snake their way between the two tables of bone. If eschars (ie as of a burn) or frank necrosis of bone appear—by reason of exposure to air or to the cold metal of the burin—they will slough away painlessly of themselves. There you have it, a quick and easy treatment.

In such cases as above, to determine whether or not the fracture has penetrated both tables of the skull, use a quill-pen and ink. Write (ie apply ink) on the fracture line. Then scrape the surface near the line (ie to jostle the ink) and look for traces of the ink elsewhere along the fracture. thereby to tell its true depth. If the fracture goes through both tables a sure sign is this: after the initial application of ink and scraping, apply a second aliquot and wipe it away with some oakum or lint. If you no longer can see the black line or if it remains only as wide as a nearby hair, the ink has drained through. But if you continue to see it (ie when the fracture is only through the outer table) scrape it all away with your burin. Next apply a compress soaked in warm oil of roses and cover it with lint and over it all you apply black ointment. I described that ointment in Chapter 8 where we treated bosses and wounds. It is a good medicine to use in all fresh wounds because it promotes granulation tissue and beneficial pus and, at the same time it cleanses the wound.

Many practitioners apply oakum soaked in mothers' milk. I have never used it because I deem it contraindicated. My reasoning is that mothers' milk being intrinsically cold also is wet and is viscous as is its butter. On the other hand, the skull also is naturally cold. Cold things are not properly perceived by the scalp (ie it is not sensitive enough to protect against excessive coldness) and, as a consequence the harmful effects of cold are transmitted through the cranium to the marrow (the brain) which it encloses.

Here is a good ointment advocated by William of Congenis (ie offered as better than mothers' milk): Take some olibanum, that is, white frankincense and mastic and grind them finely. Mix with goose or chicken fat. If you want it yellow, add some saffron, if red, add a little dragon's blood. Spread the ointment on a plaster to be laid on the wound.

And here is another good ointment: Take some fresh lard and boil it with green parsley. Add five pounds of white resin and one and one quarter pounds of wax. After all are completely blended, pass it through a cloth and stir until cold enough to prevent the wax from rising to the surface. This is my ordinary ointment with which I have helped Nature to cure all kinds of wounds. Some surgeons as well as lay practitioners erroneously call this ointment Popoleum (365) simply because it also is greenish.[51]

Oh, well! If you eliminate the parsley and use saffron the ointment becomes yellow and they call it the Golden Ointment. Those people know not of what they speak, although they make a lot of golden money with it. For my part, I call them (ie green, yellow and red) my Barber's Ointments.

CHAPTER 13.
HEAD WOUNDS INFLICTED BY THE SHARP CORNERS OF THE BLADES OF CLEAVERS, KNIVES OR HATCHETS, OR BY THE POINTS OF SWORDS

When you encounter persons with a wounds of the head caused by the points or sharp edges of swords or other cutting weapons (ie puncture wounds) examine them carefully to determine the direction that a wound takes, and also determine if it penetrates the dura mater, the outer membrane, using the diagnostic signs described in Chapter III.

In such cases (ie when the prognosis is bad) take care to avoid those treatments which will call down upon you the accusations of your colleagues. That is most important if there is fever. Alternating chills and fever foretell a fatal outcome.

But, if you detect no such symptoms, curette the surface of the

51 Pierre Pigray (Des Preceptes des Medecine et Chirurgie, Lyon, 1652, p 719) described Unguentum Populeum as containing poppy (320), mandragore (263) and many other leaves. Also, see Chapter 17 of this book (LDR).

wounded bone with a burin while you hold the patient's head between your knees, enabling you to work from above. Take your time in
scraping your way through until you see the pulsating dura mater.

Galen taught us to make the opening through the bone as small
as possible, just large enough to allow the escape of the blood that has
accumulated between the cranium and the dura mater. But if you are
concerned that the membrane itself has been torn or that there is a
(ie subdural) collection or that the dura mater is adherent (ie to the
bone), then make your exposure through the bone as large as you
deem it to be necessary, especially in the most serious wounds. Some
surgeons make their way through with a chisel and lead mallet. That
is a cruel maneuver. In addition to terrifying the patient it puts him at
grave risk for cracking through the skull and causing a stab into the
brain creating an even more serious wound than the original one.
Therefore, I advise you not to use that technique.

When you recognize that the brain, or rather its membranes, are
inflamed, apply egg-white as you were taught in the chapter on wounds
caused by sharp weapons. Instead, you may use one part of oil of roses
(388) and add 1/2 part of honey of roses (ie rosamel, 390). Equally
good is an oil pressed from unripe olives (318), the greener the
better. If that is not available, use oils from rich nuts. Avicenna commented that the green olive oil is best, and he called it Oleum
Onfacinum.

This is how to make oil of roses: Take two pounds of ordinary oil
(ie perhaps rape seed oil (377) or ripe olive oil) and process it so:
Pour in fresh water and whip it and the oil with a special spoon. Pour
it into a jar with a trough in its lip or, better, with a narrow neck with an
opening a finger-breadth in diameter. Uncork the jar and let the
water settle at the bottom as the oil rises to the surface. Repeat this (ie
the whipping and the decanting) ten times.[52] After the last, carefully
pour off the water and add ten pounds of crushed rose petals selected from the centers of the flowers, meaning that they are of medium size and have good color, for every ten pounds of oil. Mix them
well with the oil and pour it all into wide-mouth glass jars to be ex-

---

52 The water takes up soluble impurities from the oil before the roses are
    steeped (LDR).

posed to sunlight for forty days. Stir the contents with a rod every day. After forty days filter it through a cloth. Then you may keep it in the sunlight for as long as you wish. That oil is better than what you find at the pharmacists' shops because they boil the mixture in a water bath (ie rather than use sunlight).

In the same manner one may prepare all the aromatic oils of herbs and delicate flowers – violets 486), elder tree leaves (165), lilies (248), camomile (76) etc.

Another method: put the oil in a metal pot and cover it with a lid which is larger than the pot. Bury it for forty days. Disinter it, filter the mix and expose it to sunlight in a glass jar. The result is good.

The Greeks used rosamel, made as follows: Take ten pounds of very white and pure honey. Warm it and skim it before adding one pound of freshly crushed roses and bring it all to a boil. When it reaches that point add another four pounds of roses from which you have completely trimmed away any white stem material. Mix it all and boil it over a low flame while you continuously stir with a spatula until the watery part evaporates. Filter it and add an equal amount of oil, which serves to preserve the mixture, which improves and becomes sweeter as it ages. Use it in the morning or forenoon, and use it in preparing Diamargaritum and Rubea Troscicata (154).

When you use it with warm substances, it refreshes and softens the body; when given with hot things it is suitable for dry breasts (ie not explained whether to promote lactation or to suppress it).

Now let us return to our proper subject.

In all cases you must smooth the uneven surface of the bone and suture the wounds, as we described in the chapter on wounds with loss of tissue.

As for me, Master Jean Yperman, I assure you that I always prefer to scrape the access (a hole or a trough) through the cranium using instruments with curved handles (ie to provide a secure grip) which are much less dangerous than a trephine. But, in all cases, before you make your opening—whether with a trephine, a chisel and mallet or a burin—cover the wounded man's ears with wads of cotton or the like, and give him a glove to bite on. That is how you control the disturbing noise that is part of the operation and how you prevent the chattering of the victim's teeth.

Avicenna and Galen were insistent on that measure and of their desire to remove as little of the bone as possible. Other practitioners to the contrary remove large amounts of bone, a foolish practice. Galen never made the hole larger than necessary to drain the pus from the membranes, because the calvarium, as I have said, is the guardian of the brain.

Do not use a lot of egg-white on wounds that are no longer oozing blood, because that takes away the natural heat and leads to necrosis. In addition, it decreases the normal pliancy of the tissues and inhibits suppuration. However, one may safely apply it directly on the inflamed dura mater for the initial forty days after the injury. Although you may use it on other soft tissues of the head, I repeat, do not put it directly on the bare calvarium when you can avoid doing so.

CHAPTER 14.
SERIOUS SWELLINGS ON HEADS INJURED BY BLOWS OR FALLS.

Occasionally, after contusions caused by blows or by falling or after being struck by projectiles, large swellings on the bones appear without lesions of the overlying scalp. Use your senses to detect the signs and observe the symptoms as we have described them to recognize a fracture. If there is none, act according to our instructions in Chapter 10. If you confirm the existence of a fracture, you must free the bone and remove the badly bruised tissues.[53] Then dress the wound as best you can with narrow strips of oakum soaked in egg-white. Lay dry oakum over that and bandage it in place. Leave it for three days unless there is hemorrhage. In that event, you use styptics to control it as we have instructed. On the third or fourth day place the patient in the position I described, putting his head between the operator's knees. Use a curved burin to scrape your way through bone until you recognize the pulsating dura mater. Make an opening only so large as necessary, not losing sight of your goal of making it no larger than required to obtain free drainage of pus and blood from the brain. You

---

[53] Yperman abandons the subject in the Chapter Heading and goes on to scalp wounds with fractures (LDR).

must be sure not to leave behind any splinters of the fracture or bone dust produced by your burin.

After the dura mater has been exposed and when the irregular edges of bone around the defect or on the surface require correction, protect the dura mater with the previously described strips of lead pushed ahead of the burin. When you have finished, treat the defect as we have taught, using warm wine to keep the wound moist. Wipe it clean and apply the capital powder and lint fitted to the defect. Then apply the compress and continue the dressings until all is healed.

I will describe the Capital Powder in a later chapter (ie 16).

CHAPTER 15.
FRACTURES OF THE CRANIUM WHERE ONE FRAGMENT SLIPS UNDER ANOTHER

In some cases of fracture a fragment is depressed and it slips under another. You can best diagnose that by using the delicate senses of your fingertips which Nature had provided you from birth. After you have found it, shave the patient's head and make a cruciate incision through the scalp, sponge it clean and do as follows:

When needed, use Lanfranchi's technique, which he borrowed from Galen, and make a narrow opening through the bone to allow the escape of pus. Lanfranchi himself thought that he could provide drainage through the fracture defect or via the commissures, as one may be forced to do in patients who are struggling (ie and cannot be restrained). In those cases, Galen first applied oil of roses and a little vinegar, which allows the oil to seep through the commissures, there to enter and to stimulate the brain (ie to alleviate the frenzy). Lanfranchi, as did Galen, had the scalp shaved in the area of the bony defect, and even further beyond. Then he made a u-shaped incision at the edge of the shaved field, and he separated the flap from the bone.[54] He then took some warm oil of roses and rose honey and

---

54 The apex of the flap being over the subduction Note that Yperman describes a depressed fracture but defers his discussion of the treatment for it to a later chapter. In Chapter 16 he discusses the wound per se rather than techniques for reducing depressed fractures (LDR).

55 The so-called Head Melon (LDR).

spread it on oakum and laid it as a plaster on the fracture line. He added a compress wet with egg-yolk and oil of roses folded three or four times. In addition he placed on top a pad of lint. Take note that after all of the above, he applied on the surrounding scalp an ointment that we described in the chapter on incised wounds. Furthermore, he recommended the use of lard or other animal fat on the rest of the head which he bandaged with many turns of a long bandage, masterfully wrapped so it would remain in place.[55] He followed that regimen until he observed a good sprouting (ie of granulation tissue) between the fragments. If you wish (ie other than Lanfranchi's medicines), you may use Bruno's powder which he called Theodoricon (see above, Ch.5).

When the dura mater is inflamed you must try to prevent the formation of abscesses, which are life-threatening. If your treatments have induced the inflammation by the use of excessively irritating medicines, discontinue at once. If after that you see no improvement you can offer a prognosis of impending death. In those circumstances, I suggest that you look out for your own safety.[56]

CHAPTER 16.
CRANIAL FRACTURES WITHOUT SCALP WOUNDS

Now I shall give you a good lesson about head injuries with cranial fractures. This material was garnered from the personal experiences of Master Jean Yperman and from what he had learned from Lanfranchi, and as taken from reading Galen, Serapion, Hippocrates and other writers.[57]

All of them agreed that whenever that will be necessary (ie to expose the dura mater) you should remove as little of the cranium as possible. As I have taught, the cranium is the shield of the brain, which is the source of all of our faculties. For that purpose, leave the brain covered to the extent possible, protected by Nature's design. The teachings of all the Masters hold especially true when there are

---

56 When you stand to receive the blame cast on you by your competitors. See Chapter 13, par. 2 (LDR).

57 This is another confirmation of Yperman's direct experiences as a pupil of Lanfranchi, whereas he had knowledge of the others only through reading and hearsay (LDR).

punctures or fractures without displacement of the fragments. In such cases all that is necessary is to keep the pieces together, meaning on a level with each other. Lanfranchi of Milan said that was the best treatment. However, he recognized the threat in all cases of cranial fractures, especially with depressed fractures, that splinters of bone can tear the dura mater.

Keep those fragments and splinters in mind and avoid them when you perform scraping or perforating maneuvers. They are always risks for complications especially in those who are frail—women and children—who become feverish from fear alone, and then can relapse. Again, I add a comment about surgeons who are in a hurry to trephine and who lack forbearance and cause the complications.

Now I will continue with Lanfranchi's method which I use. Begin by shaving the head and removing the damaged portions of the scalp. Fill the wound with narrow strips of oakum soaked in egg-white over which you lay an oakum plaster, held in place by many turns of a long bandage. Renew the dressing after three days, or four if the wound continues to seep blood. If the hemorrhage is brisk, use the methods previously described. Extend the wound by incising as necessary to expose the entire fracture-line.

The first subsequent dressing uses two parts of oil of roses to one part of honey. Immerse the strips as usual and place them on the fractured bone. Atop the injured scalp apply strips wet with two parts of oil of roses to one part of egg-yolk. Over all lay a plaster of rose honey thickened with a little wheaten flour. That will cleanse and fortify the wound. After the wound is clean and all the inflammation is gone, and it is suppurating nicely, and the fracture-line is filled with granulation tissue, apply lint that was shredded from an old head-scarf. Put some black ointment on the scalp around the wound. At every change of dressing, irrigate the wound with warm wine and sponge it clean before you replace fresh lint. With God's help you will cure the patient. I recommend this method of treatment without perforating the bone as the most successful.

If the cranium is fractured through to the dura mater, treat as I described in the chapter on wounds caused by pointed weapons. Place some sindon or white linen between the dura mater and the bone (ie under the overhanging perimeter). Even better, use red sindon.

If the brain tends to bulge through the opening in the dura mater and bone and rises above the level of the wound-edges—an occurrence more often at times of a waxing or full moon—do this. Pack the wound with sindon and add a plaquet cut from a sheet of lead to a size no larger than the opening. The lead piece should have two holes through which you pass a piece of twisted cord with which you can manipulate it. Put the plate so its edges are between the sindon and the bone at the margins. A better plaquet is made of a thin, but not too thin, piece of maple wood. It works better because it is warmer and less heavy than the lead.

Keep the plaquet in situ until the herniated brain recedes, renewing the dressing twice daily, using clean sindon and washing the plate clean of pus.

Wounds of the head are more dangerous when the moon is waxing or is full than when it ebbs. In the full phases the brain and its membranes directly abut the (ie inner surface of) the bone, whereas in the waning times one can insert a finger between the bone the dura mater. So it is that the brain swells and recedes according to the moon's phases. Be aware of that when you treat head-wounds.

Take notice of what I have written about what the astrologers say about the signs of the moon. They say that the very worst time to suffer a wounded head is when the moon is in Aries, a zodiacal sign. That is when the moon has the brain in its empire, which lasts about two hours and five minutes at every lunation. That is why the astrologers divide the body in twelve parts, according to the twelve zodiacal signs. Aries controls the head, skull and face; Taurus controls the throat and nape; Gemini the arms and hands; Cancer the chest down to the epigastrium; Leo the upper abdomen and the regions of the flanks; Virgo the lower abdomen and intestines; Libra the hips and buttocks; Scorpio the genitalia and anus; Sagittarius the thighs; Capricorn the knees; Aquarius the legs and ankle; Pisces the feet.

Some of the Masters stated that the Signs had evil effects that may be observed in the wounds. They insisted that surgeons at least learn those parts of astronomy that have to do with the phases of the moon and its signs in the various periods. Accordingly, one should avoid lancing, incising or performing other operations in the parts of the body which are influenced by their signs. Therefore, I advise as follows, these being the signs of the phases of the moon, according to the teachers of astronomy (ie astrology).

A head-wound during the month of Aries is influenced by the moon during two days of its fulness and for three days before and after. Taurus dominates shoulders; Gemini the arms and hands; Cancer the chest; Leo the stomach and the heart; Virgo the belly and the intestines; Sagittarius the pelvis; Capricorn the knees; Aquarius the legs; Pisces the feet. This is how the moon figures in those twelve signs of the Zodiac; (for example) you should avoid touching the head (ie surgically) when it is influenced by Aries. Every surgeon should know the moon's signs in all the different zones of the Zodiac because of its great influence. (See Plate)

When the dura mater has been damaged, use Bruno's and Lanfranchi's dressing containing Capital Powder, prepared as follows: Take 3 scruples each of sarcocolla (410), frankincense and myrrh. Sift them through a sieve and pulverize them in a mortar. Sift again, this time through a cloth. Then dust the powder on a piece of sindon.[58] As soon as the dura mater is discolored (brown) by the powder, replace the dressing with one part of rose honey and three parts of onfacium placed on a cloth (ie not directly on the wound). When granulation tissue appears, use fresh lint made from a cloth used in head-scarves. Continue until healing is complete.

Now give your attention to my own procedures, and to the story of how I discovered them. First I shave the scalp around the wound. Next I enlarge the wound to the extent of the fracture. Then I apply strips of cloth dampened with oil of roses and rosamel, all this to repeat what we have already taught.

One day I happened to treat a soldier who had been injured by a blunt weapon that caused a depressed fracture of his skull. The victim had lost consciousness. I incised the scalp with a razor to expose bare bone. In that way I was able to diagnose the fracture and determine that there was a depressed fracture. I began my treatment with dressings of oil and honey, as stated. I fed him yolks of chicken eggs,

---

58 A scruple was about a third of a gram (LDR).

milk whipped with wheat flower and cooked sour apples. For a beverage I provided barley broth. I hesitated to use even those in view of his age and the seriousness of his condition.

The fracture line sprouted proud flesh and he regained consciousness. He began to speak after six weeks and he called me Uncle. Gradually, his speech improved and he asked me how he came to be wounded; he planned his revenge on the perpetrator, using a sword and a shield. But, as the healing progressed he pardoned his enemy.

The edge of bone that extended over the depressed fragment and even beyond underwent sequestration through both tables and

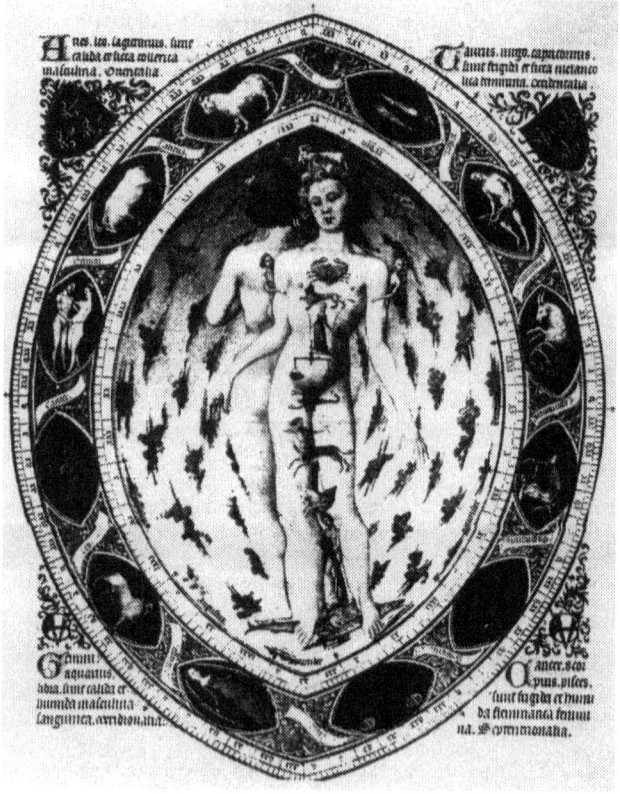

The Zodiacal Man's Anatomy
From The Très Riches Heures of Jean, Duke of Berry
Ms of Musée Condé, Chantilly
George Braziller, Inc. New York. 1969

Nature separated it from the healthy bone, while new granulation tissue was provided by the arteries from the diploe between the tables of the calvarium. In the end, the wound healed solidly without much depression or irregular projections.

Another soldier was kicked by a horse which struck him in the occiput. I removed the damaged scalp over the fracture and treated him as in the other case, and the fracture healed. He lost only a bit of the bone, the size of a finger nail, which had been exposed to a gust of air.

I also cured a young woman who suffered a horse's kick to her forehead, using the same method. Similarly I was successful in the case of an old soldier who had been struck along the commissure of the skull (ie probably the sagittal commissure). And there were many others wounded at Ypres, Flanders and thereabouts.

The incisions that you make in the scalp should be precisely aligned and sutured in quarters, using one linen or silk thread for each portion. Bring the edges together to touch each other and you will obtain pretty scars. Do it that way for all large wounds and incisions. If in spite of your good efforts the result is an ugly scar, try to get by with it but never commit the folly of re-incising.

Chapter 17
The Methods Of The Four Salernitan Masters And Of Roland And Others

Attend now to what Roland and others have taught and to the gloss (ie on Roland) compiled by the Four Masters. Roland's Latin text began thus: "Medicina equin. vocatur ad nomin." Roland had added to what Roger wrote "Post mundi fabricam". The gloss of the Four Masters began with "Sic dixit Constantinus".[59]

Roger and Roland made cruciate incisions in the scalp over the site of a suspected cranial fracture. Once that diagnosis was confirmed, they removed all the fragments, at the same intervention unless pre-

---

59 Constantine Africanus (1020-1087) translated the Greek and Arabic authors at Salerno and Monte Cassino, thereby opening the doors to the classic world and its medical practices (LDR).

vented by hemorrhage. In that event they delayed the extraction of the bony fragments until a later dressing, but made as brief a delay as possible before undertaking that delicate maneuver. At the time of the initial exploration, if they deemed it necessary to perforate the bone, they made an opening and smoothed the edges all around with a burin. Then they laid on red sindon or a linen cloth with with egg-white, and overlaid it with lint from an old fine linen cloth.

If the wound oozed blood and if the scalp was inflamed (ie edematous and red) they bled the patient from a vein in the temple, unless the patient was too weak or too young or too old to withstand it. Those authors suggested that one should bleed from a vein close to the source of the inflammation, or in the general region.

If you see that the lips of the wound are pink and turgid and that they begin to show pus, those are good signs. They show that Nature has been able to nourish the wound. But if the wound-edges are shriveled and discolored, those are unfavorable signs and they may prognosticate that death is near.[60]

The Four Masters recommended that we close the nostrils and mouths of patients with skull fractures. If his skull is fractured one may see a vapor or blood spilling from the meninges, giving indication to go ahead and trephinate, using the proper instruments.[61] They drilled many small holes around the stellate fracture site and then enlarged the holes and cut the bridges of bone between the holes. For the latter they used a small punch and mallet and lead strips (ie pushed under the bone to protect the meninges during the cutting). They removed the central piece of bone and allowed free drainage of pus and blood from the meningeal surface.

Take note that the Four Salernitans' Gloss on Roland states that if a fragment had slipped under the intact bone, one need not trephinate

---

60 The medieval surgeons, adopted the methods they learned from the Ancients, and they offered prognoses as necessary parts of the management of their patients. It seems to have been especially important that bad prognoses should be offered to the family of the patient, to protect the surgeon, both his health and his reputation, after a fatal outcome (LDR).

61 De Mets' (and probably Yperman's as well) wording is unclear. I interpret this passage as follows: The surgeon pinches the nose and covers the mouth as the victim performs the equivalent of what we call the Valsalva Maneuver, exhaling against resistance to increase intracranial pressure (LDR).

the bone on top but that he should perforate the depressed piece. Furthermore, they observed that when a surgeon knows that he must operate on the head, he should abstain from sexual activity during the night before, that he should avoid any contact with a menstruating woman, and that, during the entire preceding day he should not eat garlic, onions and spicy sauces. And he should take care to wash his hands before the operation.

After he extracts the bony fragments and before he reapplies the dressings, the surgeon should have the patient cough through his mouth while he looks to see if pus appears on the meninges (ie see footnote 36). That is a bad sign. If the patient is not already feverish, you can expect that it will happen soon.

You clean away the pus with a moistened sponge and then apply a fine powder made of the olibanum variety of frankincense directly on the surface of the brain (ie the meninges). If the surrounding scalp is inflamed cover it with the Popoleum ointment which you keep at hand or can obtain at the pharmacist's shop. That ointment is made by taking five pounds of poplar buds (364a), four ounces each of white and black poppy leaves (320), mandragore leaves, ripe blackberries (393), bella-donna leaves (217), morel (232) and money-wort leaves (290), and three pounds of lard. Crush the poplar buds with the lard and make small balls (ie to store) for future use. Set them aside for nine days. Afterward break them up and choose some of each variety of the leaves and mash them all with the balls. Put it all in a copper pot and add aromatic wine. Bring it to a boil and evaporate the wine until the mo-ment when the leaves settle to the bottom, all the while you stir with a spatula. Pour it through a cloth and place it in a jar.

The Populeum ointment is good against spiking fevers and against insomnia. Mixed with oil of violets and rubbed over the pulses at the wrists and to the palms and the soles of the feet it works well against the high fevers. When applied to the umbilicus it brings on sweats.

Now to continue with the Gloss: When the depressed fragment has been completely detached, remove it with a forceps. Do it with a steady hand and without dilly-dallying, taking care lest jagged edges of the fragment do not lacerate the dura mater. That will greatly complicate the wound. However, if that does happen, maintain your composure, search to find the splinters that remain between the calvarium and the dura mater. If the edges of the remaining unfragmented cranium are spiky, smooth them at once (ie lest they cut into the meninges and brain if and when herniation occurs). Afterward cover the exposed brain (ie the meninges) with sindon or fine linen cloth soaked with egg-white. Complete the dressing as already described.

Theodoric and Hugh of Lucca, who were both Masters of equal merit in their era applied the following plaster on wounds which had become red and swollen or were forming abscesses, especially in wounds of the head or of regions that are rich in nerves.

They boiled mallow leaves before mincing and crushing enough of them to make one plaster. That aliquot was boiled in wine as they added finely milled wheaten flour, enough to produce a moist paste for the plaster, neither too wet nor too dry. They applied it rather warm on the wound, changing it daily until they had achieved a healthy suppuration with moderate edema. After that they used warm wine with occasional applications of the ointment (ie the paste).

Theodoric wrote that he had seen Master Hugh treat a man whose occipital brain had herniated through a cranial wound. The wound healed and yet the man retained his memory. He was able to continue his trade as a harness maker as efficiently as before the injury. Hugo was amazed at the success, which was so in contrast with the observations of the Old Masters who stated that a man whose brain had been so badly damaged could retain his intellectual faculties only if the meninges had herniated and not the brain. When other practitioners objected to the report by Hugo that the brain itself had herniated, they claimed that he had seen only the meninges covered with inspissated pus which had taken on the texture and the whiteness of brain. After Hugh assured them that it really was brain, they were as astonished as was he by this never-before-seen case. Bear in mind that Hugh was no ignorant dolt; he was both a physician and a surgeon as well as a naturalist. On that occasion he commented that every surgeon should remember his (ie

---

62 Hugh's case is cited by Theodoric. (The Surgery of Theodoric, translated by E. Campbell and J. Colton, New York, Appleton-Century-Crofts, 1955. Vol.I p.109). Note here the reference to the occipital brain being the seat of the memory, an ancient conceit transmitted during many centuries before Yperman and beyond. See Chapter 1 of this book. Also note how Yperman qualifies Hugh by referring to his status as a physician and a surgeon, although in Italy in Hugh's day there were no such French qualifications as Surgeons of the Long Robe (LDR).

Hugh's) case when he was about to deem a wound unsuited for treatment (ie beyond a possibility of recovery). He should not accept as definite the signs that prognosticate a fatal outcome as the only basis for that decision.[62] That statement also is found in Roland's *Treatise on Surgery*. He, too, was a fine surgeon and he attested that the surgeon must depend on God's help. Even in situations that seem desperate all may not be lost. Therefore, have faith in God and in the powers of Nature which stem from him.

Hugh of Lucca followed a dietary regimen for wounded patients that offered scanty feedings to the robust and the healthy, whereas to the debilitated he offered more nourishment in easily digested form. In all cases of head wounds, whether or not there was a fracture, he applied a pad of oakum soaked in warm wine after having squeezed out the excess, and he put dry oakum atop that, as a measure to conserve natural heat. He wrapped the pads in place with many turns of a long bandage. Finally he gave the injured man the following potion:

Take one ounce each of fresh cannelle (79) and white ginger (301); one dram each of galigan (394), cardamone (86)—all retaining their sharp tang—and some long peppers (341). Also take some fresh and fragrant cloves (202), in the amount of about twelve to fourteen wheat grains (494); and a bit more of cumin and green pepper. Grind it all to a fine powder in a metal mortar. Sift it and place in wooden boxes for later use (ie in the wine, v.i.).

Here is how he made his claret wine: Take four pounds of wine and add one pound of white honey that has been whipped to a froth. Mix them well over heat. Remove from the flame and sprinkle on the powder, to taste and until the brew is thickened. Filter it through a cloth to make the wine very clear. Take about the same amounts (ie as in the powder) of valerian (475), gentian (199), mace (261), pimpernelle (348) and piloselle (342). Dry them and grind them to a powder and pass them through a fine sieve. Add them to the clear wine that you had

---

63 Campbell and Colton translate Theodoric's version (op.cit.Vol I p.112) as follows: "In the name of the Father and the Son and of the Holy Ghost, in the name of the Holy and Indivisible Trinity; the right hand of the Lord hath done valiantly, the right hand of the Lord hath exalted me; I shall not die but live and I shall tell the works of the Lord. He has chastised me with chastisement and He has not handed me over unto death. I shall not die but live and I shall tell the works of the Lord." (LDR)

made while making the sign of the Cross and pronouncing the following prayer:

"In nomine Patris et Filii et Spiritui Sancti individuae Trinitatis. (here Make another sign of the Cross). Dextera domini fecit virtutem, dextera domini exaltavit cos rationem meam. Non moriar sed vivam et narrabo mirabilia domini. Castigans et castigavit me dominus et morti no tradidet me."[63]

You address that prayer to God while you stir the powder into the wine. Thus, you will show your good intentions to cure the wounded patient with God's help.

That is what Hugh of Lucca taught us. He spoke the same prayers and he preferred the same claret while treating wounds of all parts of the body. He began the claret when he thought the patient was ready for nourishment, that usually being at the first dressing or after the first change.

Gilbert[64] used another method which the rhenish surgeons use regularly According to them you must say this prayer over the wounded man while placing unwashed wool soaked in warm olive oil directly on the wound. Surgeon's in the East say that although this prayer is effective on its own you should expect extra payment for what is accomplished for sake of the Lord. They speak that way because they keep tight fists on their money.

Here is the Latin text:

Tres boni fratres per viam unam ibant, at obviavit eis Dominus noster Jhesus Christus et dixit eis. "Tres boni fratres, quo itis?"

Unus ait: "Ymus ad montem Oliveti collogendas herbas ad percussiones et plagas."

Et dixit Dominus Jhesus Christus: "Venite post me, mei boni fratres, et jurate mihi per Crucifixum et per lac mulieris et virginis in abscondite dicatis nec inde mercedem acceptite et accipe lanum siccadam ovis et oleum olivarum et ponite in plagis, credite et dicite sicut Longius ebreus in latro Domini nostri Jhesu Christi pulsavit me nec non sanguinavit nec rei luctavit, nec doluit, nec putridinem fecit nec faciat ista plaga quam carmine. In nomine et Filii et Spiritui Amen.

Et dictatis ter unum Pater Noster et Ave Maria.

While there are doubters, others would have it that only when the

64 Gilbertus Anglicus fl.@1180-90 at Salerno (LDR).

prayer has been properly spoken is the result good; they add that when it does not succeed, it proves that someone prayed badly and that the Lord did not lend an ear.

Anyhow, I will translate it here:

Three good brothers met our Lord Jesus walking on a road. He asked them, "My three good fellows, where are you going?" One answered," We go to the Mount of Olives to find some herbs that are good for treating wounds." Jesus told them, "Come to me (ie use my powers), my three brethren and declare your faith on the Crucified Lord and on the milk of his Virgin Mother. Say it aloud. Do not accept payment. Take unwashed wool soaked in olive oil and place it in the wound, while speaking these words, 'Just as Longius the jew stabbed the Lord in his side and the wound hardly bled, nor did it suppurate, nor was it painful for long, nor did it putrefy, just so let this wound be.'

In the name of the Father and the Son and the Holy Spirit, Amen."

After that repeat three times the Pater Noster and the Ave Maria.

Gilbert said that you can use olive oil on all wounds except those of the head, because oils and fats do not agree with the brain (ie itself is fatty) (see Chapter 1). In those cases oil of roses is better since it is a stimulant, a natural property of roses. As a result, it is not a softener, because the oil which goes into its composition (ie oil of roses) is from olives not from mulberries.

Here we reach the end of our Chapter on head-wounds. We now go on to other Chapters in my Book I.

CHAPTER 18.
HOW TO SUTURE WOUNDS OF THE FACE

First examine a wound made by a sword or another sharp weapon to see if it is straight or oblique (ie at right angles to the surface or as an undercutting slice). Use the shortest of your three triangular (ie cutting edge) needles and thread it with a fine silk or waxed twisted linen thread. Sew the wound-edges together taking bites that are not too far back from the edges nor so deep as to reach the fleshy tissues underneath, lest you produce an ugly scar. You suture that way wherever it will show on the body—as on the face, ears, hands and on a man's penis, if such are wounded.

In an oblique or vertical wound of a lip bring the edges together, then sew them a little more deeply (ie than noted above). Then use the powder prescribed above which contains fresh lime, olibanum and sandragon; or, equally well use red powder. Over the powder, which you should renew daily for nine days, place leaves of plantains or red cabbage.

When the nose suffers an oblique cut leaving an attached piece, sew it back in place with sutures precisely edge to edge. Then dust one of the two powders cited above on the suture-line. Place tubes made of goose or swan feathers wrapped with oakum in the nostrils. That will allow the patient to breath. Then place small bolsters alongside the nose to gently push the alae inward to support the sutured wound-edges in proper position. Do that carefully and you will succeed. Use a long bandage to hold everything in place leaving an opening over the end of the nose. Prevent the bandage from coming too low on the face by passing the ends behind the ears and the head, where you fasten them.

The tubes or the wicks that are in the nares will be conduits (ie along their outer surfaces) for black ointment or the oil of roses used to moisten the wicks. They will splint the nose (ie the alae) from being pushed too far inward and as serve as a means of respiration, until the wound heals. After nine days, apply a small plaster covered with black ointment. Every time you change the dressings wipe clean the wound with warm wine, blot it dry with soft linen and reapply a plaster. In that way, with God's help, you will end up with a healthy repair..

Lanfranchi advised the use of an additional bandage placed crosswise to hold the small bolsters after he sutured the fragment in place. Further, he recommended that you use, in addition to our powders, an oakum pad wet with oil of roses and beaten egg white. He placed a wax bougie (ie as a stent) in the nostrils, a necessary means of keeping the sutured edges in close contact. Without the stent the wings of the nostrils can curl inward (ie a contracture during healing) and obstruct respiration through the nose. That obstruction prevents nasal breathing and keeps air from reaching the lungs in the normal way and results in pulmonary complications. The lungs are responsible for maintaining the normal temperature of the heart by directing to it the air which is breathed through the nose as well as through the mouth. The heart is so warm that if it failed to receive air from the lungs it would use up the moisture of the whole body (ie evaporating it); the result of the wasting and dehydration is what we call phthisis. But remember this, phthisis can be caused in two ways. I will not discuss that here because it is not in the domain of surgery.

Another comment: there are some surgeons who bring together the wound-edges by perforating them (ie across the wound) with many needles. Then they wind threads over their (ie protruding) ends. They leave in the needles for nine days and remove them when the edges are united by scar.

Chapter 19.
Babies Born With Cleft Lips Or Hare Lips

On occasion a baby is born with a cleft in a lip below one nostril, or even beneath both. We call that affliction a hare-lip. We treat it as follows:

Incise with a bistouri along the margins of the cleft, only as far as necessary to raise a flap of skin and expose a raw surface. Then bring the edges together with sutures, inside and outside (ie the mouth), as accurately as you can. Then pass a long needle crossing through both sides of the defect, inserted a good distance away from the sutured wound. Wind a thread around (ie the exposed ends of) the long needle and apply some of the lime powder or red powder and cover it with a plaster of egg-white and oil of roses.

If the wings of the nostrils also are cleft you must repair them at the same time. If you do not do that you will cause harm, since the cleft lip is an extension of the cleft in the nose. Therefore, do it all as instructed and use the same dressings. When you see good union remove the needles.

Some surgeons use no sutures. Instead they close the incision with needles alone. Others cut flaps from the cheeks to replace the defects of the cleft. They use that operation when the defect is large, for example when the central furrow of the upper lip is missing. However, it

---

65 They are stubborn in their own evaluations of what they believe to be a satisfactory outcome (LDR).

seems to me that the operation is wrong because it badly disfigures the face. I advise against any kind of operation that casts a bad light on the surgeon. Besides, when that operation does not have the desired result, as judged by various people (ie other than the surgeons who did the operation), even then the surgeons do not want to listen to reason; they see things only according to their own ways of thinking.[65]

Take notice: You can bring about nicer healing when the defect is insignificant than when a lot of tissue is lost.

CHAPTER 20
TREATMENT OF TUMORS OR BOSSES OF THE HEAD

If lumps persist after blunt trauma to the head be they soft or hard, treat them by applying, as hot as the patient will tolerate, oakum soaked in warm wine to which you add a small amount of salt.

If that is not effective and the mass persists, dose the patient with colchicum pills to the amount of about five, doubly wrapped in wafers that were soaked in claret (ie see Chapter 12 for Hugh of Lucca's recipe), given one hour before nightfall. If the patient suffers from headache, shave his scalp and apply a plaster for pain which you make as follows:

Put some ground salt into some good wine, heat to boiling and then add this powder which you had prepared in advance: Take three ounces each of bay-berries (238) (separated from their pericarps), cumin and anise from which you have stripped the skins and stems. Dry them all in a pan over a flame and then grind them in a mortar. Equally good is this recipe: Use one ounce each of powdered mastic and frankincense which was kept in a box until called for. Add that to the powder described above and some wine. Mix well and then add fine wheat-flour to reach the correct consistencey for a plaster. Then remove the pan from the fire and add an equal amount of honey. Mix all well by stirring. Apply this as a plaster on the injured part, as hot as tolerable. Keep it there five days. If thereafter the tumor persists, repeat the five-day treatments with plasters until it is cured.

Chapter 21.
Penetrating Wounds Across The Forehead Above The Eyes

When you encounter a transverse wound above the eyes with damage to the bone, first determine if the bone is penetrated. If so you must treat as described in the chapters on cranial fractures. If there are splinters of bone detach them and remove them. Then suture the wound, leaving open the lower part to allow for drainage of pus. The dressing should not dam back pus in the depths of the wound

I must inform you again that the bone behind the eyebrows really is not part of the cranium but was put there by Nature to adorn the face. God so adorned Adam and Eve, the first humans, and he endowed them with the ability to produce children who resembled their parents. However, if the father has too much semen, then the limbs of his children will be overdeveloped. In contrast, if the child is rachitic and knock-kneed, that indicates that the mother was in disgrace during her pregnancy or had some abnormality of her uterus

Children frequently inherit their parents' defects, yet sometimes the contrary also occurs (ie congenital defects without inheritance). That is not to be a cause for wonderment because one often encounters women who fail (ie to carry through a successful pregnancy. For example, children often are born with defects that are caused by a woman's fantasies during the procreative act. Hare-lip is in that category. Some others believe that it is the result of something she ate during her pregnancy such as rabbit or barbeau de mer. That is a gross misconception. There have been many babies born with hare lips whose mothers had not eaten rabbit during their pregnancies, let alone those women who had never even seen a barbeau de mer.[66]

Chapter 22
When An Ear Is Partially Sliced Off.

Once in a while you will encounter a patient whose ear is almost completely detached from the head, as when the head is caught be-

---

66 Barbeau de Mer was the red mullet, Mullus barbatus, with a forked extension from the lower jaw, vaguely suggestive of a cleft lip. (LDR)

tween two fence-posts. You should examine the remaining attachment to see if it is viable and if it is adequate to carry nourishment to the detached ear. If that is so, lose no time in reattaching it with several bites of a (ie running) suture. Sprinkle over the sutures a powder compounded as we have taught, or use red powder and lay an oakum plaster over that.

If the ear remains warm it will heal in place. You must keep it moist with warm wine and renew the dressing with the red powder every ninth day. The final dressing should be some wine-soaked oakum.

Many surgeons use ointments in such cases. I advise against that, and the Old Masters agree with me, stating that the only useful kind of ointment is 'contradictory', that is both a stimulating and an astringent preparation. Most ointments lack that property. For example, that is the case for black ointment and most ointments based on oil of roses, oil of mastic or oil of myrtle. Those materials do not combine with astringents, as when you add mastic or frankincense to sangdragon or hepatic aloes or cypress berries (149) or with powdered galls (195) or with balaustia (47) and the like. Those medicines which are digestives, such as those made with olive oils, both green or ripened, or with other fatty materials are harmful when applied to cartilaginous or nerve-bearing tissues.

I mention this in the context of the region of the ear to show you why you must always consider the individual characteristics of the various parts of the body that you are called upon to treat. You must evaluate that information and deal with each region according to its own properties.

If the ear is cut by a sharp weapon such as a sword or a dagger or a knife, and it dangles from the cheek, held only by a small flap, with or without a bone fragment, replace it promptly and suture it. Always insert a wick into the ear canal lest the process of healing will close it off and impair the patient's hearing. That would make you a laughing stock. Be very exacting about restoring everything to its natural position.

There are some folks who try to inflate their reputations by boasting to an audience that they had seen a case where the ear had been completely sliced off and the victim had retrieved the specimen and had taken it to a surgeon who reattached it in its former place and it healed. Oh, well! Those are fables. Any part of the body that has been completely cut off immediately loses its vitality. What is dead does not return to life, unless there are miracles and in our work we do not make miracles. You will encounter examples that will confirm what I say. In this sort of situation when a part of the face or some other region has been sliced off, leaving a slim flap which is not adequate to supply the rest of the detached tissues, that part will wither and die. However, it may happen that even a very tenuous flap may be sufficient for survival if an hepatic vein[67] traverses it to serve the tissues or an artery survives to carry the body's vitality and heat.

Also, it may happen that the reattachment may strangle the flap and gangrene will ensue. That is the fault of the surgeon. I advise every surgeon for the sake of his own reputation and self-interest and that of the patient, to avoid that error and avoid censure.

Chapter 23.
Wounds Of The Face And Nearby Regions Caused By Projectiles

Wounds of the face often are caused by arrows or other projectiles with metal tips that can penetrate the skull. That is a frequent occurrence in wars along the Mediterranean Sea coast and in the Roman States (ie Holy Roman Empire), Spain, France, England, Scotland, Wallonia and Flanders.

This is how I manage such cases. First I examine the wounded man, placing him in the posture he was in when he was struck. If the arrow-shaft has already been removed, I ascertain if the metal tip also came out. As a rule, wounds are more serious if they were directed upward from below, reasoning as follows. Suppose one is shooting from the base of a wall of a castle or a fortress, aiming toward the top. The weapon reaches the defender's head or body. In the first case the concern is whether the projectile reached the brain; in the second, whether it struck an internal organ—liver, lung, urinary bladder, spleen, stomach—and whether the direction of the wound of entry is downward (ie the external opening is higher than the internal) which favors collec-

---

67 Here as elsewhere in the anatomic lore of the classic and medieval eras we find the claim that the liver is the source of venous blood, and that the hepatic segment of the inferior vena cava was the root of the system rather than the right cardiac atrium which was considered a tributary of the vena cava carrying nutrition to the heart (LDR).

tions of pus. But there are, however more serious consequences with such wounds, as we will show you.

If the arrow remains in situ when you arrive at the scene, determine if the metal tip and the wood shaft are still attached. If so, pull them out together; use great care and avoid censure if only the wood comes forth. Search for hooks (ie the barbs) that may have broken loose and remain in the wound. That would run later risks of having to make painful incisions to recover what was left behind.

However, it is better to make those incisions than to leave the pieces. Nature abhors foreign materials left within the body, although the body itself may extrude them if it retains enough vitality to do so. Not infrequently one encounters people who have harbored pieces of projectiles or other foreign bodies which were extruded a year or more after the wounding. Then the muscle or fascia or bone where the foreign material has lodged will undergo liquefaction (ie encystment) more or less rapidly. When it 'points' the victim then will suffer intense itching and an urge to scratch at the center of the old wound, near the object. Thus he will cause the liquid to be expelled, allowing the escape or the removal of the foreign body. Then the wound will heal.

If the person has been shot with an English arrow, one that has two barbs on each side (ie of the arrowhead), or with a javelin (ie probably here a dart) with hooks along its side, do as follows. Slip a tube made from a goose's or a swan's feather over the barbs or hooks and withdraw the weapon. Failure to do that allows them (ie the hooks and barbs) to remain in the tissues and cause serious complications. The wound is worse off than before (ie the treatment). Those objects can be removed (ie by withdrawing them with the tubes) and large and deep incisions will not be necessary.

The process of pulling out the projectile must be fearless and resolute; pull parallel to the direction of the wounding (ie the course traversed by the weapon) or else you will damage more tissue and create complications. Whether done by hand or with a forceps guide the arrow with the thumb and two fingers of your right hand (ie delicately).

If the arrow was shot (ie with the force of) a bow or a cross-bow and is buried in a bulky part of the body, for example, the thigh, you must grasp the projectile with a forceps that has a serrated jaw so it will not slip when you pull with it.

If even then you fail to remove the projectile, get some help and advice from your colleagues, and follow the consensus of the recommendations. But, before going ahead, see to the needs of your patient for his general support. If the weapon is large and has been shot into a fleshy limb with sufficient force to imbed all of the barbs or hooks and you find that you cannot pull it out in reverse, then you must push it through the tissues and out the opposite side.

If the victim suffers a wound in which the metal tip of the arrow is attached to the wooden shaft by a pin through the heft, as is in common use in Hungary and among the pagans (ie the Saracens), almost certainly you can extract the entire arrow and its tip in one piece. After that extraction, treat the wounded man with a potion described here. You can treat all such cases (ie after complete and uncomplicated extraction) without drains.

Take a pinch each of tansy (454), clove, orties (326), red cabbage (71), plantain (353), sour red blackberries. Boil all together with three pints of wine until it is reduced to two pints. Filter through a cloth and add some frothy (ie whipped) honey to sweeten to taste. Allow to cool before adding five beaten egg-whites, stirring continuously. Now bring it to a boil, without further stirring, and pour it through a cloth. Give the patient one table-spoon-full, morning and evening, and lay red cabbage leaves on the wound.

In that way you may treat the wounds that we have described without drains. The same method is good for wounds made by other projectiles provided that the flesh is not mangled. You may treat wounds made by sword points and daggers in the same way.

Avicenna prescribed a potion with which I personally achieved a nice cure in a patient whose arms and a thigh had been perforated, through and through; the wound had been suffered 17 hours before. This potion also was described by the Four Masters in their Commentary on Roland's Chirurgia. Really it is the best potion when you treat wounds without drains. Here it is:

Take some garance root (197) and equal amounts of large and small plantains, cannabis seeds (78), red cabbage and lady apples.

The amount of red madder roots should be twice that of the amounts of each of the others. Mix with wine and boil down to one quart. Add more wine, boil again. Repeat three times and then pour through a cloth. Set aside for use as desired.

Give it three times daily, morning, midday and evening. Do not use drains in the wound, which you cover with red cabbage leaves.[68]

Another potion: Take equal amounts of cloves, absinthe, pigle wheat (494), consoude (128) and Robert's herb (6). Use wine and boil-down as above. Dose the patient in whom you do not use drains.

And yet another potion: Take a handfull each of hemp buds, blackberries and tansy. Grind together with some red madder root, using a pestle. Mold into small balls the size of a small coin, taking care not to squeeze out their juices. Set them in sunlight to dry. When you wish to use them, wet a ball down with wine and give it to the patient if he is not feverish. If he has fever, wet the ball with syrup of violets or water instead of wine. The dose of this potion is three full table-spoons daily. Apply red cabbage leaves on his wound.

Another similar potion: Take hemp, seeds or leaves, tansy and red cabbage, in equal amounts and red madder roots in an amount equal to the sum of all the others. Grind in a mortar. Moisten with wine. Filter. Dose the patient three times daily in amounts equal to a boiled egg. Use red cabbage leaves on the wound. If the patient refuses the potion (ie any of them) that is a sign that death is near.

CHAPTER 24
REMOVAL OF THORNS AND OTHER PROJECTILES WITHOUT INCISIONS

Since many wounded persons are fearful of being cut for removal of arrows, thorns and fragments of other objects that remain in wounds, you may try to eliminate them (ie by extrusion) with the following plaster:

Take fraxinelle (189), polypodium (362) and coudrier (hazel) sap (136a). Grind them all and add lard to make a plaster. You may

---

68 The use of potions by surgeons was limited, to be used only as part of treatments for open wounds, especially of the head and the thorax. Laxatives, lozenges, gargles etc. were not classed as potions (LDR).

use this plaster even if the foreign body is metallic (ie iron) and the victim refuses to allow the removal.[69] However, I prefer to use a maturing plaster which, by provoking suppuration in the region of the wound, causes the foreign body to be discharged with a flow of pus. A better method (ie than when an abscess is allowed to necessitate) is to drain the abscess with a deftly performed incision.

If you must use the plaster method for eliminating foreign bodies you should explain to the patient that it will take a long time. He will lose his confidence in your ability if you promise a rapid delivery of the object and it is not forthcoming,.

The plaster is successful for spontaneous extrusion only if a foreign body is buried in soft tissues. If it is embedded in a bone, you must use a forceps or other techniques that you may have to devise.

If an arrow has pierced the scalp and the skull you must incise from the wound of entry to the wound of exit. If is not a through-and-through wound you must incise to the bottom of it. If you happen to encounter a fragment of something, remove it, clean the wound, and dress it as a for a simple wound.

If the wound penetrates the bone and the dura-mater, you must incise the scalp, following the track of the projectile down to the bone. Elevate the skin and the deeper layers of the scalp over the bone which is scraped bare to allow you to inspect it and to remove any foreign material, avoiding injury to the dura mater. If (ie while you are removing the unwanted bits), there are untoward symptoms, and if the victim's friends strongly abjure you, leave the scene. In that event, inform them, as I have taught you, of your concern for the outcome of his case.

CHAPTER 25
THE DIET REGIMEN FOR WOUNDED PATIENTS

Attend now to my suggestions for diets to be given to the wounded.

If he has lost a lot of blood, restore his losses with food and drink. For example, if he is almost bled out but remains lucid, give him almond milk and wheat gruel. However, those foods are contraindicated if he had suffered a head-wound, because the milk of oily nuts

---

69 The usual objects were splinters, thorns, bits of wood darts, etc. (LDR).

and of hazel nuts, being less digestible are harmful to the head. Give those patients cooked sour apples or a puree of shelled white peas.

In addition you may give consomme acidified with a little vinegar, and boiled milk beaten with a small amount of flour. As a beverage, prescribe tea or small beer without herbs, or milk of almonds prepared with boiled water. Those drinks are good for the mentally intact as well as for delirious patients.

The following beverage strengthens the stomach and blocks the bad humors from rising to the head and from obstructing the body (ie constipating). Also, it lessens fever.

Take two drams of barley (orges,323), one dram of wheaten bread crumbs, ten Damascus plums (355). Boil all in ten pounds of water until it is reduced by half. Filter through a cloth. Keep in glass jars. Serve it cold.

Another beverage: Take fifteen pints of pure water, three drams of hulled barley, five drams each of jujubes (230) and sebesten plums (421), one ounce of damson plums and one ounce of plum pits, three ounces of rosamel (385). Boil all until reduced to about five pints. Serve cold.

If the wounded man has lost blood and is not feverish you may offer him boiled chicken, game birds and pigs' feet, but be sure all are well cooked. You may also give boiled eggs. For beverages, use watered wine, but not enough to make him drunk. Inebriety is contrary to nature; the drunken patient cannot generate energy where it is needed nor can he assimilate what he needs, nor can he relieve the heat of the liver. The corrupt humors then produce fevers.

You should forbid the following from wounded persons: pork, beef, venison, rabbit, goose, swan, duck and all kinds of web-footed birds, eel, carp, trout and all fish that are bottom-feeders. You may allow him to eat small fish with scales such as roach, gudgeon, perch and young pike. You may allow the meat of hens, chicks, capons and boiled young roosters, partridge, finch, lark and all small birds with spread claws or with mixed or fawn-colored plumage (ie pigeons and doves).

CHAPTER 26
SPASM (TETANUS), THE CRAMPS THAT BESET VICTIMS OF WOUNDS.

Spasm is a terrifying malady when it attacks a wounded person, and usually it is fatal. It manifests itself in either of two ways: by plethora or by atony. Two examples of the first are a wounded plethoric person who has not lost enough blood to lose his plethoric appearance, or if indeed he has lost enough blood but the wound was caused by a sharp edged weapon, a sword or the like. In the case without excessive blood loss, if he is otherwise not played out, you should bleed him from a vein close to the wound. Thus, if he suffered a head-wound, bleed him from a vein on the same side of the head. If the wound was caused by a blow from a cudgel or other blunt weapon, you should remove a large amount of blood. A large amount of (ie vital) humors are carried toward the bruise (ie by the blood). Hence, by phlebotomy the blood is attracted from the site of injury to where it is being removed. Such (ie the foregoing about plethora) is the first useful lesson about wounds associated with tetanus.

If spasm appears after atony, it is incurable because the body cannot restore itself. In that situation the stomach no longer can digest raw foods and the liver is enfeebled and chilled and consequently it cannot absorb the nutriments contained in the stomach nor remit them back to all the parts of the body that remain viable.

Emprosthotonus, Episthotonus and Tetanus (ie opisthotonus) In emprosthotonus the muscles bend the head forward, bringing the chin down toward the chest. The jaws are clenched so that you cannot slip even a knife blade between the teeth, and the fingers are flexed into the palm so that you cannot straighten them.

In episthotonus, the head is pulled back. The mouth is held agape, the cheeks and the teeth do not meet and one cannot close his mouth. Finally, the fingers are held stiffly extended and he cannot make a fist.

Tetanus is the prototype of Spasm. Every part of the body contracts all at once such that contrary movement is impossible. The body, from the top of the head to the soles of the feet is rigid, as if it was impaled on a rod. This is the last of the affections which properly are called the spasms of the wounded. Here are the five principal causes:

1. After plethora. 2. After atony. 3. Nerves are immersed in pus which infects the wound, and irritates them. 4. Following the application of rancid fatty substances on wounds. By that I mean rancid fats or oils such as appear in fetid ointments, especially those that were made according to the instructions of Avicenna who used (ie only fresh) oil of roses or, preferably, drawn butter, olive oil or the like (ie and the fresh preparations had been allowed to spoil). 5. Spasm that comes after cold air has affected the nerves in a wound. That could follow exposure to a cold breeze or to a cold medicine. Those are the five principal causes of tetanus in wounds.

I explained that the signs of plethora show themselves promptly and they are obvious, whereas for atony it is different. The other three causes frequently are the results of mismanagement by ignorant surgeons, usually they are lay practitioners who were the students of other laics, who boast that they have forgotten nothing, simply because they had learned nothing. For my part, I do things as I saw them done by my surgical masters who taught me what I know. You can be certain that none of them was a laic. Now, let us get on to the treatment of Tetanus, as the Great Surgical Masters recommended in their books.

Spasm caused by the first and the by the last three causes (ie of the five) is treated by bleeding. You rarely will need to use phlebotomy when spasm is caused by atony.

Pour warm oil of roses into all wounds in regions that contain many nerves; all medicaments that you use in those wounds should be warm.

Massage the neck, the nape, the vertebral column and the flanks, using the oil of laurel—also known as oil of bay-berries—or oils of euphorbia (173), castor (95), nard (302), rue (394), lily (348), oil bénite (ie sacramental oil, 344), petroleum (ie mineral oil, 344) or any other warmed oil. Holy oil is better than mineral oil because of its natural warmth.

Also, you may use this ointment advocated by Master Bruno: Take three ounces each of castor beans and euphorbia seeds; five drams each of pyrethrum (371), frankincense, myrrh, aloes and mastic; one dram each of the oils of laurel, elder tree, tussilage (470) and lapatum acutum (395); wax in amounts as needed. Grind the solids in a metal mortar and then mix with the oils. Heat over a flame and add the wax. It is an excellent oinment for treating tetanus.

Have the patient drink the following potion: Take equal amounts of castor beans, cinnamon, lavander aspic (240), pepper, calamus (sedge, 74), marjolaine (270), sage (400) and rue. Master Hugh of Lucca made a clear wine (ie claret) with those herbs (ie see Chapter 122) and he gave small doses to his patients. He vouched for its benefits.

In addition, you may use this gargle (ie throat-rinse): Take seeds of mustard (297), pyrethrum and staphisaigre (445). Boil them in wine with some honey. Strain through a cloth before giving it to the patient.

Use the following sneeze powder (ie sternutatory): Grind castor beans and pepper in a mortar. Put a little of the powder in the nose to make the patient sneeze.

To provoke a sweat, place the patient in warm bath best prepared as follows: Boil these herbs in a tightly stoppered jar (ie in water): absinthe, sage, rue, fennel and mint (288a). Pour the decoction into the sick man's bath. Keep a fire going under the tub until he has a good sweat and then apply the ointment given above. After the treatment you must see to it that he does not take a chill. Place him in a soft bed. After he has rested a while, repeat the above baths until, God willing, he recovers.

In cases of emprosthotomnus, take the precaution of putting strip of wood between his teeth to prevent him from biting his tongue during a fit.

Here is another excellent ointment to use when tetanus occurs with plethora. Take some pouliot (367), absinthe, laurel and cumin. Grind them to a fine powder. Mix with honey by stirring and apply— neither too hot nor too cold—on the affected parts to ease the pain.

And here is another, which Avicenna advocated for use in children with spasm: Take anise, saffron and honey. Make an ointment (ie with oils and wax) to apply to the affected parts.

Finally, let me admonish you that spasm caused by atony may follow excessive hemorrhage (ie including phlebotomy), excessive diarrhea (ie including purging) and prolonged fevers.

Chapter 27.
Tinea Of The Scalp. The Teachings Of The Four Masters

Some cases of ringworm can be cured, others not. In the last group the scalp is adherent to the cranium: indurated, fixed, released only by applying a lot of sulfur which dissolves the hair. If you are willing to accept any cases of tinea in your practice, avoid the incurable patients.

There are two categories that are curable. One occurs when the growth of hair is normally abundant, the so-called purulent tinea. The scalp is healthy, soft and not adherent to the bone. In the other, the scalp is healthy and dry, but causes much itching and tends to baldness. In treating both kinds, first soften the scalp by rubbing it with butter before scraping away pustules, as I will instruct later on.

You may use the following ointment (ie instead of butter) to soften the scalp. Take one ounce each of white ellebore (164) and the flowerheads of lapatum acutum; four ounces each of soft ship tar (455), walnut shells and oily nuts (309). Grind all and make an ointment. In winter time before you proceed to remove the hairs with their roots, you should devote eight or nine hours, or even longer, to the softening of the scalp with the oils of nuts. Then after the hair is removed, you continue, using the scalp softening ointment. When the hair grows back, (ie during the long course of treatment) wet the scalp with a strong solution of lye. Wipe dry and rub in the preparation called cylotrum (327), prepared thus: Take four ounces of quick lime (251), stir in some water and add two drams of orpiment and boil until (ie when tested) the plumage is easily pulled from the shaft of a briefly dipped goose-feather. Rub the scalp with the medication until depilation is complete. As the hairs grow back repeat the process until the scalp is no longer red (ie inflamed by tinea) but remains pale. You are assured of a cure when the new hair is soft.

When the scalp seems too dry, that is, if the tinea is the dry type, add a little olive oil to the cylotrum to preserve the natural turgor of the scalp. However, if the tinea is the moist type, use the cylotrum undiluted, without the oily supplement.

We learn from the Gloss of the Four Masters that tinea often appears after improper treatments by surgeons who apply plasters on scalps which are too hot and too dry. They diminish the natural turgor of the skin and cause dryness where Nature prefers moisture. In their ignorance they bring on a hardness that causes the hair to fall out and prevents re-growth. Really if hair is to be restored one needs a moderate degree of warmth and a proper moisture. Excessive heat and excessive wetness submerge and drown the hair.

In addition the Gloss states that tinea can be produced if one leaves plasters in place for too long, causing injury or an ulcer. That kind of tinea also is caused by sour humors. When they are too large the plasters cause intense itching and the shedding of large flakes or scales.

There is a variety of tinea caused by melancholy or atrabilia (ie peevishness, and splenic disposition) which does not cause much itching as a result of its own coldness and dryness. Rather its humors are dirty and from them come large pustules, especially in persons who over-eat, who are indolent and who do not bathe.

Tinea manifests itself in many different ways, according to the various different constitutions of the patients. The precepts which I give here concerning the constitutions were defined by the illustrious Old Masters: Hippocrates, Galen, Avicenna, Rhazes and many others.

The sanguine group: They have a lot of blood; they are obese or robust; they are ruddy in complexion; they have happy facial expressions. When pustules appear they are filled with a good kind of pus. Their urine is dark and dense. This constitution (ie sanguine) is mostly found among young people below age thirty. They love meat and substantial foods and good wine. Those are their salient characteristics.

Those with bilious constitutions are lean; they have large and red hands; they eat sparingly and are not choosy about food. Their pustules are yellowish and dry. So much for the bilious.

The phlegmatics have pale skin. Their pustules are colorless, or more precisely, are as pale as their skins. They are overweight and they move sluggishly. They produce a lot of sputum and their urine is white, pale or cloudy and dense.[70] Their digestion is slow. Parts of their bodies are soft and yielding and blanch when touched. Their personalities and their humors are cold.

The melancholics and atrabilious are skinny, but dark-skinned. Their urine is brown or pale and clear, or occasionally greenish and clear. They eat well and their blood is brown and thick. They reject beef, goat's meat and soups of cabbage and red beans considered to be causes of dark and spleeny bile. When affected by tinea the skin of the region turns brown or reddish and it hardens.

With those facts in mind and if the tineal humors are of the atrabilious sort, you must further soften the scalp with compresses of water in which you had boiled violet leaves (486) and leaves of of fumitory (191). After that, anoint with oil of violets until the skin is soft and moist. Feed the patient good fresh food: game, boiled chicken, roman soup, hen's eggs, boiled milk whipped with barley. All raw foods, except those that I have listed, are contraindicated as causes of melancholy and peevishness.

Now I will list the varieties of pustules to be found on the head and in other parts of the body.

Those that are like bubbles rising in boiling water were called water blisters by Master Gilbert. When the blisters were hard he called the disease spedecie, and they were like bony tents (ie capped by hard crusts).

Occasionally, here and there on the scalp, small pustules form, from which thick hairs, like pig bristles, emerge. That illness is called caries (ie rot). When the pustules are gone small cavities remain which emit a honey-like purulent matter. They are called alveolae. Frequently the skin grows over them or in many spots there will be scurfy flakes with intense itching. Scratching produces scales, and there may be tufts of about four long hairs. That disorder is called tines.

If the scalp is red, the malady is sanguine. If it is hot and yellowish, it is by nature bilious. If it is brownish and the scurf is the color of lead

---

70 Urinoscopy had scant mention in the surgical treatises of the era (LDR).

then it is atrabilious (ie spleeny). If it is white and edematous and if it discharges oily matter it is lymphatic.

Now let us go on to the treatment according to the specific indications, which we must ever keep in mind.

For children and for those who have recurred after more than a year, begin with the medications described at length. For oldsters and prime adults you first must establish the category of the disease and the constitution and other indications. If you know the underlying causes try to get rid of them beforehand (ie before treating the tinea).

If the tinea is of the sanguine variety, first dissolve the foul matter by having the patient use three large spoonfuls of osisatum (330) and honey in three large spoonfuls of warm water taken morning and evening. Bleed him from a medial antecubital vein and give him this potion: Take one ounce of violets, twelve damson plums, fourteen sebesten plums, and twenty jujubes. Boil them all in four pounds of water until that is reduced to one pound. Strain through a cloth before adding one ounce of cassia pulp, five ounces each of tamarind (452) and manne (265), one dram each of ground yellow myrobalans (298) and rhubarb (382) and five ounces of rose honey. Offer it as a beverage, a little hotter than just tepid.

The next evening have the patient take a hot bath which will bring on a sweat. After that he should take a daily dose of syrup of Grisecon (ie like yerasimum, 502a) or of fumitory

If the tineas were sustained by sour humors you should first digest them with oximel. If the patient is constipated purge him with two to five gros of yerasimum. You may use that as a purgative even if the patient is not constipated because it will rid him of sour humors. On the third day when he is in the bath for his sweat you shampoo his head with brine. When he is clean, dry him. Again on the fourth day bleed him from a medial antecubital vein. That is the initial treatment when there are sour humors.

After that you soften the scalp with the following medicine: Take a sufficient amount of mauve and roots of guimauve. Boil them in plain water and apply to the scalp. You may also anoint the scalp with those herbs mixed in fresh butter.

Use the bath treatments frequently. After a bath pull out the diseased hairs with a forceps and rub with cylotrum which will heat and inflame the scalp. For relief, rub in this ointment: Mix oil of violets and oil of roses and two egg-yolks and fresh lard. That mixture will relieve the excess heat and inflammation. Then apply this drying ointment: Take some mustard and staphisaigre seeds. Grind them and add some honey. Rub that on the scalp but do not leave too long lest it bring on a fever.

Here is another prescription: Take equal amounts of soap (430c), sulfur (450), pepper, pyrethrum, staphisaigre and half that amount of mercury (283) (ie the sheen of) which was dulled by exposure with a fasting man's saliva (403). Grind it all with some lard and rub it into the tinea.

Here is prescription to be used against moist tinea because it is a drying agent. Take equal amounts of fresh lime and orpiment. Grind. Dilute with some soap and olive oil and rub it in the region of the tinea.

For use against humid tineas and all cool discharges: Take two ounces of litharge and grind it well. Mix with olive oil and vinegar. Pour into a metal mortar and grind while adding more vinegar until it has the consistency of a sauce or, better, of honey.

Another good one: Pulverize fresh lime and orpiment; dilute with vinegar. That ointment can cure tinea without loss of hair.

To make a molded cap for removal of the hair, take melted ships' tar and add finely powdered white frankincense, mastic and a little red honey. Mix. Spread it on a piece of leather or toile or hemp cloth to which you have fastened several lengths of ribbon. Apply the bonnet when warm and tie it in place for three or four days. Seat the patient on a chair and attach a strong cord to a ceiling beam and tie all the ribbons securely to the cord. Then, very suddenly pull the chair out from under the patient. The cap will be wrenched off (ie with the hair!). That procedure is called The Molded Cap.

Observe well the exact position of the tinea on the scalp and just where you must first soften the scalp before using the cylotrum . Failing that you will not be able to pull out the bad hairs. After softening you can use the molded cap as above or with another medicine.

Take ship's tar, colophane and terebinth. Melt all together and spread it on a leather or heavy cloth sheet.

CHAPTER 28
VERMIN (IE LICE) IN THE SCALP AND IN OTHER PARTS OF THE BODY

Lice that grow on the body produce excrement that lodges between the skin and the subcutaneous flesh, and when shed it becomes nits or lice.

If it develops in people with hot temperaments use the following: Take some mercury or ashes of burnt felt; add vinegar and olive oil and make an ointment. Rub it into the verminous regions. You also may use this ointment: Take litharge and mercury, dilute with oil and vinegar and apply it.

If the patient has a cool temperament use this : Take white hellebore, staphisaigre, pastel (497). and red orpiment. Dilute with vinegar and rub it in. You may obtain similar results with red orpiment and oil. Also, you may use sea water (492b) or brine mixed with vinegar.

Another recipe: Take mercury altered with a young person's saliva and lard; add wood or felt ashes and add some powdery granules of staphisaigre and put it all in a folded waist band, or better, on a woolen strip to be wrapped around the body. You will soon observe that all the lice are attracted. The same result is obtained by placing on the chest a folded envelope of cotton containing powdered staphisaigre and terebinth. As a final measure you may use mercury diluted with ashes of burned human hair.

Master Gilbert taught the same lesson that we do, that lice produce corrupt humors. He also said that in persons with atrabilious complexions the vermin are blacker, in those with lymphatic complexions they are whiter, and in the sanguineous their color is redder.

Sometimes the lice are caused to multiply by sweat and by filthy clothing, or they develop in the course of other illnesses. The latter is a prognosis of impending death.

There is a variety of vermin that is indestructible. It is a precursor of leprosy.

CHAPTER 29
WENS OF THE SCALP

A type of tumor which the Picardese-Flemish call warne or overbeene—in our terms it is a wen—often appears on the scalp. Not infrequently it is quite hard. It derives from the hair pore rather than from the hair itself. The tumors produce dense humors mixed with the spleeny kind. If you are asked to treat a patient to rid him of such a wen, make a superficial incision with a razor, taking care to avoid cutting through the thin capsule of the cyst. Then you can dissect it intact and easily shell it out with a blunt hook. The incision must be longitudinal (ie parasagittal) in the direction of the hair rather than transverse. After assuring yourself that all of it has been removed you may, if necessary, suture the defect using a cutting-edge (ie triangular) needle mounted with a waxed thread. Dress it without a drain, carefully observing it to detect (ie and drain) a pocket of pus. That is how you treat wens anywhere on the body, always making the incision in the direction of the tissues.[71] However, when a wen is near an eye you must not incise at right angles to the orbit, but transversely—in a direction from the nose toward the temple, parallel to the eyebrows. For wens on the cheek, incise vertically, that is from above down, from the eye toward the cheek. Always try to obtain the smallest possible scar.

After suturing the incision, Albucasis applied on but not into the wound the powder we have described in a previous chapter on wounds. Let me call your attention to avoid leaving any of the debris of the cyst (ie cyst wall) in the wound. Even the smallest remnant will regenerate a wen.

If the wen is so adherent that it is torn (ie during the operation) and cannot be removed all-of-a-piece, you must not suture the wound. Dust into the wound a powder to be described below. That powder works well anywhere when you have some matter that must be eliminated. If there is a lot of it to be destroyed use a large dose; use a small

---

71 This certainly anticipates "Langer's " lines (LDR).

dose when the need is small. The slough of the wen will come away after nine days. Then apply lard or fresh butter twice daily.

Here is the recipe for the powder: Take equal amounts of iron filings (limaille, 249a), vert-de-gris, yellow orpiment, vitriol (490) and couperose (136a); take twice as much quick-lime as each of the aforementioned; pulverize in a metal mortar and pass through a cloth sieve. Dilute with frothy honey and form into small balls which you set out to dry in sunlight. Re-pulverize and again add honey. Repeat the operation three times and store the little balls in a dry place. When needed, pulverize one ball at a time and apply the powder on the retained matter in the wound.

Here is another powder with similar actions: Take four drams each of the juice of chelidonium (109) roots and of the urine of children at age five or thereabout. Take three drams of fresh lime and one dram of orpiment. Pulverize separately the lime and the orpiment. Mix the powdered lime with the urine and the juice. Bring it to a boil over a low flame stirring continuously while you add the orpiment, only just to the point of boiling. The orpiment will lose its effectivenenss if it is allowed to boil. Form balls as already instructed and dry in sunlight. Store in a dry place until used.

If the patient wants to get rid of his wen without incision, lay on a cloth dam with an opening to expose only the skin over the wen. Apply the following epispastic (ie vesicant): Take some soap and add one part each of orpiment and fresh lime to reach the consistency of an ointment. Apply it on the surface over the wen. Then lay on a cloth folded in four plies and hold it in place for a full day with a suitable bandage, not too tightly wrapped. The skin will be corroded and necrotic. Apply fresh lard or butter which will cause the damaged skin to slough away. Then apply the powder as given above to the exposed wen, leading to its rupture. Continue the applications until you cannot detect any remnants of the sac in the wound. Then treat the wound as we have instructed.

If the wound is on the vertex of the calvarium and it adheres to the skull, be sure that no rootlets extend through to the dura mater (ie it really is not a wen). In that event you must be exceedingly circum-spect. If you should incise and you rupture the membrane, then, by your imprudent action, you will cause the death of your patient. I advise you, therefore, that this matter deserves your full attention and that you be on guard should you encounter such a case.

CHAPTER 30
THE TREATMENT OF THE TUMOR OF THE HEAD CALLED TESTUDO

A tumor of the head which in Latin is called Testudo (ie turtle) appears frequently.[72] It is an aposthem that develops between the scalp and the cranium and penetrates the scalp as it continues to grow there (ie it necessitates as an abscess). It favors the very fibrous skin that is found there (ie in the scalp) rather than in other parts of the body, as I described at the beginning of this book in the chapter on the structure of the head. It is found most often in children under the age ten.

Treat it as follows: Incise the skin and the abscess in the direction of the hair, the full length of the abscess. Empty the pus and curette the sac in the depths of the accumulation. Pack the cavity with lint and place atop that a pad of lint bound in place until the next day. Then remove the lint and dress the wound without more lint. If the abscess cavity is very large and if there are retained pockets of pus that one cannot expose to evacuate, then you must accomplish the debridement with a cruciate incision. Then dress the wound as I have already taught. If you can manage to treat the abscess without a cruciate incision, using only a linear one, you will obtain a cure with less pain and with a smaller scar.

If the abscess had already ruptured, that is, the affected tissues had been eaten away, discharging foul pus, then you must destroy them with previously charred blue couperose which you had ground into a powder. That (ie corrosive) substance destroys carbuncular tissue anywhere in the body, and allows subsequent healing. But, in

---

72 De Mets suggests that Yperman's abscess was a form of Anthrax. I disagree. All the texts of that epoch and of earlier centuries describe it as one of the class of aposthems which we know to be a very large sebaceous cyst. They called it Testudo, the Latin 'turtle'; it was frequently infected. The Romans also gave the name 'testudo' to a siege device, covered with a protective lid. The word comes from 'testa' meaning 'shell' (LDR).

women, although it destroys the foul flesh, it does not heal the wound. That is because women have colder and moister complexions than adult males.

You must not allow pus to form pockets; that will happen if you pack in the lint (ie too tightly) and not permit free drainage. The pus will liquefy and form sesspools.

The hair usually is lost (does not grow) in the region over the purulent collection. Usually it will re-grow unless the suppuration persists for too long a time and the roots are damaged or destroyed.

Let the foregoing material on the head and its diseases be sufficient.

BOOK II: THE EYE AND THE TREATMENT OF OCULAR DISEASES, ACCORDING TO THE INSTRUCTION OF MASTER JEHAN YPERMAN.

CHAPTER 1.
THE STRUCTURE OF THE EYE

Let us first examine the structure of the ocular apparatus.

The eye has very nearly the shape of a pine cone.[73] The posterior part is drawn out, the front is flatter and the central part is quite round. Thus, it is better able to radiate its perceptions inward.

At the rear there is a tubular nerve that enters the brain and carries to it the optic images. When the nerve is blocked by (ie diseased) humors the person is blind yet the eye itself is beautifully intact.

Inside the globe there is a very pure fluid that we call the fluid of the compartments or chambers, which receives the light after it passes through three transparent membranes. The first, the uvea lies closest to the aqueous humor. The second is called crystalline, and outermost is the cornea.[74]

The innermost, the uvea, resembles the skin of a raisin; in Latin it is called *uva passa.*

The middle membrane is called the crystalline for its resemblance to a crystal. The third membrane is called cornea for its resemblance to (ie a flake of) horn; in additon to being transparent it is flexible.

Those membranes from front to back are penetrated by light which

---

73 The eye and the attached orbital contents (LDR).

74 At this point, Yperman does not distinguish the aqueous from the vitreous, both being very clear. The anterior surface of the crystalline lens here is considered as a transparent membrane, one of three anterior to the vitreous. The refractive functions of the lens were not recognized at that time. The gelatinous contents of the lens were a third humor for other medieval writers. See Mondeville, 'humeur albuginée'(LDR).

is transmitted through the aqueous humor and from there to the nerve which is found at the conical part of the eye. That nerve is attached at the rear to two fibrous membranes which enclose the entire eye. One is called the sclera and derives from the dura mater. The other is called the secondine because it derives from the first. The two together enclose the various elements that make the eye. The inner one is in contact with the aqueous humor, the outer one is in contact with the muscular tissues and is called the white of the eye. In its substance are the arteries and the veins which nourish the organ.

There is yet another membrane, called the small one, which arises from the pia mater as well as from the sclera. It is very thin and surrounds the vitreous body.[75] Between these membranes there are many others that are loosely arranged and which form a diaphragm which can dilate and contract. More will be said about that later on.

The tubular nerve is formed by three components, the dura mater, the pia mater and the arachnoid network which covers and isolates the lobes of the brain.

Between the window (ie the cornea) and the aqueous humor we find a circlet (ie attached) at the edge of the cornea, bearing the name Iris. That membrane contains the principal colorant of the eye, differing, person to person, from gray to blue to brown or to mixtures thereof. It traps the blood that otherwise would flow directly into the lens or the cornea, as is sometimes seen after blows or contusions incurred by falling, or from other causes—for example, after rheumatism (ie iritis) or after other serious diseases.

Attached to that ring you find another membrane called *aranea* in Latin and in common language the spider-net. That very thin and subtle membrane is quite tough. Attached to the arachnoid network at the periphery of the cornea it covers the inner surface of the eye (ie as the choroid-retina) excepting the cornea.

Nature has provided an additional layer, the outer one (ie the most exposed) which covers the (ie the face of) globe, excepting the cornea. It is called the conjunctiva. If that would cover the cornea, the

75 The finer anatomy of the eye could not be determined without magnifying lenses. I think that Yperman describes the "membranule" being the same as what he called the secundina, and that it probably is the choroid-retina (aranea) (LDR).

pupil could not receive light. But it (ie the conjunctiva) is attached to the (ie periphery of) three transparent membranes that lie in front of the aqueous humor (ie cornea, uvea, lens).

The nerves that enter and leave the eyes, right and left, differ from other nerves of the body. They arise from the anterior part of the brain along with the two nerves that enable the nose to transmit the sense of smell, and which end like the milk ducts in a woman's breasts. The optic nerves cross each other while passing from the eyes to the brain. Nature had many good reasons for that. If vision in one eye is obstructed, the other eye will be able, by reason of the crossed nerves, to see for two. Aristotle said that what was lost in one eye was duplicated in the other.

You can demonstrate the faculty of transmitted vision via the crossed optic nerves when the condition exists that in Latin is called *limpinositas* and in Flemish is *drope,* (ie conjunctivitis) which results from a catarrh flowing from the brain and which befalls sometimes one and sometimes both eyes. When only one eye is affected, the suffering is felt in both eyes via the crossed nerves. Furthermore, Nature has provided the crossing to allow one eye to come to the aid of the other (ie in providing vision). The effect of the crossing is also observed in this example: when you stare at an object with both eyes you see one. But if you displace one eye by pushing it with a finger tip, you see two or even more. That means that you have pressed one nerve and prevented it from transmitting normal vision. Now we have completed our description of normal eyes.

CHAPTER 2.
NOW WE PROCEED TO KNOWLEDGE OF THE DISEASES OF THE EYES AND THEIR CAUSES

Afflictions of the eyes are numerous—be they sui generis or caused by corruption of the humors. The causes may be internal or external. The latter are more common and they derive from the heat or coldness of the air, from dust, from vapors, from wind and the like.[76]

The internal causes may come from corrupt humors, from a bad

76 Vapors probably include steam and emissions from acrid sources, such as onions (LDR).

constitution, from repercussions (ie as complications of other diseases) or as a result of contact with somebody who has a contagious ophthalmia.

Among the diseases that affect the eyes and the surrounding region we list ophthalmias, pustules (ie styes), ulcerations, red or white blotches, pruritus, psora (ie pruritis with eruptions), grit (sabel), specks and films, ocular consumption, cataracts, sicoen (ie dryness), inflammations of the eyelids, irritations by defective eyelashes and, lastly, lacrimal fistulas. There are many other ocular afflictions, such as blindness, but they are not for the surgeon to treat.

In the following I will offer some instructions and prescriptions with which to cure those diseases or simply to offer relief. I will begin with ophthalmias, simple inflammations which come in three degrees: benign, intense and grave (ie threatening).

Chapter 3.
Treatment Of Benign Ophthalmia

Benign ophthalmia is redness accompanied by mild discomfort, with slight or no puffiness of the lids. It may be caused by too hot or too cold winds, by vapors, dust, excessive insomnia, laborious work or by exposure to too bright light.

If the symptoms—local redness, heat or pain—are mild, simply use beaten foamy egg white (163) and drip the clear liquid exuding from it into the eyes of the patient who lies supine with face up. That collyrium is known to be very good and it may be used safely without restrictions. It is glutinous and it adheres to the eye for a long time, and it cleanses while relieving the inflammmation. If the ophthalmia is caused by exposure to cold, in addition to the collyrium have the patient drink some good wine and then submit to fumigations with vapors arising from boiling rose petals (389), camomille (76) and fenugrec (181).

If those measures fail to give relief, you should bleed from a vein in the temple in order to lessen the congestion that accompanies the inflammation. At the same time, apply the white collyrium, the composition of which will be included in a chapter to follow.

Chapter 4.
Ophthalmia Of The Second Degree, A More Intense Variety

In the more intense ophthalmia the white of the eye and the cornea are redder and the scleral vessels are congested with blood. The caruncle over the tear sac is severely inflamed, causing much discomfort and the agglutination of the lids. In some cases you may see small whitish patches (ie probably exudate) on the cornea. In the very severe cases the cornea seems hidden under a veil of reddish discharge. The lids also are inflamed: puffy, glossy and often covered with pustules.[77]

As in all cases of ophthalmia,, here, too, the treatment first should be directed against the inflammation (ie infection), as I will indicate later.

When the inflammation has subsided a bit, bleed the patient from a vein on his temple or from an arm on the side of the affected eye if only one eye is affected. If both eyes are involved, bleed more copiously in young and sturdy patients and less in oldsters.

When the patient is young and sanguine (ie constitution) show-ing a great intensity of redness, apply cups between the scapulas. However, if he is rather bilious (ie the constitution) and he has only a little edema and less pain (ie than the sanguinous patient), but he has a degree of yellowness of the eyes, then a small bleed will suffice. Afterwards, purge the patient with yellow myrobalans.

When the discharge is bilious and mixed with some thick green-ish matter, and the condition has become chronic, there is no better treatment than Rhazes' pills, so-called Rhazes' nuts.

Now let me describe the best Prescriptions for use against the more intense ophthalmias (ie see footnote 8).

a. Take one egg-yolk and amounts equal to them of oil of roses
   and verbena (477). Add one scruple each of saffron and
   opium and make a plaster (ie with added wax and olive oil).
   Put a previously prepared cloth over the eyes and spread the

77 A 'Pustule' in the medieval texts is any vesicle, often crusted. The contents may be any liquid or oily matter, not necessarily pus. (LDR).

paste on it. Before that, drip into the eyes some of the white
collyrium diluted with breast milk (486) from a young
woman.

b. The white collyrium of Galen is called the great remedy
because by itself it leads to cure within a few days. It is made
this way: Take three drams of céruse (105), ground and
sifted and grind it in pure water using a special stone such as
scribes use for grinding their coloured ink-powders. Let it
stand covered, for six days, not to be contaminated by dust or
anything else.

Then dissolve two and one half drams of gum arabic (212) in
clean water and mix it with the white lead. Then add the
following fine powder: Three drams of amidum (21) and
one fourth dram each of sarcocolla gum, parsley and saffron,
and make pills the size of peas. When dried they are kept for
use. When needed, crumble a pill in some young-mother's
milk, working it to a consistency of wine-must. Apply this
collyrium into the eye over which you lay the plaster (ie
described above in a.). Repeat twice a day until recovery.

c. Master Lanfranchi said that Master Bevenoud prescribed what
he (Lanfranchi) used to his own satisfaction. He made it so:
A small amount of powdered sarcocolla sifted through a
cloth (ie a head scarf) folded two or three plies or through
sindon. He applied the powder three times daily into the
eyes of the patient who lies supine with his face up until the
powder is dissolved. Then he placed over the lids a pad of
oakum wet with cold water. That reduced the inflammation
and allowed the patient to rest comfortably. He called the
powder "God's Powder". Bevenoud used it and omitted
bleeding and purges.

The Regimen (ie the general care of the patient):

Feed the patient broths, milk of almonds, soft boiled eggs, baked
potatoes and dry raisins. Abstain from beef and other heavy meats
which are difficult to digest. Avoid such spices as pepper, garlic and

mustard. He must not drink wine unless it is thinly diluted with water. Also, avoid hydromel beer (220) (ie mead), herbal decoctions and some clarets.

When cure seems near, allow him to eat soups of bugloss (69), beets (54) and parsley. Allow boiled chicken and birds with tawny feathers, boiled pigs feet and some fish such as sole, perch, sea-pike, gudgeon and other small fish with large scales.

The sick man should avoid stooping forward and sleeping face-down. He should sleep with his head elevated on pillows and as much as possible, in the dark. He should avoid staring at a light-source.

CHAPTER 5
ON GRAVE OPHTHALMIAS AND THE VARIOUS DISORDERS THAT ENSUE

Some writers describe the serious complications caused by Grave Ophthalmias as a subsequence of poorly treated milder ophthalmias at the hands of certain surgeons whose ignorance led to the aggravations. Thus it happens that an eye may become completely white, and the globe as well as the lids are covered with pustules, and the vision is lost.[78] That condition is beyond cure; the blindness is permanent.

Some eye doctors blame bad diet as cause for continuous discharges from the eyes. In those cases, treat by purging the head with these medicines: Take one dram each of the milky sap of beech fern (362), myrobalans, mastic, cubeb (143), spikenard, nutmeg (308), and cinnamon. Mix with the sap of sycamore trees (450b). and make small pills. Administer in amounts needed (ie to purge). Also, morning and evening give dialibanum (316), which you will find in the third chapter on cataracts.

You may also instill in the diseased eyes the powder of Nabete (448) [79] or the Alexandrine powder, also to be described.

Treat the eyes until the cure is complete, taking heed of proper diets as we already have advised.

---

78 Probably panophthalmitis with corneal ulcers and scars or herpes zoster (LDR).
79 Nabatean Powder (448) was finely powdered sugar, often exposed to smoke (LDR).

Chapter 6.
Pustules Of The Eyes And The Whiteness Called Ungula In Latin (ie Pterygium)

Excrescences appear on the surface of the eye in the absence of inflammation (or ophthalmia). If such a patient has not been treated before he comes to you, have a confectioner make this collyrium from frankincense: Take ten penny-weights of very pure frankincense and five pennies of antimony and sarcocolla. Mix with a mucilage of fenugreek and make pellets. Store them dry. For use, wet one in some of the mucilage and saturate a long strip of cotton which you lay on the eye. Renew it three times in twenty four hours, continuing until the cloth becomes soaked with pus and the inflammation is well established. Then use the following collyrium:

Use eight penny weights each of burnt lead (354), antimony (28), ground tuthie (471), copper oxide (121), gum arabic and adragant (8); and one obole of parsley. Pulverize all and make pills, using rain water or well water or rose water. Keep them dry. To prepare for use water down a pill with the same type of water you used before. Soak a cotton pad and apply to the eye. That collyrium cures and stimulates the granulation tissue.

If, after healing, there remain some white spots, called macula in Latin but more commonly simply called spots, which usually are the result of chronic ophthalmia, treat them with the white collyrium which I described before, composed so: Take eight penny weights each of hepatic aloes and saffron; sixteen penny-weights of ground copper oxide, gum arabic and opium; twelve pennies of myrrh. Grind them well and make up small packets of the powder. Add a packet to some sweet wine to make a collyrium.

Those substances mixed together are good for getting rid of films of recent origin.[80]

---

80 An obole was a farthing weight, a fraction of a penny-weight. The penny (denier) was about 1 1/2 grams.
Note that Yperman mentions Ungula in the Chapter Heading but does not include it in the text until Chapter 13 (LDR).

Chapter 7.
The Opacity Called Pannus Which Completely Obstructs Vision

Once in a while you will encounter a different sort of blemish, which we call a pannus in Latin and in ordinary argot is called a torn piece of a curtain. At times the coverage is only partial while at other times it completely covers the cornea, such that vision is limited or completely obstructed (ie probably Trachoma). We will limit our discussion in this chapter simply to mention causes.

The chief cause is bad eye care (ie uncleanliness). Another cause is open drainage from infections of the head (ie scalp) whence come discharges that drip over the temple and over the eyes. Those inflammations make the temples throb and affect the eyes, where the blemishes form which often block the vision.

Chapter 8.
The Varieties Of The Types Of Blemishes And Opacities

The first kind of speck to be seen on the cornea forms as a small sand-like grain (ie pingueculum). It comes from the coexistence of congestion in the vessels and inflammation.

The second variety resembles a fish scale.

The third is seen on one side of the eye, resembling a snowflake falling on water.

In the fourth type the entire cornea is covered by a white veil, a completely unnatural color.

Now we will deal with each of those cloudy veils in detail.

Chapter 9
The First Variety: They Resemble Grains Of Sand (ie Pinguecula)

The first variety of spots, those that appear like grains of sand, require no treatment, that is, no purgative medicines, no powders, no collyria, no electuaries and no cauterization. The last often is more harmful than beneficial. However, you may use this remedy (ie if the patient demands some sort of treatment):

Take five ripe blackberries and crush them and mix them into two liters of a good white wine, using a new jar. Add (ie after grinding) a pinch of rue, a half pound of gypsum (214), six ounces of fennel seeds and a pound and a half of oil of roses. The grindable materials are pulverized and then boiled with the wine in the new jar, using a low flame, until the wine is almost all evaporated. Then take four ounces of camomille leaves, dry or fresh, one ounce each of powdered camomille flowers and fresh wax. Add them to the jar and again bring to a boil for a short time before adding six egg-whites. Mix and pass through a cloth. What comes through is called the Precious Ointment.[81]

The ointment has many virtues. It cleans wounds and leads to rapid healing by preventing infection. It quickly relieves toothaches and sore gums when rubbed on the affected parts. Women afflicted with vaginal discharges and inflammation of the uterus are soon relieved of their ailments by using the ointment in the form of an electuary. It favorably affects fevers when applied over the belly, feet, hands and the flanks. When rubbed on the forehead and the temples, up to the eyebrows, it cures all kinds of headaches.

Chapter 10
The Second Variety: They Resemble Fish-Scales

This is what I have to say about the spots that resemble fish-scales.

If they are not cured by the treatments already described, you should proceed to another lest the scaly matter harden and degenerate along with the cornea under it. If you try to lift the spot with a hook or slide a sharp blade under it you will cut the cornea and you may destroy the eye. Be forewarned and be mindful of your reputation.

Therefore, use this treatment. Apply a small actual cautery to the temple just as I describe here: Use a disc of iron with a small hole drilled through. The second part of the apparatus is an iron wire

---

81 The Precious Ointment contained, in addition to the others already described, gypsum. I assume some of it was crumbled and dissolved in making the ointment. The electuary recommenmded for'female disorders' was for intravaginal rather than oral use (LDR).

attached to a ball about the size of a pea (ie a little larger than the hole). Heat the ball to redness and apply it through (ie over) the hole in the disc to the skin of the temple. That will soften the humors and cause the matter of the blemish to be absorbed and it will prevent its extension over the cornea.

Since the cautery acts only to dissolve and to absorb the humors, you must clarify the eye with the medicines I will describe. After the cauterization apply in the eye some of a powder of crystallized sugar, called the powder of Nabete. The second part of the treatment uses a baked sour apple from which all of the burned skin has been removed. Mash it all and add enough egg-white to make the consistency of an ointment. Apply that over the shut eyelids twice a day. Before every application of the cataplasm of apple put in more of the powder of Nabete. Keep the medicines in place with a loose, soft bandage.

This treatment will enable you to get rid of the spots of recent origin (ie not chronic).

CHAPTER 11.
SPOTS THAT RESEMBLE SNOW-FLAKES

The third variety of blemish resembles a snow-flake that falls on water. Here, too, you use the cautery and apply the powder as in the preceding chapter. In addition, do this: Take a new terra cotta jar and put in some charcoal embers which you have stirred to life. Let them burn four ounces of aloe wood. Place a basin over the opening, large enough to collect the smoke. Then put in the basin (ie atop the soot) some crystallized sugar which you have crumbled with a metal rod.

Place the fine powder of Nabete in the eye after cauterizing the temple. Then lay on the sour apple cataplasm and, as instructed above, renew it twice a day. That is how, with God's help, you treat the third type of blemish.

Now I want to describe the virtues of the Powder of Nabete, composed of finely ground pure, transparent crystallized sugar. First of all it is good for removing corneal spots, as we have shown. Second it calms inflammation. Third it eliminates it. Fourth it absorbs the humors which cause the blemish (ie it is hygroscopic). Fifth it strengthens the eye and its cornea. Sixth it controls the tears which produce cold humors. Furthermore, the powder never harms the eye and it is useful in nearly all ocular disorders. And to all the listed qualities we may add that it dissipates the redness and hardness of the white of the eye. Withal, it fortifies vision, and it reawakens it (ie after a period of obstruction).

Do not forget what I have taught about preparing the powder for treating the third type of blemish. You must let the smoke of the burning aloe wood permeate the other ingredients.

CHAPTER 12
THE FOURTH VARIETY, THAT WHICH COVERS THE ENTIRE EYE

The fourth type of veil covers so much of the cornea that light cannot penetrate. It seems as if a white plate covers the cornea (ie ? trachoma). In such a case the real white of the eye—the sclera—is reddish (ie by comparison). The victim believes everything is white.

This is the treatment: Cauterize the temple. Take a flat dish with a dozen egg whites and whip them with a rod with a feathered end until they are completely foamy. After the mound of foam stands a while, a clear liquid will collect beneath. Soak a strip of cotton cloth in it and lay it over the shut eye-lids. Repeat five times, day and night, until cured. Bevenoud stated that this procedure was sufficient treatment of itself.

CHAPTER 13.
THE OPACITY THAT IS CALLED UNGULA IN LATIN [82]

The cloudy opacities or films that form over the whole globe are of two sorts. The first is like a spider web anchored at the medial commissure of the lids. In Latin it is called *Pannus*. The other kind of film is formed of denser and fleshier tissue, called *Ungula* in Latin, and ongle (ie finger-nail) by us.

Treat both types first with the collyria which I describe here:

Take six penny-weights of hematite (216) and burnt vitriol; four

---

82 Pterygium (LDR).

penny-weights of cupric oxide; ten penny-weights of myrrh and saffron; one penny-weight of long peppers. Pulverize all in a metal mortar and sift finely. Make pellets using a good old wine and save for later use. When you wish to use the collyrium, dissolve one pill in a good old clear wine. That remedy works against pannus. Against ungula (pterygium) use instead the stronger green collyrium.

Take three penny weights of the Spanish Green, so-called verdegris; six penny weights each of red arsenic (24), borax (63) and spuma maris (163). Add ammoniacum dissolved in enough juice of rue to make pellets. For use, dissolve a pill in more of the juice and make a collyrium for frequent applications in the eye. The oil of rue should be made from rue water which is prepared in the same way as we made rose water in buried urns. All the other collyria should be as thin as hydromel.

If those measures do not destroy the pterygium, go on to the following procedure. Lift the lesion with as small a hook as you can fashion and cut it away with a sharp blade. Take care not to cut too deep and too close to the lacrimal caruncle. If you undercut the latter you may cause continuous tearing.

When treating most ocular disorders it is worthwhile to rid the eyes of their warm humors by bleeding. Also as part of the treatment avoid feeding the patient exciting foods, because nearly all the diseases cause too much warming of the blood, and exciting foods (ie as have been listed) produce the same warming effects.

After the pterygium has been cured, apply the sugar-crystal powder or one of the collyria that we have described.

CHAPTER 14.
BROWN OPACITIES OR PTERYGIA IN ATRABILIOUS PATIENTS

The opacities over the cornea may be black or brown, indicating an atrabilious etiology and therefore an incurable condition. That is because the cornea has been completely destroyed by a chronic process. It is even more incurable when it is caused by chronic ophthalmia, because then it is not just pannus or pterygium or some other common lesion. That opacity is truly a scarred cornea (ie not just a membraneous overlay).

Avoid those incurable cases unless they are of recent origin. Master Bruno (ie da Longoburgo) used this treatment (in fresh cases): Take some oil of roses with juice from ripe poppies, such as grow in wheat-fields and which bear red blossoms, in Latin called *Papaver rubrum* and the same amount of oil of wild thistle (102), called *Virga pastoris* and apply them in the eye. It works well in fresh cases.

Another good collyrium is made from copper filings (249a) moistened with a strong white vinegar and set in the sun for seven days. Then let it dry (ie as pellets?).

If you need a more energetic collyrium, take equal amounts of sarcocolla and crystallized sugar and camphor (77) and make a fine powder.

CHAPTER 15.
LESIONS THAT APPEAR AS A RESULT OF BLOWS OR AS A SEQUEL OF 'BLACK EYES'

Sometimes tiny red spots persist after the other effects of local contusions have healed.[83] They also appear after grave ophthalmias and after congestion of blood vessels when a small artery ruptures and blood extravasates in the outer layers of the globe. In such cases blood from young pigeons may help. Insert a needle into the artery that courses beneath a pigeon's wing and allow the blood to drip directly on the patient's eye. Instead, you may use milk from a young woman's breast squeezed directly on the eye.

N.B. Dryness may cause itching which may be relieved by applying beaten egg-whites. Or you may use Rhazes' collyrium, which we described earlier.

Itching may be relieved with powdered hepatic aloes placed in a small sack and suspended in white wine. Drip the wine from a spoon on to the globe.

CHAPTER 16.
ON SCRUFF, REDNESS AND INTENSE ITCHING OF THE LIDS

This chapter offers treatments for the psorophthalmia and the

---

83 Telangiectasias (LDR).

accompaning redness and itching of the inner surfaces of the lids and the accompaning swelling of the lid margins. Occasionally that malady causes ophthalmias in which cases the entire globe (sclera) is red and the eye seems misshapen.

Treat first with the collyria and the other preparations which you already know. If the malady is mild you may cure it this way: Put verdigris in white wine and daub the eyes with it, as a lotion. If that doesn't give relief use the red collyrium, as you already know it. If yet a more energetic collyrium is needed, use the green one.

CHAPTER 17.
SEBEL OF THE EYE [84] [85]

Sebel results from swelling and engorgement of the veins at the corneal-conjunctival junction, causing cloudiness and pterygium.

Treat it with red or green collyria. Sometimes you will have to hook and and then remove some of the veins with a sharp blade. After that little operation continue with the collyria.

I will not discuss the case of complete corneal opacification. That would lead us too far (ie away from our main subject). Besides, nearly all our surgical remedies fail, and the remedies of the greatest Master Physicians (ie on blindness) have no bearing on this chapter. I will not discuss them.

I will go on to other ocular disorders. First, consider those that are accompanied by watery eyes.

CHAPTER 18.
WATERY EYES—THE STUFF OF THE DISCHARGE—ITS TREATMENT

Now I shall discuss the fluids that drip from the eyes. First, harken to and remember what the Old Masters, especially Bruno, taught.

84 De Mets appended this footnote: "Sebel, or Sabel in Arabic, is a very vague term, inexact. It may describe obstructed of vision from any of many causes. Yperman states naively '...the best Masters' teachings have no bearing on this chapter, and I do not wish to get involved.' Let us, also, not ask for more."

85 Sebel was mentioned (by Guy de Chauliac (p 477) as being a congestion of veins at the edge of the cornea with a cloudy opacity. He may have taken his description from that of Yperman (LDR).

There are two kinds of humors that come from the eyes. The first derives from the veins that course between the skull and the dura mater. That fluid is of no concern to surgeons, but it is a proper subject for the Doctors of Medicine who must give their advice on how to treat it. In brief, their recommendations are for drying by purging the tears by diverting what overflows the eyes and disturbs vision.

The discharge also may derive from the vessels which run in the space between the two tables of the calvarium (ie the diploe) and which nourish the bone, as we taught in the special chapter on the anatomy of the head at the beginning of this book. Those vessels frequently are congested and they attempt to decompress their plethora (ie by means of the watery discharge). In such cases (ie of plethoric and congested vessels) their recommendation for drying is the same.

Now we come to speak of the vessels within the eye itself. We diagnose them as the cause of the tearing when what appears as a swarming of insects inside the eye [86] accompanies the external discharge and interferes with vision, in the absence of any external engorgement (ie scleral and conjunctival). Those symptoms lead us to diagnose an internal plethora. But when the watery discharge comes from the vessels that run in the tissues inside the bony orbit, the patient sees an irregular pattern as of one insect walking in front of the eye.

The watery flow sometimes is brought on by the inward growth of eyelashes that irritate the globe and the lids and produce tears. When that happens, pull out the lashes with a small forceps. The lacrimation will stop when the cause is eliminated.

When the flow comes from the fleshy tissues (ie periorbital muscles etc.) and cause the symptoms described above, apply plasters of eggs and the red powder, which I described in the chapter on hemostasis. Add to that a little finely milled wheat-flour that you will find on the walls of mills (ie so-called mill-dust). Make it of the consistency of honey and put it in on a cloth the size of the forehead and cover both eyes with it. Bandage it in place for three days. Repeat that step-by-

86 Many scintillating scotomata, as different from a single wandering spot (LDR).

step four times and (ie each time) apply in the eyes some saliva produced by chewing cumin.

If that remedy fails apply an actual cautery above the eye, or on both sides if both eyes are affected; the same holds for the use of the plasters for one or both eyes.

If even then you are unsuccessful, take a hand towel and tighten it around the neck and throat in order to distend and dilate the vessels on the temples and forehead. Then use a needle armed with a waxed silk thread and pass it through the skin and under a vein, avoiding injury to the deeper layers of the scalp. Do it twice for each of two veins, placing the bites a finger-breadth apart, and do the same for a forehead vein. Use long threads to make it easy to tie knots.

Then incise the veins with a sharp knife and let flow as much blood as you deem advisable. Then ligate the veins, using the threads already in place. During the ensuing three days lay on the wounds an oakum pad soaked in egg-white and a dry pad on top. After that dress the wounds as ordinary. Cut the sutures and remove them after nine days.

That is how to treat lacrimation caused by external vessels. However, Avicenna said that the method is improper for use in patients whose ocular tissues are loose and weak.

The principal causes of excess lacrimation often are augmented by too frequent sexual intercourse with women and with excessive reading of fine script and in retiring to bed with a full belly. It is better to wait until the initial phases of digestion have been completed.[87] The treatments which I have described are equally effective in cases of watery discharges caused by rheumatism.

In all cases there are contraindications (ie to therapy): constipation, overindulgence in foods that thicken the blood and which disturb the functions of the head.[88] Baths, such as are used to treat sanguine plethora, are harmful to the eyes. Similarly harmful is weeping and excessive bleeding, especially if that is performed with a scarifier (ie a scraper instead of a razor).

All foods that irritate the key to the stomach (the cardia) also

---

87 This passage could be understood to mean waiting until after a postprandial defecation (LDR).

88 We note Yperman's emphasis on vascular congestion and plethora - especially in sanguine persons - in his management of excess lacrimation (LDR).

harm the eyes: strong wine, garlic, onion, leeks, dill, red cabbage, beans and peas. Also contraindicated are exposure to steam, wind, (ie blowing) sand and prolonged staring at tiny or white objects. The patient rather should gaze at dark-colored objects.

Do not use the cautery in excess of five days (ie consecutive).

CHAPTER 19.
THICK AND STICKY EYELIDS

You will encounter patients with eyelids laden with gummy matter. This develops when tears and sour humors meet. The result changes the appearance and causes the edges of the lids to be crusted. The crusts then degenerate into moldy matter.

The treatment is this: pass a needle into the moldy matter. Do it very delicately so not to injure the underlying tissue. Then lift the deposit with the needle and cut it away with a lancet or scissors. Remove what remains of the debris and apply a strip thoroughly soaked with egg-white directly on the globe, preventing further contact with the eye of any irritating substances.

For patients who cannot be persuaded to allow the cutting, use the following, even though it may mean a prolonged course: Take a small rod and place it obliquely under the eye so to fold back the lid. Then take some goose-fat and rock-salt (404) and sal ammoniac (424) and apply large amounts of the mixture to the (exposed inner surface of) the lid, five times a day for as long as is necessary. That method will destroy the fungous matter. After every application moisten the lid with cold oil of fennel. As a general rule use cold collyria in the eye. The eye itself being naturally nervous and gristly will warm what was injected.

If the lids are gummy after the healing of negligently treated wounds or ulcers ,[89] treat them as follows: Cut away the scar with a scissors and treat the new wound as a simple (ie fresh) one. Even better, incise transversely (ie across the old scar) beneath the lid and dress the wound with packing. Then pass a thread through the lid and draw up the thread attached to a bandage wrapped on the head.

---

89 A contracture causing ectropion (LDR).

Continue the dressings using a small plaster covered with a bland ointment and dipped in breast milk. Continue until healed.[90]

Note: One meets patients who have traveled all over the world seeking relief from crusted lids, whereas there are others who care little about it.

Chapter 20
Bags Under The Eyes After Blows Or Falls[91]

When the pouch under the eye of a patient is full of blood, bleed him from the large brachial vein on the same side as the affected eye. Before that, apply plain egg-white, not beaten, because that lessens its glutinous quality and its freshness. Afterwards soak a cloth in the sap of joubarbe (229) and apply it to the eye, renew it frequently.

If the treatment fails and the blood does not dissipate, take fresh wax and powdered cumin and make a paste by kneading it near a fire. Use it warm over the entire eye. That kind of plaster favors the dispersal and the absorption of the hematoma.

However, here is the fastest treatment: Mix soap and populeum and put it on a plaster of oakum or lint, cut to the dimensions of the region of the hematoma, and set it there. The remedy will lessen the dark discoloration but will cause the region to become red and hot. Treat that with cold water. During the entire treatment warn the patient to keep his eyes shut lest it be irritated by the soap, which would interfere with the cure.

Afterwards use oil of roses mixed with breast milk. Soak a wick of oakum or lint in the mix and lay it on the eye. That will disperse the blood and heal the eye.

90 To convert a contracture of a vertical scar to a transverse one (LDR).

91 Yperman refers to hematomas that drift into the loose suborbital tissues. In other words the "black eye" (LDR).

CHAPTER 21.
THE FOUR CATARACTS IDENTIFIABLE AS TREATABLE[92]

Of the seven types of cataracts, four are curable and three are not.

The affliction called *Cataract* in Latin and *Sluus* (ie sluice-gate) in Thiois is a common one. If some of the humors which naturally reach the eye via the same nerve that carries visual sensations to the brain are blocked at the pupil, they become opaque and disturb vision by displacing the aqueous humor normally there.

The natural (ie terrestrial) circulation of waters may be dammed by floodgates (ie sluices), as you find them at mills or at millponds. When one wishes to release the waters he raises the sluices. That (ie the sudden spill of water) explains the word cataract.

The surgical treatment of a cataract should be undertaken only after you have determined its hardness and its opacity. You may judge that by using the following surgical test. Close the lids of one eye and press (ie hard) with your thumb on the lids of the other (ie the one with the cataract) and suddenly let go. If the aqueous humor had been displaced and returns from all directions toward the point of dispersal, then the cataract is ripe and is suitable for operation. If that does not happen, it means that the cataract is not fully formed and that you should do nothing for it.

The first type of treatable cataract is as white as chalk. It is caused by a blunt injury, as by a club or axe-handle or some other tool, or by a missile such as a rock or a snow ball or the like. That cataract is easily and quickly treated (ie by couching), but the patient will not see as clearly as he did before the accident. The fluids which normally flow between the three membranes behind the cornea now cannot be completely dispersed and some cloudiness remains between the layers, which ordinarily are clear and transparent.

The second curable cataract is bluish-white and is caused by faulty alimentation, which gives rise to bad substances. They are carried from the stomach to the brain and then to the eyes where they inter-

92 Yperman found little counsel from contemporary surgeons, and little more than that from the Arabs. He seems to consider as cataracts all opacifying lesions behind the cornea, and, as will be noted, he included blindness even with clear media, and hypopyon. No surgical operations for cataracts are given in the text. DeMets offers no explanation (LDR).

fere with the fluids and cause the bluish whiteness. If you decompress this sort of cataract by needling it,[93] clear vision, equal to that before the injury, can be restored. The result is better here than for the other three types because the aqueous humor remains clear and the optic nerve can easily produce the desired effect (ie restored vision).

The third curable cataract is grayish white and follows cerebral disorders such as a too cold brain or excessive weeping or insomnia. It does not persist as such for very long because it soon becomes completely opaque (ie the fourth type) unless it is treated with the following electuary, taken morning and evening in doses of about the size of a chestnut. The patient should avoid improper foods such as the meats of cattle, she-goats or rams, eels, peas, etc. Also, abstain from wine, baths (ie therapeutic) and fumigations. Rather, let him eat light, succulent and naturally warm foods, avoiding those which are naturally cold.

This is how to make the electuary: Take two ounces of olibanum; a half-ounce each of cloves, nutmeg and saffron; one ounce of ripe castor beans. Grind all and sift it and make electuaries of proper size with foamed honey.

In winter time the patient should drink small amounts of warm white wine with added bits of sage and rue.

This electuary is useful not only in these cases but also in all cases of afflictions of the head that are caused by catarrhs from the brain or brought on by cold. Also it is effective in treating watery eyes.

Chapter 22
The Three Incurable Types Of Cataracts

There are three types of cataracts which are incurable. The first is called *gutta serena* (sic)[94] It is recognized by the black and shiny pupil as if there was no opacity, which reflects an ever-changing silvery sparkle. That (ie cataract) is a product of a corruption of humors during pregnancy, and the children are usually blind at birth. A few

---

93 This 'cataract' probably was hypopyon treated by needling and draining (LDR).

94 'Gutta serena' probably is a copyist's error for 'Notte serena' an Italian expression meaning a clear night (LDR).

may have some vision, poor at best but allowing them to get around during their lifetimes. They are called myopes. Others (ie of the few not totally blind at birth) rapidly lose what little vision they have, becoming completely blind as if they had no eyes. Indeed, unless God in his pity makes a miracle, they cannot be cured. In those eyes the nerve-conduits are blocked. The serene cataracts are beyond our surgical skills.[95]

Another type of incurable cataract exhibits a bright color. It develops rapidly, derived from the brain as a result of prolonged insomnia, great worry, excessive tearing and great privation (ie poverty).

The third incurable variety of cataract typically reflects the same color as the iris.

CHAPTER 23.
WOUNDS OF THE EYES.

Eyes are injured in careless accidents. Children often are exposed to pointed articles including their own finger-nails. The best treatment is beaten egg-whites. Even better are the liquid drippings from that. Renew such applications four times daily and twice during the night for fifteen consecutive days.

However, if the vision is impaired you must use the 'supreme treatment', as given here: Take one dozen eggs of white ducks. Mash them in a lead mortar with a lead pestle until they have the consistencey of a pomade (ie a thick cream). Introduce it under the lids three times a day. When the worst symptoms abate apply compresses of cotton soaked in egg-white (ie hen's eggs). [96] Bevenoud called it the 'divine' method for three reasons: it lessons inflammation, it removes pus and it dissolves bad humors. It is the sovereign treatment because, of its own nature, it is mollifying and it is very gentle. The liquid part of egg-whites has special benefits when the vision is altered. Do not do what some masters practice and apply

95 Yperman suggests that what he called the serene cataracts was the bright reflection from the insensitive retinas in cases of congenital amaurosis of central rather than ocular etiology (LDR).

96 Oeufs De Canard Blanc. Observe how frequently Yperman uses eggs, whole or parts (whites or yolks). Hens' eggs appear in many recipes, less frequent are the mention of eggs of the goose and the duck – as here (LDR).

pomades directly on the eyes.[97] It is a bad practice because it deprives the eyes of important substances. They produce excessive lacrimation thus causing the eye to overheat and to depress the cool humors. The latter really require cooling medicines.

Again, I must caution you that some masters use treatments that heat the eyes. You must eschew that practice and instead use only beaten egg-whites. That is the excellent remedy which I recommend.

CHAPTER 24.
LACRIMAL FISTULAS

Pay attention to what I have to say on this subject and understand that these fistulas are caused by fluid (ie pus) trapped in the region (ie lacrimal sac) which cannot be eliminated. It follows that the best treatment is making a tiny opening to let out the pus. Very often you can see the abscess in the corner of the eye, the swelling and the persisting redness. When you press it with a finger tip pus will drain out the nose.

Now I will explain how to treat it and again tell you to mark well what I teach. The treatment consists of enlarging the wound (ie the fistula) using the peeled twigs of an elder tree or the dry roots of gentian. You cut thin strips (ie and insert them into the opening). When the opening is sufficiently dilated, insert a wick of oakum dipped in the powder we described in the chapter on wens (Book I). Avoid an excess of the powder lest you make the opening too large and thereby disfigure the face and cause an uncontrolled running off of the tears.

Master Benvenoud [98] made his incisions (to make the opening mentioned in the first paragraph above) with the tip of a razor paral-

----

97 This caveat against pomades seems contrary to what Yperman recommended in the previous paragraph about a duck-eggs. However the latter were eggs alone, whereas the dangerous pomades were compounded of several ingredients. (LDR).

98 Yperman's frequent references to Master Benvenoud (see Appendix) suggest that he may have known him personally. DeMets suggests that Grapheus Benevenutus was a Palestinian who had moved to Europe. A more reliable source (S. de Renzi, *Collectio Salernitana*, Bologna, Forni Editore, 1855, Vol. III, p 335, identifies him as a member of the college at Salerno in 1300. (LDR).

lel to the nose, trying to avoid injury to the nose adjacent to the lacrimal sac. He was careful not to slit the edge of the lid and to allow the tears to spill out of the eye. After he made the incision he placed a pea in the defect until the following day. Then he replaced it with the cited powder, not too much of it. If that eats away too much tissue the face would be disfigured. The golden rule (ie for surgeons) is to treat all wounds so to achieve healing with the smallest possible scar, especially in the face.

After the above, use plasters smeared with melted lard or melted fresh butter. Then insert a bit of sponge in the defect. Treat it twice a day until the wound is nicely cleansed. The sponge serves two purposes: it keeps the wound open and it soaks up the pus and other fluids.

Afterwards, dress the wound with lint from an old linen cloth coated with the ointment of the Twelve Apostles, which Avicenna first made and named it *unguentum veneris duodecim apostolorum.*[99] The ointment is useful in fistulas (ie chronic) whose edges are eburnated and mummified. It cleanses as well as it gets rid of the redness and the slough. Make the ointment so: Take fourteen drams each of naval tar, poix, ammoniac; two drams each of opoponax, vert d'espagne; eight drams of litharge; six drams each of birth wort, frankincense, mastic, and orpiment and bdellium. Melt gently in strong vinegar the ammoniac, galbanum (ie not in the list above) and opoponax. Then take olive oil , two pounds in summer time and three pounds in winter, and melt in it the wax, the naval tar and the poix and add the gums dissolved in the vinegar. Put in all the other ingredients. Grind it and pass it through a sieve.

Put some of the ointment in the wound and, if you deem it necessary, also put in a wick. As I have stated, Avicenna approved of this method.

However,. Master Benvenoud advised against cauterizing fistulas [100]

---

99 Ointment Of The Twelve Apostles, see Book I, footnotes 20 and 22. The description here differs slightly from the earlier version. That is another indication of the time-lapses between Yperman's writing his various chapters. Substances not included in the earlier version are ship's tar; poix (360), a shoemaker's wax or pitch; verdigris; orpiment, yellow arsenic (LDR).

100 Here the cauterization is by caustics rather than heat (LDR).

because it risks exposure and drying of the nerve which transmits visual sensations from the eye.

Master Roland differed. He advised using a small iron or copper tube, pushing it through to the bottom of the fistula after he had enlarged the opening with wicks as above. Then he took an iron wire, heated it to redness and he thrust it through the tube to the bottom. The operation must be done quickly, because the hot iron left in too long risks injury by drying the nerve, as Benvenoud had warned. After the operation place a wick wet with egg white, then with lard to cool the burnt tissues. Then insert a sponge-wick. Continue with the ointment of the Twelve Apostles or with the ointment described below, found in the *Gloss of the Four Masters* on Roland's *Chirurgie*.

Take one ounce of verdigris and one half ounce of rock salt, and two pounds of rancid lard. Melt the lard and filter it through a cloth; add the other ingredients which you had ground together beforehand; make an ointment (ie with the usual wax and/or olive oil) and put it on a wick for insertion in the fistula. Use it until the treatment is complete.

Here is another prescription from the *Gloss*: Take myrrh, aloes, euphorbia sap, celandine and rancid lard. Combine them; make an ointment; use as above.

The Herb of Robert (6) placed on the fistula or its juice dropped into it, and caryophyla (93) have similar effects and may be used alone in treating fistulas of recent origin.

Another collyrium, introduced into the fistula or into the eye, is very useful for treating the redness: Take one half dram of verdigris and a half pint of white wine. Shake well until it is uniformly green. Use it in the sick eye.

William of Congenis offered the following collyrium to cauterize the fistula, stop the overflow of tears, destroy the sticky matter on the lids and much more: Take one pound of white wine and one dram each of verdigris and rock salt. Grind the solids and add to the wine. Shake well.

Lanfranchi and Avicenna prescribed this collyrium: Take 2 drams of pure myrrh and one dram of gum arabic. Grind them and mix with beef bile (57) to make an oily product. Pass it through a cloth and put some on the fistula. This remedy cleanses, cures and prevents the accumulation of bad humors.

If you cannot cure the fistula with this treatment and the drainage recurs in the face of it, that indicates caries (ie osteomyelitis) of the underlying bone. That condition must be treated with a cautery inside a hollow tube, as described above, followed by the measures used there. Avicenna and Lanfranchi both recommended the actual cautery rather than caustic medications, because the former burns the tissue that it directly touches whereas the latter must eat through from a distance to reach the target.[101] Furthermore, in cases where the fistulous opening is ulcerated you must avoid them because their actions are unpredictable and they may cause grave and persisting complications.

CHAPTER 25.
FORBIDDEN LESIONS OF THE FACE AND LIPS[102]

The *noli-me-tangere* is a kind of ulceration that can be anywhere on the face, from the chin to the forehead. Some say that it is contagious (ie but not Yperman).

It is caused by two different types of bile: One comes from hot bile, the eruption (ie ulcerated tissue) of which is of a dark color throughout. The other comes from bile of normal temperature and it is reddish right down to its roots.

You will find no disagreement in the general rule that when the interior surfaces of the perforating lesions are purulent and erose, those are signs of chronicity and refractoriness in treatment. That also is true for fistulas for noli-me-tangere and for cancers. The cancers are more bilious and more from hot bile than are the ulcerated noli me tangere .

Here is the treatment for this serious affection (ie for the noli me tangere lesions): During the first month direct your primary attention to stopping the advance of the ulcer by using oxysaccharum and

---

101 The two types of cauterization, Actual with hot metal and Potential with caustic chemicals were discussed even in 'classic' times (LDR).

102 The Forbidden Lesions remain to be defined. Some of the ulcerating lesions here may have been herpetic, others basal cell or epidermod carcinomas and, perhaps even nomas. (LDR).

by cleansing the patient with cholagogues which attack the bad humors where they become overheated. Oxysaccharum and the cholagogues both are medicines that work to purify the blood and the bile.

On the third day, bathe the patient in a steam bath containing herbs of the cool variety, using a terra cotta tub with tubes, constructed as I taught at the beginning of this book (ie not in the Ms. translated by Dr. DeMets). When he leaves the bath have him rinse in a basin containing water in which you had boiled some linaria (420).

The following day, bleed him from the liver-vein (ie basilic), because the evil humors take origin at the liver. Then bleed him from the head-vein (ie cephalic). Then go ahead and treat the lesion.

On the outer surface (ie of a perforating lesion) do this: Lift and cut away the crust over the lesion and apply ashes from burned grape-vine wood to which you have added equal parts of powdered salt, quick-lime, sulfate of iron (228a) and cream of tartar (456), making the ashes (ie as a plaster) suitable for an overnight application, putting popoleum ointment all around the lesion (ie to protect the normal skin).

The next day, use angled instruments to dissect and remove as much of the diseased tissue as will come away, then apply rancid lard and the juice of the plantain.

Later, for ten or twelve days, lay on crushed leaves of the plantain reddened with its own juice and some lye made from the ashes of grape-vine wood.

After the lesion has been destroyed and purified you will see healthy and beautiful granulation tissue. Then, for one day, lay on crushed linaria with some of its own juice. Then wash it every day with a lessive (244a) and wipe it with an old cloth of proper size and softness on which you have sprinkled a powder of mastic, frankincense and rose petals. When all the perforation is filled with new tissue, refresh the surrounding area.

During the period of treatment, the patient must abstain from spicy and salty foods and all other things that can stir (ie excite) the blood.

EXPLICAT

Finito libro sit et gloria Christo

(Let this book end here with praise and glorification of Christ)

BOOK THREE: THE NOSE

INTRODUCTION[103] AND ANATOMY

There are six chapters: Nasal Polyps, Nasal Pustules, Nasal Ulcers, Proud Flesh (spongy) in The Nose, Nosebleeds and Bad Odors in The Nose.

We begin this treatise on the Nose with its anatomy. First be reminded that a hollow nerve (ie optic) leaves the anterior part of the brain. Also exiting from the brain are two small nerves, resembling the fibers in a woman's breast (ie Cooper's Ligaments). They are the instruments of olfaction. When exposed to excessively cold or hot humors, a person loses the sense of smell, and it may persist as a complete anosmia.

The cavity where the little rootlets appear is called the nasal fossa. Air collects there so one can recognize odors. There, too, excess fluid is released from the brain; we call it morva in Flemish.[104]

The nasal cavity opens lower down into the mouth. The highest part has two triangular bones which make contact with the undersurface of the frontal bone of the cranium, and at the sides they meet the orbital bone, near the corner of the eyelids.

Each bone has a cartilage and they meet another cartilage in the center. That divides the nose in two. It is firmer and tougher than the others. By this division Nature anticipated the availability of one respiratory passage when the other has been obstructed.

When the two bones come together they shape the nose, and they provide the means for its functions. One: it can rid the brain of its discharges. Two: it captures the air and transmits odors to the brain. Three: most of the inhaled air is carried to the lungs, even when the

103 Tabanelli took Book III from The Cambridge Codex and the French translation by Carolus. I have limited the English translation to Tabanelli's Italian version of the Mss, excluding most of his comments about the text (LDR).
104 Nasal catarrh is discharge from the brain (LDR).

mouth is shut.[105] Fourth: the nose modulates the voice, which is less intelligible when the passages are blocked.

The usefulness of the cartilage is evident. If the protruding nose were bony , it would be easily broken and the face would be deformed. The elasticity of the cartilaginous structure spares us from that. However, that benefit does not hold against slicing weapons or an erosive ulcer caused by bad humors which affect the cartilages, especially the cold and dry black-bile that eats away the tissues.

The principal lesions of the nose are polyps, cancers, pustules, ulcers, fungous flesh and nosebleeds. We will deal with each in turn.

CHAPTER 1. NASAL POLYPS

Nasal Polyps are an affection derived from humors that seep from a catarrh of the brain. The result is a fungus-like excrescence which may occlude the nostrils and obstruct the nasal passage. The name, polyp, comes from its resemblance to an octopus, which can grasp a person and not let go.

Sometimes the polyps resemble mucoid lumps when they are cool and moist. At other times, when they are cool and dry, they derive from black bile; those polyps may degenerate and become cancerous.

When the polyps grow larger they may also impair mouth-breathing. The polyp itself may outgrow its own nutrition. That should alert us to the possibilities of phthisis and leprosy.

Polyps may be unilateral or bilateral, and they may be malodorous (ie to the victim). They may extend forward to and through the nostril, even to reach the upper lip. They may expand in bulk and distend the and deform the nose. They may become fatty and firm (ie grape-like) and take on a brown color and be quite insensitive. That type is caused by black bile and seldom grows as far as the nostril.[106] When that is the case, my Son, you must not be aggressive in your efforts to cure it; as I have said, it has become a cancer. However, when it is pedunculated and soft and it does not discolor the nose, then you may be active in your efforts and you should intervene early.

First clean out the nose. Then grasp the polyp with a forceps and

105 There is no concept of the lungs providing air for respiration as we know it. The lungs service the heart only by keeping it cool (LDR).
106 It is not pedunculated and it invades a broad base (LDR).

Pull it forward while you cut it on both its sides, removing as much as possible until you expose the base. Control the bleeding by packing the nose with oakum pads. When some of the polyp remains, try to destroy it by scraping it with a curette; take away some of the tissue surrounding the base. Then burn the roots with a red-hot cautery, being very careful not to char the cartilage.

Another method: Destroy the polyp by applying our 'wolf powder'.[107] Be very careful; if you expose the cartilages or bones, their covering (ie perichondrium or periosteum) will not regenerate and they may slough. The nose will be deformed and the face will be disfigured.

After applying the corrosives, lay on strips of cloth soaked in tallow or fresh butter. Continue the treatments until you can see that the polyp has been completely destroyed. Then discontinue the corrosives.[108]

When the polyp extends upward (ie into the nasopharynx) and tends to obstruct nasal breathing, treat it this way. Insert a strip of oakum, its tip covered with a corrosive powder, and make contact with the polyp. Afterwards apply the fresh butter or lard, as above. Repeat until the polyp has been destroyed.

Another method: Insert a long sturdy thread through a nostril until you can catch it in the pharynx and bring it out through the mouth. Tie a series of knots in the thread. Saw to-and-fro and use the knots to cut away and eliminate the excrescence. Then use a drying powder or ointment such as the Apostolicon, as it was made in The Glosses of the Four Masters.[109]

After a good clean-out, douche the nose with a good wine or warm vinegar and insert a drain to remain all day. Repeat the measure until the passage is open and the bleeding has ceased. Thus, the exposed lesion will have been dissolved and the discomforts thereby are relieved.

107 One of the several corrosives described in Book I, Ch. 29 (LDR).

108 A fair 'anticipation' of the modern chemosurgical procedures as introduced by Mohs (LDR).

109 See the Pharmacopeia in the Appendix, Item 30. The Apostles' Ointment (containing 12 substances) had several different formulas as made and used by various authors. The formulas in the text as cited by Yperman or a later copyist (see Book I, Ch. 8) differ from that in my copy of The Glosses – see Bibliography (LDR).

Afterwards use this ointment: Juices of blackberries, plantains, cynoglossus (148a), parsley (344) and artemisia (35), 1 dram of each. Mix with honey and boil away the fluid until it is thick. Then add 1 dram of ferrous sulfate. Boil until it becomes an ointment. Apply it in the nostril which you stopper to retain the medicine. Repeat as necessary.

Take note that the juice of the small scammony (416) will cure polyps and cancers if it is applied when they first appear.

A properly fashioned drain, made by a competent surgeon, and covered with powdered antimony will cure early polyps.

CHAPTER 2. NASAL PUSTULES

Humors cause these lesions which are accompanied by acute pain and heat. The treatment includes bleeding from an arm vein and purging with Galen's pigra (344c) or hieralogodon. First apply ossisacara or similar to bring the pustule to a head. Then apply eggwhite with oil of roses. When the pustule is open, use Rhazes' white ointment (381a).

CHAPTER 3. NASAL ULCERS

When hot humors cause the ulcers, treat them as we do the pustules. When cool humors are at fault, use lotions of wine and honey which are brought to a boil before adding the Apostolicon or the surgeons' Green Ointment (210) as Roland made it: Take a pinch each of rumex (395), chelidonium, dried leaves of sage, cinnamon (117a), lovage (256), scabious (419) and agrimony (13). Grind them and mix with one pound of oil of aloes and allow it to sit for nine to eleven days. Then simmer it in a tin pot until the leaves settle at the bottom. Filter it through a cloth sieve and reheat it before adding one ounce of wax. Then add a half-ounce each of mastic, olibanum and verdigris. The last-named should be added only when the mixture already is thick. Take it all from the flame when the color is uniformly green. Then add one half-ounce of hepatic aloes. Stir and filter again. Now it is ready for use. The ointment is good for chronic ulcers, because it regenerates the healing tissues.

Chapter 4. Spongy Tissue in The Nose[110]

Eliminate the fungous tissue with one of the powders described in Book I, Chapter 29. Follow that with the Green Ointment or the Apostolicon or with Rhazes' white ointment as we formulate it. The last-named is good in all parts of the body which are naturally warm and when they are inflamed by open pustules. Make it so: Take four ounces of oil of roses, a half-ounce of fresh wax, one ounce of ceruse (so-called Spanish White Lead), one dram of camphor and the whites of two eggs. Grind two or three shelled almonds (17) in a metal mortar. Empty the almond paste and clean the mortar before putting in the camphor. Now melt the oil and the wax and mix everything with an iron pestle. When it cools add the egg-whites while stirring vigorously. The more thorough the mix the better it will work.

Some authorities make it differently. They take six drams each of white lead, oil and camphor and formulate in the order given above. It is an excellent desiccative ointment.

Chapter 5. Nose Bleeds

As we stated above, many people suffer from repeated epistaxis. Often the bleed may be harmful rather than acting as a beneficial therapeutic phlebotomy, as in cases of chronic fevers (ie malaria) or to calm violent agitated states or to correct amenorrhea in women or treat cataracts due to warm humors or simply to relieve plethora. A patient should undergo phlebotomy to relieve the effects of hot weather, when his blood boils and its vapors rise to his head as if to overfill it and its blood vessels, threatening to burst them.[111]

Now consider treatments for nose-bleeds. Sometimes the distended vessels will leak. If the hemorrhage is profuse and comes from the right nostril, open the right brachial vein and bind off both arms and legs with cords (ie tourniquets). If the epistaxis continues, incinerate some egg-shells and make a powder to insufflate into a nostril. Or: insert a cloth wick wet with ink made from oak galls and vitriol. Or: take a warmed string vinegar and bathe the bleeding

110 Probably granulation tissue in ulcers (LDR).
111 See fn. 198, Book VII, Ch. 21B (LDR).

region. If the patient is a woman, massage her chest and then her
arms and legs.

Another remedy: Take some powdered red rose petals (389)
mixed with barley-flour and moistened with vinegar. Add the juice of
plantains and the serum of egg-whites. Apply the paste over the forehead and temples if the cause derives from humors in the head. But
if the source is from the liver, put it on the right side of the head (ie
that of the liver). If the source is from the spleen put it on the left
side. If the source is from the uterus, apply it over the navel and on
the suprapubic surface. Whatever the source may be in a woman,[112]
bleed from a vein over her medial malleolus at the ankle, or apply a
cup without scarification over her umbilicus or under her breasts.
Take care to limit the blood losses. Have the woman hold some leaves
of a fruit tree; that alone often will stop the epistaxis. Another: catch
the blood from the nose on a hot tile. Pulverize the desiccated clot
and insufflate it into the nostrils. Often that is successful.

Sometimes an ointment with added vinegar applied over the nostrils as a plaster will arrest a nose-bleed. Galen's secret remedy was
this: Place the nude man supine and drip water and vinegar on his
up-turned face. That will stop the bleeding. Another: Take some
hare's foot clover (344a) and roll a leaf to make a drain. Dip it in the
water-vinegar mixture and insert it in the nostril. It works.

The bleeding will stop if the patient vigorously chews the roots of
nettles or fennel. That measure may help to distinguish a bleed caused
from the head or eyes from that caused by the liver (ie or spleen).
Observe the following to diagnose an hepatic source: While chewing,
the patient will feel pain over the right hypochondrium when the
bleed is from the right nostril. When the source is the spleen, the
pain will be on the left side when the blood comes from the left
nostril.

When the bleeding is a useful treatment for chronic fever, frenzy
etc., let it continue at length, unless the patient is feeble or very sick.
When the epistaxis occurs in a young woman at puberty, let it continue as long as her vitality will allow.

---

112 The source of the offending humor (LDR).

CHAPTER 6. BAD ODORS IN THE NOSTRILS

Galen said that bad odors in the nose are caused by humors that descend from the head into the nasopharynx and are corrupted there when they are not dispelled before they come in contact with air, and may be caused by nasal pustules when the humors are acrid. That matter may cause polyps and proud flesh, all of which we can recognize by their own symptoms.

When the humors are corrupted, the bad odors can be detected even when the nostrils are blocked. We can tell when the malady is pustular by the accompanying heat (ie inflammation). You know a polyp or proud flesh when you see them. So, when it is the odor alone, consult a good physician for his suggestions how to control the bad humors. He may prescribe a hierologodon (ie a laxative), or a plaster of cashews (25) used by Theodoric, which contains aloes, ginger, cassia and myrobalans. Or he may use a pill (ie oral) made with the same simples. The sources for the bad odors will be macerated (ie by a plaster) or digested (ie by the pill). Then massage the head with olive oil and introduce some pure (ie filtered) oil into the nose after you have cleaned it well. Prescribe some pills of castoreum (96) mixed with vinegar. Then use some Alexandrine gold (composed of many simples) boiled with oil as an incense, known as olibastro when it is burned to make fumes. If all those measures fail, wash out the nose with a medication made from the roots of a plant [113] mixed with oil-lees (175). Rub it over the nose and drip some into the nostrils, to remain for two or three hours. That will do it.

HERE ENDS BOOK III.

---

[113] The copyist did not name the plant (T).

BOOK IV THE MOUTH AND ITS CONTENTS
THE ANATOMY OF THE MOUTH AND ITS CONTENTS[114]

The oral cavity is lined entirely by a soft membrane which extends to the stomach. That explains why some people vomit when the palate is touched.

Two passages lead from the rear end of the oral cavity; one is for swallowing, the other is for respiration. The latter opening allows the transport of air in and out, and provides for speech. The passage itself is cartilaginous and is called the larynx. The first-named opening lies behind it. Together they rest against the cervical vertebrae, and lack a common name.[115]

Another structure is a cartilaginous lid over the larynx and is attached to it. It is called the 'comele'[116] because its nerves (ie ligaments and tendons) allow it to move and to cover the food passage called the esophagus while a person speaks. Sometimes food slips into the larynx if he swallows when he speaks and causes violent coughing.

The uvula is suspended from the upper part of the mouth. Behind it you find the openings unto the two nares. The uvula is thick at its base and slim lower down. It produces the rumbles and other throaty sounds that begin at the lungs.

Some persons have so-called nasal voices because their uvulas carry an excess of humors from the brain.[117]

---

114 For his Italian translation of Book IV Prof. Tabanelli used the Cambridge Codex from the texts of Carolus and Broeckx, and refered to the French translation of Lonneville in The Belgian Journal of Stomatology (see Bibliog. in the Introduction of DM and T) (LDR).

115 Our pharynx (LDR).

116 Tabanelli could not find that name for the epiglottis. Perhaps a copyist meant to write 'comete', meaning a companion or coworker (LDR).

117 This simply repeats the ancient concept that catarrh (rheum) was formed in the brain and reached the nasopharynx via the olfactory foramina (LDR).

The tongue is attached to the floor of the mouth. It consists of soft muscles and veins. You will find there more veins (ie blood vessels) than in any other (ie muscular) organ in the body. At the base of the tongue there are two hollows wherein saliva forms; it keeps the tongue moist.

The tongue serves to move the food about in the mouth and to push it between the teeth for mastication. That allows one to taste what he chews. Also, the tongue clips sounds as they come up through the throat and thereby forms our words. Persons with fat (ie swollen) tongues cannot speak as clearly as those with slender ones.

The mouth contains teeth: thirty-two in most people, thirty in others, as few as eighteen in some. Among those with twenty-eight teeth, fourteen are in the lower and fourteen in the upper jaws. The teeth have a common origin with the bones, but they have a special sensitivity which bones lack.

The lips lie outside the teeth and are the portals through which many diseases gain entry.

Chapter 1. The Uvula And Its Connections

According to Master Platearius [118] the uvula often enlarges when it is inflamed. That inflammation is caused by an excess of humors or by heat or by frigidity. When it is caused by heat, you must perform phlebotomy from the blue veins beneath the tongue. Then provide a gargle of sumac (449) balaustia, bile and rose-petals. Boil them with diamoron (155). Use it when the uvula be elongated, or if it is inflamed by cold humors that provoke excessive salivation or because the region has been bled out by the phlebotomy. In that case, purge the patient with this: Take one part of vinegar and one-half part of honey and boil them. Then add some roots of pyrethrum, some ginger and some rose-petals. Or: insufflate the mouth through a tube with this powder: Take equal parts of black powder (?soot) and ammoniacum (424); make a fine powder and blow it on the uvula. If warm humors are at fault, use this powder: Take equal parts of bile, balaustia and sumac. Macerate them in rain-water and heat them. Add diamoron to a moderately hot solution and use as a gargle.

118 Platearius: see Appendix II (LDR).

If all the above fail, you should cut away some of a uvula that is too long or too fat. But when it is too dark or too red, especially if the dark predominates, avoid cutting.[119] Use a scissors to cut a slim or cord-like uvula that looks like a mouse's tail. Or: take a long tube with side openings like a flute. Plug one end with a bit of sheet-lead. Let the uvula droop into one of the openings near the end. Insert a sharp iron chisel-knife into the tube (ie and slice off the dangling piece of uvula). Have this powder ready at hand before cutting: Take equal amounts of mastic, cinnamon and lime, all pulverized. Apply it with your finger tip to the cut end of the remaining uvula to coagulate the blood and heal the wound.

Be careful not to cut off too much and do permanent harm to the deprived patient. Avicenna said that a hoarse voice and a persistent cough will be the results.

Chapter 2. The Tongue And Its Disorders

The following chapters deal with ailments of the tongue, such as have been described and discussed in many books by physicians and passed down to us. The tongue is subject to many disorders, especially buttons (ie aphthous ulcers), swellings, fissures, short frenulum, ranula, spasms, elongation and blisters.

Chapter 3. Abscesses Of The Tongue

When hot humors cause a swelling or an aposthem of the tongue, you will find it to be hot and red. Treat it so: Bleed from a vein on the head and apply leeches under the chin. Allow them to suck out a lot of blood. Then have the fasting patient drink the following laxative in a single dose: yellow myrobalans mixed with the serum of freshly made cheese. Those measures will purge the inflammation from below.[120] Afterwards rinse the mouth two or three times a day with the following: Take equal amounts of aquatic moss (243a), balaustia, pomegranate bark (364), roses and sumac. Boil all in equal amounts of water and vinegar. Rinse. Then apply and retain this powder on the

119 Engorged with blood (LDR).
120 Below : From beneath the chin as well as by laxation (LDR).

palate: Equal amounts of red rose petals, powdered red and white sandarac wood and balaustia and a pinch of camphor. It will relieve the discomforts of an elongated uvula.[121] Or: rub this powder within the mouth: Take equal amounts of spode (439), leaves of sumac, coriander and dried peeled lentils, and seeds of portulaca (366), and a pinch of camphor. Pulverize all and apply after rinsing the mouth with equal parts of warm rose-water and pure vinegar.

CHAPTER 4. FISSURES OF THE TONGUE

For these lesions apply a powder of tragacanth mixed with a mucilage of mauve and millet seeds or take some finely ground slips of mauve and make a broth to apply as a rinse. The patient should drink warm broths and chew boiled pig's and ram's feet. Also, he may apply a lotion made from the their boiled tendons.

CHAPTER 5. THE FRENULUM

When the frenulum beneath the tongue is overly thick we call it the shortened frenulum. We see it most often in the newborn. We cut it with a special knife. If the bleeding is excessive, apply a gold (ie wire) cautery. That seldom is necessary except when we delay the incision until the child is older.

CHAPTER 6. RANULA[122]

A ranula is a mass under the tongue. When it is caused by cold humors, the saliva is white. When the faulty humors are melancholic, the spittle is dark. In the latter cases do not intervene with the knife. First treat by rubbing salt on the tumor until it bleeds. When that fails, use a powder of green vitriol. That, too, may fail if the mass is too large or too full of humors. In such cases incise and apply a mixture of yellow and red orpiment (327), alum, ginger, salt and pepper. Make a powder and cover the wound with it. If you succeed in eliminating

121 'Uvula': This is so out of place in the text that I insist it is an error of a copyist. The proper reference is 'a swollen tongue' (LDR)

122 A subungual cystic mass (LDR)

the mass, irrigate the wound with vinegar containing the powder. Soak a strip of cotton in the fluid and let the tongue move it over the defect. Then have the patient retain a mouthful of warm oil of roses until the inflammation subsides.

Chapter 7. Spasms Of The Tongue

The tongue in spasm is a complication of a syncope. It is caused by a contraction at the base of the tongue. Treat it so:

The patient should retain a mouthful of oil of roses containing camomile (76) for as long as he can. Then apply the same mixture to his head and neck, with added pyrethrum and powdered mastic. The mouthful of the medication will draw out the faulty humors from the mouth and the tongue (ie to be expectorated).

Chapter 8. Buttons (ie Small Sores) On The Tongue

These aphthous sores are caused by warm humors. Treat them with phlebotomy from veins on the head and apply leeches under the chin. When you realize that hot humors are involved you should use bleeding until the patient's vitality is sufficiently depleted. Then apply the medication used in Chapter 7.

Chapter 9. Ailments Of The Gums

The malady (ie gingivitis, pyorrhea) is called a cancer of the mouth. The usual cause is a descent of humors from the head into the mouth. The sore gums are soft and bleed easily. The palate often is inflamed and ulcerated and the breath is foul.

From the outset, discourage the patient from biting.[123] Rinse his mouth with a boiled mixture of water, wine and blood. Vinegar is not used because it damages the teeth and is corrosive, and because it is thin and can work its way down to the roots and penetrate into the teeth. As I have explained it, hot water purifies the mouth. Wash it out repeatedly until all the blood and and bits of matter are gone. Then use your fingers to apply this powder directly on the inflamed

---

123 Chewing may dislodge a loosened tooth (LDR).

gums three times a day: Take equal amounts of the roots of consolida, slips of caryophyla (93), cinnamon, rose petals and pomegranate bark. Make a fine powder which will dry and heal the sores.

When the patient ignores the problem for too long a time, often it becomes a cancer or a fistula. In such cases use the mouth washes as above and then apply this powder:

Take equal amounts of cinnamon, caryophyla, nutmeg. red rose petals. alum, pyrethrum, the heads and arms of marine crayfish, calcined seeds of dates and pomegranate bark. Make a fine powder.

Overgrowth Of Proud Flesh In The Mouth (ie Epulis) Not infrequently, clumps of granulation tissue will grow like little teats in the gums. You should cut them away and let the wounds bleed. Then use our first powder (as above) on the defects. If you fail to do that, the excision will be of no avail. My old Master (ie Lanfranchi) taught that we should cauterize twice and to do it vigorously to prevent a recurrence.

CHAPTER 10 SPLIT LIPS

Potent humors and local inflammation together are the causes of chapped lips; they cause the outer skin to peel and crack. This is the treatment:

Take tragacanth (466) and anoint the lips, or use warm oil of roses. If those are inadequate, try others like them.

CHAPTER 11. SWOLLEN GUMS[124]

Sometimes the swollen gums fall way from the teeth and bleed. The breath is nauseating and the discharge is purulent Use this medicine: Grind equal amounts of thin strips of caryophyla, cinnamon, alum and sugar. Mix and filter through a cloth. After applying the product on the gums, rinse the mouth repeatedly with this wash: one part each of wine and vinegar, and three parts of honey. Add small amounts of roots of white radishes, pomegranate bark and peppers. Bring all to a boil. Filter and use it to irrigate the gums. Then apply the powder..

---

124 Tabanelli quotes Lonneville who blamed scurvy for this (LDR).

Chapter 12. How Dental Abscesses Form

Dental abscesses are provoked by humors either from the stomach or from the brain, and they may be hot or cold. The humors arise from drippings that are carried to the teeth by the nerves that confer sensibility.

When the source is in the head, the pain is more severe and lancinating, there is much local heat and the overlying face is red. When the faulty humor is cold, the cerebral-source abscess is less pronounced. When dental caries are involved, as is often the case, have the patient chew cheese or raw portulaca or warm wax.[125] If the cerebral-source humors are hot – recognizable by the heat and the local redness of the gums and the tongue – bleed the patient from a vein in the head, and the next day, from a dark sublingual vein. That especially holds for persons who use routine phlebotomies (ie prophylactic) and for patients who are neither too young or too ill. After the bleeds, the patient should swish and hold in his mouth some of the oil of roses and vinegar. That treatment usually is successful.

While above measures are in progress, instill into the ipsilateral ear canal a three-to-one mixture of oil of roses and vinegar. When the bad humors are hot and the abscess is very bad, use this tried and true medicine: Take two parts each of hyoscyamus seeds, the heads of white poppies and of marsh-apium (29), and three parts of apium seeds. Grind them with some vinegar made from a fine wine, enough to make an oil as thick as honey. Make small balls, the size of fava beans. Pack a ball in and around the affected tooth to abort the abscess. After four days of treatments, the patient should retain mouthfuls of warm oil of roses containing some bits of mastic.

When the faulty humor is cold, the region around the tooth is pale, as is the face. Here use purges: Rhazes' pills (344c) and, if the patient is very pale, use Galen's theriac (462c). Another treatment: Have the patient chew pyrethum directly over the affected tooth. That will open the tooth and allow the abscess to drain. [126] The patient must expectorate the pus and not swallow it.

Another effective powder: pyrethrum, seeds of staphisagre and

125 Materials suitable for plugging the caries (LDR).
126 Via the root canal! (LDR).

verdigris. Pulverize them and place the mixture in a sack of new cloth, about the size of a phlalanx of the thumb. Place it over the bad tooth. Biting down on it will release the juices. Frequent spitting will prevent the bad humors from re-entering the body.

All the preceding measures also succeed when there are no caries.

CHAPTER 13. DENTAL ABSCESS AND PHLEGMON

These lesions often form around teeth. [127] They are caused by cool rheumatic humors and are favored by caries that contain worms. You know that only mobile worms cause dental abscesses. In the case of a carious but not abscessed molar tooth that is not loose (ie movable) an attempted extraction carries great risks. A failure leads to serious and incurable complications and much suffering, even to death. That complication is a phlegmon in the cheek which contains and discharges bits of sequestrated jaw-bones. The phlegmon becomes a fistula and the cheek will remain puffy. When the tooth is movable, there is little risk in removing it. When the patient refuses extraction and the tooth remains in place, do this, as was taught by the old-time Masters. Take one scruple each of marjoram (270) and seeds of cicuta (115). Boil them in water. Take a metal tube and insert through it a wire cautery, heated to redness after you had dipped it in boiling oil. Go right to the bottom of the cavity, and do it twice, taking care not to touch the lips or the gums. This maneuver will produce a watery discharge from the tooth and out the mouth.[128] If still you are not able to remove it and you wish to avoid cutting it out, do this: Take equal amounts of mulberry tree bark and pyrethrum. Combine them

---

127 Pyorrheaas distinct from dental root abscesses (LDR)

128 This ancient treatment for toothache depends less on the burn than on the smoke! It appears before the end of the 12thC in The Salernitan Regimen. A lovely English version in verse was created by Sir John Harington early in the 17thC. I quote it here. The Elizabethan English spelling has not been changed. "If in your teeth you hap to be tormented, By meane some little wormes therein do breed: Which paine (if heed be tane) may be prevented, By keeping clean your teeth when as you feed. Burn Frankincense (a gum not evill sented) Put Henbane unto this, and Onyon seed, And in a *Tunnel* (italics are mine) to the Tooth that's hollow, Convey the smoake thereof, and ease shall follow." From *Regimen Sanitatis Salerni* , the English version. Rome, Edizioni Saturnia. So.Gra.Ro.,1959. p 66. (LDR).

and mix with a fine wine vinegar. Put it all in a sack which you hang exposed to sunlight. When you are ready to extract the tooth, put some of the substance around the tooth when you separate the gums with a dissector.

Yet another way: Take powdered pyrethrum wet with a strong vinegar. Hang it in sunlight for forty days. Place the powder between the tooth and the gums. That will loosen the tooth and permit a risk-free extraction.

CHAPTER 14. HOW TO BLEACH AND CLEAN DARKLY STAINED TEETH

When the cleaning and the whitening of a patient's stained teeth has been requested, scrub the teeth frequently with this: Take some barley flour (323) and salt and add honey to make a paste. Spread it on a sheet of paper and roll it before incinerating it in an oven. Make a powder of the ashes (38) and take three parts to mix with two parts each of powdered calcined crayfish (138a) and egg-shells or alum. Mix the powders (three parts to two). Scrub the stains until they whiten.

HERE ENDS BOOK IV

To Follow Is Book V On The Ear

What is there, How it is formed and the Ailments which beset it

BOOK V THE EAR
The Anatomy Of The Ear[129]

God created Man's ears and placed them on his head to enable him to hear from both far and near. He led the ears into the cranial canals on both sides of the head. The canals are curved at the Lord's behest, not only in men but in all animals. The brain is part of the auditory apparatus.

As stated in Book I, there are four principal organs, the brain (ie the first of the four) is the seat of the five senses: vision, audition, olfaction, taste and tactile sense. In addition to those senses, the brain is the site of the memory and of ideation.

The curvature of the canals protect the ears from violent winds which could damage their nerves and impair hearing. The nerves, as do all others, arise from the brain, and form a dense membrane.[130] When the membrane is not blocked by humors (watery) and is exposed, a person can hear nicely. When the little membrane is too thick one cannot hear. Another reason for the canals' curvature is to moderate the exposure to cold and hot air, and thereby protect the sensitive nerves.

The external ear is cartilaginous – neither bone nor muscle. That allows it to be closed in emergencies, whereas if it was bone, it could not be closed off. Therefore, it is neither too soft nor to hard.

The ear must be kept open in order to hear well.

---

129 Professor Tabanelli translated his text from the Codices of Brussells, Ghent, Cambridge and London, from the Text of Van Leersum and from the French translations of G. Lonneville. see Introduction. p 39. (LDR).

130 Certain combinations of nerves and ligamentous tissues were called membranes. For example, the thinner part of the urinary bladder-wall was called a membrane and considered to be 'nervous'. Here, the reticule-wall was the tympanic membrane (LDR).

Chapter 1. Inflammations Of The Ears

Otic inflammations sometimes occur as abscesses or fistulas. Less severe inflammations are caused by sick complexions and overheating. They are manifested by heat and redness of varying degrees.

When you treat the less severe inflammations (ie due to overheating), use shucked fava beans that are thoroughly cooked in water (ie become pasty) in a tightly covered small pot to prevent the escape of the vapors. Use a funnel and a tube to guide the fumes from the pot into the ear when you boil the broth.

When the inflammation has been caused by exposure to cold, boil the beans in wine and warm the ear with the vapors.

Another remedy: Boil some oats and put the mash into very small sacks which you can insert in the ear – as hot as the patient can tolerate. That is an effective treatment.

Another: Bring water to boil and lower the flame before adding a fistful of red rose petals. As above, fumigate the ear with a funnel and tube. When the cause was cold air and pus appears, use wine instead of water. Instead of a fumigation in the latter case you can apply this plaster: Take rose petals, absinthe and artemisia. Another: Use oil of bitter almonds or oil of musk (as used by Nicolas) (96) and drip two or three drops into the ear. It is excellent.

Another: Melt and filter goose-fat and drip two or three drops in the ear. It works.

The patient should lie abed with the healthy ear down, thus allowing the drops to reach the diseased part. When both ears are sick, treat them alternatively, waiting for the upper ear to cool.

Chapter 2. Treatment Of The More Severe Otic Inflammations

This is how to treat abscesses in the ear. First examine carefully to see if the ear canal is obsructed by an abscess. If so, apply this plaster: Take equal amounts of minced fresh figs, wheat flour and some grapes without seeds (208). Add one part each of honey and butter to make a moderately thick plaster. Apply it moderately hot over the ear.

Another: Take plump figs, grapes without seeds, lard and honey. Combine them as above and apply.

If pus does not drain, use this ointment: Take small amounts of lard and a lot of honey. Mix them and cover a strip of oakum with it and insert it into the ear. It will purify, cleanse and cure the ear.

Another: Burn some ash-tree wood (189) by exposing one end of a small branch in the flames. Collect the fluid that will drip out of the other end and put it in a cupful of oil of violets. It will relieve the earache. After the abscess bursts and the pus drains out the ear, use this ointment . . . . [131]

CHAPTER 3. WORMS TRAPPED IN THE EAR-CANAL

For this grind walnut shells (309) and extract the oil and drip it into the ear. Or you may use the juices of crushed absinthe-leaves or peach-tree leaves. The acrid juices will kill the worms, as well as lice, fleas and other harmful insects.

CHAPTER 4. FOREIGN BODIES IN THE EAR

When objects such as cereal grains, pebbles et al. are caught in the canal, first have a friend of the patient breathe into his ear to barely moisten the surface of the trapped object. After a suitable delay, have the patient exhale in spurts and cough to eject the object. If it is a small nut or a cherry-pit or a pebble, irrigate the ear with oil of roses to lubricate the surfaces. But, if the object is a cereal grain, a seed, a pea or a dry bean, do not use oil. The object will expand and be impacted .

Take a long needle, bend one end as a hook and pass it to (ie just beyond) the object and rotate it so the hook will catch it and allow you to withdraw it.

Another maneuver: Take a straw or a smooth reed with a pointed tip. Dip it in a thick pine tar and lay it against the object and allow it to adhere before withdrawing it.

On occasion you will not be able to reach and remove the foreign

---

131 Here the text repeats verbatim the recipe in the previous paragraph. Probably a copyist's error. (LDR).

body and it may be impacted too far inside the canal. In such a case you may have to cut your way deeply to get beyond the object and dislodge it. That is a very risky operation, to be undertaken only when doing nothing will be even more threatening.

CHAPTER 5. WATER TRAPPED IN THE EAR-CANAL

In such cases Galen advised this: Use a very dry short length of a reed or of a lotus stem and insert it. Fill the outer end of the tubule with some wax and ignite it as if it is a candle. The heat will attract the water.

CHAPTER 6. CHRONIC MALODOROUS DRAINAGE FROM THE EAR

Not infrequently you will encounter cases of chronically draining ears which emit nauseating odors. That stench is more disturbing than the abscess itself. We call them 'otic fistulas'. The pus at the bottom is beyond the reach of a drain and the ailment is more serious when the pus resembles white paint, because yellow pus is a sign of an acute abscess (ie easier to treat). When the pus is dark it is caused by melancholic humors; when red it is cause by sanguine humors (ie bloody); when cloudy-white it is caused by phlegm.

The patient must first seek treatment by a learned physician[132] before going to the surgeon. The physician can prescribe the proper purges to clear the faulty humor. Afterwards the surgeon will know how to clear out the bad matter and prevent chronic drainage. The treatment with purgation uses the cochia pills and hierapicra. When used alone, it is a risky business and should not be managed by a surgeon who has no experience with it.

Galen recommended against the use of cool ointments, and advised we use chelidonium. Take some and macerate it in vinegar and irrigate the ear with the heated liquid.

When the drainage is not foul, you may use the juices of the leaves of white willow (402a) as an irrigant or use Rhazes' white ointment thinned with oil of roses, instilled when hot. When the drainage is long-standing, so-called 'aegritudo cronica' in Latin, use equal

132 Another bow to the 'establishment' (LDR).

amounts of myrhh, aloes, olibanum, sarcocolla and sandragon. Grind them well in a metal mortar and sieve them through a thick cloth. Put the powder on a strip of cloth and introduce it after cleaning the canal with pure honey. If the drain cannot reach the source, dissolve some of the powder in vinegar and spring-water and use it as an irrigant.

When the condition is very old and the ear has been cleaned out many times, use the following: Take some rust scraped off some old iron (419) and make a fine powder to mix with strong vinegar. Boil it in an iron pot until it is dry. Add vinegar and boil again. Repeat the action seven times, each time grinding the residue and adding vinegar. When finally it has the consistency of honey, drip it into the ear and it will penetrate to the source of the pus and attack the inflammation.

CHAPTER 7. TINNITUS

Ringing in the ears is a common complaint. The best treatment is purging the head by means of cochia pills or hierapicra. Dose the patient at night after a brief nap, when his stomach is empty. Then let him go back to sleep.

For those who are not otherwise sick, this is a good remedy for the ringing: Take oil of bitter almonds and use it along with the following pills: Take flakes of colocynth (125), one oz. each of castoreum, round aristolochium, juice of absinthe leaves; one-half oz. of euphorbia (173) and an equal weight (about fifteen grains) of wheat. Grind them and make the pills. Add the almond oil to the pills. Before putting the thick liquid in the ear, boil some marjoram , absinthe and arabian sticados (446a) in water and add one once of minced frankincense mixed with foamed honey. Drop some of it while warm into the ear.

CHAPTER 8. DEAFNESS

After anyone has been deaf for two or three years he can be cured only with great difficulty, because the faulty humors have obstructed the auditory nerves, and we cannot get at them locally (beyond the surgeon's reach) or by administering internal potions (ie beyond the physician's, too).

Although much has been written about medicines which have been touted for their good results in many patients, I have yet to see very much improvement in the cases where I have tried them. However, I will repeat what the Masters have recommended (ie and their claims!).

Take ant-eggs, earthworms, maggots and leaves of rue. Mince them all and sieve the mixture through a cloth. Put a drop in the ear and plug the exit with some cotton and anoint the outer surfaces with some of the same oily stuff. That will cure deafness. Another recipe: Core out the center of a halved onion and fill the defect with olive oil. Keep it so until you can see a small round worm with a black head appear between the onion leaves and the skin! Then boil everything in olive oil and use it in the deaf ear. It works.

Other Masters recommend the body fat of frogs used as above. And others say this: Take equal amounts of leaves of rue and fresh absinthe and boil them in wine from the Poitou. When done, decant it into an earthenware jug. Lay the patient on his side and drip it repeatedly while hot into the ear for one to two hours.

When the deafness has an internal cause, these medications will have no effect on the deafness, but there is no harm in trying them. I myself use them in treating deafness due to external causes.[133]

How To Treat Lumps In The Scalp[134]

The treatment is simple. Incise with a bistouri along the long axis of the mass. Squeeze out the 'pus' and remove the capsule. Fill the defect with powdered zinc sulfate or salt, which will eat away whatever remains of the bad matter.

Some Masters made cruciate incisions, but I think my incision

133 In his concluding statement Yperman almost admits to what has not been mentioned but indeed must be the case. All of the curious remedies will relieve deafness if the cause is a plug of ear-wax which the drops will loosen and cause to be discharged. That was the 'external' cause of many cases of deafness! (LDR).

134 These are sebaceous cysts; here the cyst has suppurated. Long before Yperman the lesion was called testudo (turtle) (LDR).

leaves a better scar. The scalp hair will fall out where it is exposed to the pus, but it will grow back if the exposure is brief, not long enough to kill the hair-roots. Treat the incision as you do other wounds. Be on guard against the bad proud flesh which will crop up rapidly here.[135] Destroy it as it appears and prevent its regeneration.

HERE ENDS BOOK V ON THE HEAD AND BEGINS BOOK VI ON THE THROAT

And

Here Ends Part I Of My Treatise Which Deals With The Head, The Eyes, The Nose, The Mouth And The Ears, And With Wounds Of Those Structures

---

135 The spongy purulent granulation tissue (LDR).

BOOK VI THE NECK AND THE THROAT
THE ANATOMY [136]

A surgeon cannot ignore the internal structures of Man.[137] He must know the risks of injuring them. Here I shall describe what is in the throat (ie gola) in front and in the neck (ie collo) in back.

First we go behind: The neck has seven separate vertebrae. Many ligaments bind them too the skull in such a way that Nature allows the head to move side-to-side, fore-and-back and to twist-and-turn as is desired. Other less tenuous (ie tougher) ligaments bind the head and the neck to prevent separation. The first vertebra is securely bound to the second below it, second to the third etc., until the seventh is bound to the shoulder and the uppermost dorsal vertebra. This last attachment is looser than the others.

A pair of nerves emerges between each pair of vertebrae, beginning between the cranium and the first cervical and continuing down to the space below the seventh. Nature distributes the nerves over the head, the neck, the chest, the shoulders and the arms. The nerves fan out and serve the various parts after dividing into small fibers that admix with those from the cranial nerves. The former are purely motor nerves and the cranials are purely sensory. The motor nerves become part of the muscles of the region which contract voluntarily.[138]

---

136 Tabanelli's sources for his Italian edition are The Codices at Brussells, Ghent, Cambridge and London (Van Leersum's text) and the French translations by Lonneville in *Le Scalpel*, 1933. see Introduction (LDR).

137 This aggregation of anatomical misconceptions was put forth even when Mondino de Luzzi was beginning his anatomical investigations which could refute some of them. Europe had to await two centuries for Vesalius et al. To 'discover' the human body(LDR).

138 These concepts are older than Galen! The nerves and the muscles together are the contractile element. The word 'nerve' may denote a tendon, a nerve or the combination of both, sometimes called a 'cord'. As noted before, a fibrous membrane was thought to be a 'nervous' tissue(LDR).

In the back of the neck (ie prevertebral) lie two large nerves behind which are large vessels which carry nutrition from the liver to the head, as I have described them in Book I. After their nutritive function has been carried out, they descend behind the ears and carry the vital part of a Man – in Latin it is called the sperm – down to the testes. If you divide those arteries, a man will be impotent.

Nature has placed organs on both sides of the neck (which we call 'cervix'). Those are the ligaments of the neck and its organs.[139] They are not very sensitive. They are attached the the skull and to the vertebrae. Over them ride the nerves arising from the spinal cord (ie the 'marrow') in the neck and within the dorsal vertebrae. Those structures (ie the marrow) are like the brain in substance and have the same two investing membranes.

Now we move up front to the throat (gola) where we find the apparatus for swallowing (the pharynx) and for respiration (the larynx). The latter extends from the level of the chin to that of the clavicle. The former is the esophagus which lies between the neck in back and the throat in front. The esophagus is a small tube attached above to the lining membrane of the mouth and below it reaches the stomach. Whatever we swallow goes through the tube to the stomach. It passes behind the larynx[140] in front of a total of fifteen vertebrae, the seventh cervical and fourteen dorsal.

The esophagus makes a gentle turn forward to go through the diaphragm toward the stomach. The esophagus consists of two membranes, a longitudinal muscle layer which propels the matter that has been ingested. At the lower end the muscle splays out so it can widen the opening into the stomach.

The larynx lies in front of the esophagus. It consists of rings of cartilage, not bone. The rings are held together by membranes, inner and outer. The inner membrane is very soft. The (circles of) the rings are closed behind and are separated from the contiguous esophagus by the membranes. This allows the tube to swallow large and firm masses into the stomach, without doing harm.

139 These are the lateral muscles and tendons which other authors call the Neck. They distinguished Collo from Nucha (nape) and divide the region in three, whereas Yperman makes the lateral structures part of the collo (LDR).
140 Yperman includes the trachea in his 'larynx' (LDR).

At the upper ends of the larynx and esophagus – which are bound together – we find a small box made of three cartilages. When one inspires or expires in breathing, the box is open, but when one swallows it closes, such that neither solid food nor drink can enter it. If any food or saliva happens to get into the little box it initiates coughing until it has been restored to its normal state.

On the surface of the throat are two arteries, called the caprine (ie goat-like), which consist of two layers. The inner layer is like cartilage to resist the hot blood within them That characterizes all arteries wherever they are encountered, after they come from the heart. The outer layer is muscular, made to resist the pulsation.

Wounds of these large arteries threaten life. If the vessels are divided the victim will die rapidly. That is because blood from the heart goes into the arteries and supplies the organism's vitality. When the arteries are opened, two things are rapidly lost, the blood and the vital spirit; the heart's blood is the gentle vehicle of Vital Spirit throughout the body.

Chapter 1. Wounds Of The Neck

Although some wounds are curable and others are lethal, all of them are life-threatening. A wound that transects the spinal marrow always is fatal. Any transverse slicing wound by a sword or sickle etc. may cut the marrow. Carefully examine such a wound and observe whether or not a vertebra is injured directly or if the intervertebral ligaments are divided. If the latter, determine if the wound enters the spinal marrow (ie as distinct from the bone-marrow). In such a case the marrow oozes and that will tell you if the wound is fatal, because the spinal marrow is an extension of the brain. However, the Master Surgeons say that if the marrow does not ooze, the victim may survive even thou he may be paralyzed below the level of the injury because the nerves which leave the marrow below that level no longer function, as we taught in the Anatomy section at the beginning of this treatise. When you cannot see into the depths of a wound but the wound is large enough to admit an examining finger, palpate to determine if a bone has been injured, When the bone is intact and inflammation (suppuration) [141] has not supervened, suture the wound with a braided waxed thread. But if the wound is inflamed, abrade the surfaces before suturing them. However, if the edges bleed too freely, and the wound surfaces are anemic (ie feeble), arrest the hemorrhage as we have instructed in the Chapter on Blood-Clotting. After the sutures have been placed, dust on the powder as in the Chapter on Powders.

If you wish, you may use Albucasis' very popular powder or those of other Masters that are equally famous. Then continue the treatments as we do for all wounds.

When the wound suppurates, use the following ointment, whether or not the nerves are damaged.[142] Take three ounces of boiled rosamel, two oz. each of wax and resin (379), 3 oz. of terebinth, 1 oz. each of mastic and sarcocolla (410) and mummy (295), 3 oz. of oil of mastic, and 3 oz. of barley-meal. Mix them and simmer until all are blended. Put it in the wound.

CHAPTER 2. AILMENTS OF THE CERVICAL ESOPHAGUS

You must examine minutely all wounds by cutting weapons or by fire-arms[143] that enter the neck or throat until you are certain about their severity. You already know about wounds that enter the spinal marrow, now learn about the wounds that enter the esophagus. You will see that they spill whatever solid or liquid matter that is swallowed. That wound is very difficult to cure, and if it is curable it will take a long time, because the organ is muscular (ie the edges move). [144]

141 The term 'inflammation' is misconstrued. Here Yperman means that the wound has been open for long enough for the surfaces to be dry, and he repeats the ancient practice of freshening the dried surfaces of a wound to make them ooze before bringing them together with or without sutures (LDR)

142 The accepted practice among most of the Masters avoided applying oily substances directly on exposed nerves (LDR).

143 Certainly this one of the earliest mention of fire-arms in medieval literature. A few notices may be found written during the third decade of the 14thC, coincident with Yperman's treatise. However, the weapons were not hand-held. Does Yperman refer here to a 'shrapnel' wound? See Sarton, Vol. III, p. 722 ff (LDR).

144 Galen had taught that wound-edges that move against each other will not unite (LDR).

Nevertheless, I recommend that you use a compressive powder [145] such as the red powder (377b). Bandage it in place so it completely covers the opening. The victim must abstain from food and beverages for as long as possible, the longer the better. Nature sometimes works strange wonders and causes the wound to seal when nothing is allowed to pass through it and reopen it. Nature works its cure by means of the paternal sperm which younger patients possess in larger abundance and when they have not wasted it or if they remain celibate.

We use no drains. When you see healing in progress continue the strict abstinence until there is no leak. When that stage is reached, offer the following beverage: Take a handful each of caryophyla, incinerated nettles (326), tansy (454), red cabbage (71), hemp (78) and add oil. Put it in a large pot with six liters of wine and boil it down to two liters. Filter it through cloth and add honey to sweeten it to the taste of the patient. Heat a cabbage leaf which you immerse in the potion before dressing the wound with it. This dressing is good for treating all incised wounds when you use no drains. If the beverage is too costly for the patient because it requires so much wine, use the above herbs and some green cannabis. Mince them all and add a small amount of wine, not much, but do not eliminate the honey. You can use this potion to replace the first, perhaps with less benefit but nonetheless worth while.

CHAPTER 3. WOUNDS OF THE THROAT [146]

When the throat is cut the air escapes from the wound and the lungs cannot serve the heart (ie by cooling it). The continuous passage of air prevents the wound from sealing. The throat (larynx-trachea) consists of cartilaginous rings bound together by inner and outer membranes. Despite all the risks, just as we described in the preceding chapter, recovery is possible if you act promptly. But be sure to give a dire prognosis to the patient's entourage.

---

145 Packed against the opening (LDR).

146 Here Yperman's term 'gola' is used instead of larynx (ie the larynx and trachea) which is the only structure dealt with. Again, we question the author as well as the copyists (LDR)

CHAPTER 4. THREE DIFFERENT TYPES OF ANGINA

Angina is an ailment of the throat, especially in the pharynx. It appears in three ways: squinancia, sinancia and quinancia.

The angina called sinancia is caused by humors working internally as well as externally. It is not as serious as quinancia because the action usually is external. Although the lesion itself may not be so serious, it may be threatening when it obstructs the air passages, or the patient may not be able to swallow. food or beverages, as he gasps for air.

Begin your treatment for sinancia this way: Perform an emergency phlebotomy from an ipsilateral arm vein or from both arms, and bleed until the patient faints. The next day bleed from the dark sublingual veins if the patient is robust and can withstand the losses. Use my gargle of diamoron (155) in which you have mixed a decoction of plantain or another made as follows: Take sumac, bile, pomegranate blossoms and rose petals. Mince them and boil them in rose-water. Cool it and add it to the diamoron for use as a gargle. That will promote the discharge of the bad humors from the aposthem. At first use the cool gargle which contains the plantains because it will cool the fricative heat usually caused by rheumatic humors. Then use the other gargle which digests and condenses.

Massage the throat with rosemary flowers applied on unwashed wool fleece. The following plaster also is good for applications on the throat: Take roots of guimauve and lentils and boil them in rain water before mashing them in a mortar with some lard. Apply as a plaster (ie on cloth).

When the uvula is acutely swollen and red, treat with phlebotomies as instructed in Chapter 1 of Book IV. Then—put the powder on the uvula (ie see below.

Another plaster for use against squinancia that is recommended by the Authorities: Take minced boiled verbena and place it on the squinancia. You may save the lives of many when you act quickly. Another good plaster: Take the roots of wild plum trees (355) and some peeled garlic and some absinthe. Mince them all and then squeeze out their juices. Mix that with some barley meal and flax seeds (252).

Add greasy drippings from roasting meats and simmer it in a casserole while adding liberal amounts of honey, cook it until it thickens. Apply on the mass.

The powder for the uvula (ie see above) is applied through a small perforated tube with many openings (ie near the end) while you use another instrument to lift the structure. Then use this gargle: Take equal amounts of sweet wine, honey and vinegar . Boil them. Pulverize finely in a metal mortar pepper, pyrethrum, staphisagre and pomegranate flowers. Boil the powder and the fluid to make the gargle to be used both in the morning and evening.

Or use this powder: Take laurel berries, cinnamon, pennyroyal (367), gum arabic (212) Mix with warm honey, spread it on oakum and apply it on the dome of the head.

Failing all the above, apply a red hot cautery on the neck.

The following powder also will cause the discharge of the humors (ie pus) : Take some pitch cintered on a broiling plate and add powdered white frankincense and make a powder of both to use in these cases. If it doesn't work, cut the tip off, after intubating it as previously described.[147]

CHAPTER 5. LARGE TONSILS

In some cses masses shaped like almonds exists behind the tongue in the throat.[148]

They derive from catarrhal humors that come down from the head. These tonsils sometimes interfere with breathing where they are at the level of the carotid arteries.

Begin your treatment with purges to eliminate the faulty humors. Then go on to their removal. Seat the patient opposite you, facing the light. Depress his tongue with a sound or a spoon to give a clear view of the throat. Have the patient gargle and look again, to see the two 'almonds', one on each side of the tongue. Catch one with an iron or

---

147 This confused and haphazrdly constructed chapter fails to define the three forms of quinsy and reintroduces the inflamed uvula, and it alternates the treatments for all the ailments without explanation. Do we blame Yperman who may have dashed off the chapter between calls to military service. Or can we blame scribes in later years? (LDR).

148 Here Yperman used his term 'gola' to mean the pharynx (LDR).

bronze hook and draw it out as you cut on each side of it with a bistouri knife or a special tonsillectomy knife. Do not cut the surrounding membrane (ie mucosa) as you shell out the tonsil. Then have the patient gargle with rose water, vinegar and juice of plantains. If the procedure releases foul odors (ie purulent tonsillitis) remove some of the membranes at its base to expose the cavity and cauterize the site with a hot gold cautery inserted through a protective tube.

A Special Note On Quinsy – Lanfranchi's Experience

I will cite at length a lesson I learned by example. It happened in Milan when Lanfranchi was called to attend an elderly lady, aged 49, who had developed an angina (ie a tonsillar abscess) caused by phlegm. Both tonsils were involved, pointing inside as well as outside the throat. She neither could speak nor swallow. She had been treated by a young physician who had been able to relieve her pain, but the masses continued to enlarge. Lanfranchi went to her after she had not eaten for nine days, and she had not slept for fear of suffocation. Her pulse was feeble. He looked for a tender spot under her jaw and he found it.[149] The pus lay so deep that everyone thought that the poor woman would suffocate before the abscess would drain inside or externally. He recommended that he incise below the jaw and the family agreed. He used a bistouri and released a jet of fetid pus, but a lot more remained inside.

After the operation, the patient began to improve; her breathing was easier and her pulse was stronger. He gave her some broth to drink and only a small amount came out the wound. He applied a plaster of marsh celery (4), wheat-flour and honey. If you do not have the recipe at hand look for it in our chapter on anthrax where I give the details. He used the plaster until he noted that the foul nauseating odor come from a sloughing piece of tough artery that had the appearance of gangrenous intestine. After the slough had passed, the wound was free of odor. Then the patient was fed a liquid which she sucked through a silver tube which reached beyond the internal opening of the abscess; it allowed her to swallow without leakage

---

149 The place where the infection was closest to the surface, indicating where he should lance it (LDR).

through the wound.

After the above, he irrigate the wound with warm wine and applied some of the black ointment which I described in the chapter on wounds of the head. I had a similar experience in Ypres treating a young man at the beginning of the year 1328.

CHAPTER 6. RANULA BENEATH THE TONGUE

On occasion you will see a fleshy swelling under the tongue, called a ranula in Latin and een-punt (ranocchia) in Flemish. It interferes with the tongue's movements in speaking and sometimes it is so large that it fills the mouth.

I suggests that you try to treat it with small amounts of this plaster: Take one-half lb. each of red and yellow orpiment, one lb. each of ginger, salt, bile and pyrethrum and let them soak in vinegar. Dip a pledget of cotton in the mixture and let it dry. Mince it and lay a bit on the ranula. Then have the patient rinse with oil of roses to calm the inflammation provoked by the corrosive substances.

If that prescription is not effective or the ranula is too large, you will have to excise it. First catch it with a hook and lift it outward. However, if it is firm and dark in color and insensitive, do not touch it, because it is caused by a melancholic humor and it is incurable.[150] The ranulas which can be excised are soft and pale. If they do not empty themselves, remove them through openings produced by the corrosives as above. Hook the lesion and dissect it away from the tongue and sublingual tissues with a bistouri. Then rinse the mouth with vinegar and spring water. Observe all the precautions that we described in the chapter on the gums.

CHAPTER 7. FOOD PARTICLES OR FISH-BONES CAUGHT IN THE THROAT

When a fish-bone or a barb of a fish is caught in the throat, set the patient facing the light or in full sunlight so you can look far into his throat. Depress the tongue with a small wood blade or with your thumb,

---

150 A caveat repeated whenever Ypres describes a malignant lesion. Here it is a cancer of the floor of the mouth (LDR).

as in the previous chapter. When you see the foreign body, remove it if you can. Or, have the patient swallow as much food as he can and have him vomit it before it has a chance to digest in the stomach. If the emesis does not bring up the bone, tie a strong cord around a piece of sponge and have the patient swallow it. Then withdraw the sponge which may catch the bone on its rough surface. And if that, too, does not succeed, have the patient eat crusts of stale bread to push the foreign body into the stomach.

Chapter 8. Goiter

A goiter is a fleshy mass that appears under the surface of the throat. It is attached to the carotid arteries and sometimes to nerves from the neck. The attachment to the arteries makes a surgical removal very dangerous; an injury to those arteries may be lethal. If the goiter is not fixed to the arteries but simply to the nerves you may not be able to separate it from those attachments without injuring them, as if you were making a wound across the neck.

Goiter is caused by catarrhal (ie rheumatic) humors from above in the head. The condition often involves a child as well as its parents, as does phthisis, leprosy, epilepsy—the so-called grand lethargy [151] — and many disorders of the eyes.

When you wish to remove a goiter, or when you simply consult re the treatment, first act to get rid of the faulty humors by natural means. Purge the superfluous humors with medicines prescribed by a competent physician. That is the proper thing to do. It is not correct for the surgeon of today to act also as a physician as it was in the times of Hippocrates, Galen or Avicenna, and as it still may be at Salerno, Montpellier, Paris and elsewhere.

Here are time-tested plasters to melt away the humors and to eat into hard flesh[152]: Take some roots of cochlearia (horse-radish, 373)

---

151 Grand mal epilepsy with post-ictal somnolence (LDR).

152 The conservative surgeon favors the use of caustic medications to eat through the skin rather than to make a clean incision. so much feared by the patients, who seemed to accept the pain and the prolonged procedures and the deprivations of sex-life and alimentation rather than the knife. The surgeon protected his reputation for eschewing the knife, both in the public arena as well as among the physicians who referred their patients to him (LDR).

wild water-melon (492) and saxifrage (413). Boil them in spring-water and then mash the pulp with lard or goat-fat. Apply it on the goiter and leave it for a long time, during which period the patient should drink the following: Strip some roots of a barren walnut tree while you chant the Pater Noster. Crush the matter with two grams of pepper and boil them in a good wine until the volume is reduced by half. The liquid should be imbibed daily on an empty stomach until the goiter subsides. At the same time he should eat some wheat-bread that is well baked and is somewhat stale. After the potion he may drink some diluted good wine.

The patient will avoid all sexual activity for one year and he should not eat cold food or drink spring water.[153] When the mass is not fixed to the carotid arteries or to muscles[154] use a bistouri to cut the skin overlying the nodule and try to shell it out without causing too much pain.[155] If you fail in that, apply a piece of realgar (380), a compound of arsenic and sulfur, on the exposed tissue. Don't leave it there too long and destroy the patient (ie as it eats beyond the goiter). Or, you may use the powder we prescribed for wens in the scalp. Then apply lard or butter as we did there. Continue the treatments until the tumor is eliminated. As the mass shrinks, use less and less of the caustic powders. If you are not careful, the medicine will erode the arteries and kill the patient.

After the goiter has disappeared, cleanse the wound and treat it as we do other wounds of the head.

CHAPTER 9 . SCROFULA OR THE KING'S EVIL

The Latin word scrofula means a sow, because the female pig bears large litters, and scrofula consists of clusters of nodules grow-

---

153 Tabanelli suggests this may imply an understanding why alpine peoples who drank melted snow, the sources for their spring-water, more commonly suffered goiter than the low-land people who drank water from streams that contained more iodine ((T).

154 Here Yperman uses 'muscle' instead of 'nerves' as in par. 2 of this chapter. Again ,we note how the ancient anatomists misconceived nerves and tendons as part of the muscular apparatus (LDR).

155 The word 'skin' may be interpreted as the capsule of the exposed thyroid if indeed the skin it had been eaten away during the 'year' of treatment with corrosives (LDR).

ing beneath the ears, near the throat, beneath the jaws, in the axillae and groins near the principal organs that we use for purging, as I will teach also in the chapter on ulcers.

There are two types of scrofules – glandules and true scrofules. A gland is a nodule that usually derives from phlegmatic humors. The true scrofule is different, caused by melancholic humors. A glandule is soft, scrofules are firm.

Avicenna advised when you are called to treat them, to be sure to ask if they are longstanding or of recent origin.

Begin with purges and a limited diet. When the purges are emetic as well as laxative, they are good for both kinds of scrofules. When the evacuations are not sufficient, intensify the use of purgatives known to eliminate phlegm and other viscous humors. Use this potion: Take equal amounts of turbith, ginger and white sugar. Make a powder and dose two oz. to the patient if he can take it. Give it at midnight or a little later. The patient will return to bed until he must get up to evacuate, and he should not return to sleep until the purgation is complete. The patient should be careful not to heed his appetite and to eat sparingly. He should not eat after early evening nor drink spring-water nor take anything cold at mealtimes. He should remain hungry. He should avoid bowing his head lest he draw the humors there, nor should he kneel and cause swollen knees. That is bad, because any swelling takes the fluid from the humors and leaves behind the harmful thick parts.

Now we will go to the treatment of glandules, scrofules and fatty tumors of the scalp. Although few people pay attention to the masses unless they are open (ie draining) or are causing discomfort, our goal is to eliminate the masses by means of plasters applied on the intact skin over them. I use this plaster: Take some small red snails (249) and boil them with some lard. Add honey and mix. Apply it on scrofules in the head (ie neck).

Another: Mince some guimauve roots with lard or chicken-fat and wine. This makes an equally good plaster. Another good plaster is made from goat turds mixed with honey and vinegar.

Another: Take equal amounts of ammoniac resin (23), bdellium(53) and galbanum (194). Macerate them in strong vinegar for three days. Dissolve some sulfur in the fluid and make a plaster.

Avicenna liked this one: Take roots of lilies (248), flax seeds and pigeon droppings (179) and dissolve them in wine. When the scrofules, glands and the fatty tumors on the head were of a cold nature – not reddened by inflammation—he added more pigeon droppings. If otherwise, he used smaller amounts. When treating children or women he used one-fourth the amount.

Another plaster was used by Avicenna and has been praised by all the Masters since; it has a very complicated recipe. Pay close attention and be careful not to burn it or to allow it to bubble over into the flames. It is called 'emplaustrum diaquilon' in Latin and is excellent against scrofules, fatty tumors and all indurated ulcers. Make its so: Take one lb. each of fenugreek, flax seeds and roots of guimauve. Place them in separate earthenware pans and cover them each with three lbs. of boiling water (ie a total of nine lbs.) and let them steep for a full day and night. Then bring each separately to a boil and strain each alone through linen cloths to yield thick liquids, the more the better. Then take one-half lb. of litharge filtered through a fine mesh to obtain a fine powder. Then take two lbs. of aged, pure and clean olive oil and bring it to a boil while stirring in the litharge over a low flame (removing it frequently so not to overcook it) until the color begins to fade. You can tell when it has simmered long enough when a drop of it on a slate or on the bottom of an empty basin does not spread. Then remove the casserole from the flame and allow it to cool slightly before adding one and one-fourth lbs. of the gelatin (the mixture of the three thickened filtered materials) which you had prepared beforehand, and put it all to simmer again slowly while stirring with a spatula until it has the consistency of wax. Quit the fire and work the paste with your hands which you keep wet with fresh oil to prevent the paste from adhering to them. The more you knead, the better will be the result.[156] This plaster is excellent for all ailments indicated above when placed on the intact skin. It is good for inflammations, abscesses and ulcers, a thousand times better than 'treyt'.[157]

---

156 I assume that this final maneuver incorporated the initial herbs into the paste (LDR).

157 Not identified (T).

CHAPTER 10. EXCISING SCROFULES AND GLANDS

When you attempt to remove them, take care that they are not fixed to the muscles or the carotid arteries; an injury to the latter could cost a life. After incising, grasp the gland or fatty tumor with your thumb and a finger and avoid cutting into the mass. Do not cut into the capsule. Dissect it away from the overlying skin and other tissues before removing the lump in toto. When dealing with a glandule, scrofule or sebaceous cyst, use a hook for traction. When brisk bleeding interferes, use the now-familiar coagulants. When a bit of capsule remains, destroy it as we have taught (ie with corrosives). [158]

CHAPTER 11. WHEN SCROFULES AND GLANDULES BECOME FISTULAS[159]

Many people believe that God endowed the King of France with the ability to halt the growth of scrofules. They believe that he can cure by spiritual means alone, with his hands and eyes. However, none of the Royal cures were incurable cases to begin with. Many authorities, including some surgeons, believe (ie another faith cure) that the patient and the surgeon should be immersed in a running stream on the Eve of St. John, and that the patient should be bled there so his blood will spill into the water. They insist that many cures have been obtained.

In spite of all such testimony, I believe that a more certain cure can be obtained with the powder we described and with the capital powder described in our chapter on sebaceous cysts of the scalp in Book I.

Put a small amount over each scrofule.[160] The next morning, take some tallow which you cooked with some red cabbage and insert it

---

158 Tabanelli notes that Yperman here repeats Lanfranchi (Book III, Ch. 2) in his nosology and treatments (T).

159 Chronic drainage characterized secondarily infected tuberculous lymphadenitis (LDR)

160 Insert the corrosive powder into the open ulcer or fistula. The tumors described here have necessitated from within or have been treated with caustics placed on the overlying skin (LDR).

into what remains of a nodule. If another presents itself in the same place, repeat the treatment. When the mass is gone, treat the wound.

After every operation for removal of a nodule, put some of the powder in the pocket whence came the tumor. Do not endanger the lives of your patients and embarrass yourselves as do many surgeons through incompetence and derring-do.[161]

HERE ENDS THE BOOK VI ON THE NECK[162]

I ask that all of you who know it and study it to translate this Latin book into Flemish. I have written it for those who will come after I am gone, whereas today most surgical practitioners cannot deal with it as it is and that is a shameful situation. They put their own souls at risk by seeking only to accumulate personal profits. But God Bless us all.

---

161 Y warns not to attempt to excise an adherent capsule when a caustic powder will do the job safely (LDR).

162 The postscript obviously was not by Yperman, who wrote his book in Western Flemish, not in Latin (LDR).

BOOK VII THE BODY BELOW THE NECK: THREE PARTS

Book VII as it follows here is a confused mixture of one hundred-two chapters, taken from three codices. All of them are in Tabanelli's Edition.

The Brussells Codex of forty chapters deals mostly with traditional 'surgical' matters: certain diseases, wounds and techniques. Chapters will be numbered 1B, 2B, etc.

The Cambridge Codex (Van Leersum's text) has fifty-one chapters that are not in the Brussells Codex. Their subject matter is very different: dermatological ailments, bites. poisons, abscesses here-and-there, hernias, etc. Chapters will be numbered 1C, 2C, etc.

The Ghent Codex (also from Van Leersum's text) has eleven chapters that are not in the other codices., and they consist only of brief statements, excepting Chapter 9. They deal with fractures and dislocations. Chapters will be numbered 1G, 2G, etc.

The Rubrics for all three parts of Book VII are placed in the General Table of Contents.

PART I
FORTY CHAPTERS FROM THE BRUSSELLS CODEX

CHAPTER 1 B. WOUNDS OF VEINS AND ARTERIES

When veins and arteries are entered anywhere in the body, the loss of blood can cause the patient to collapse. His pale face and the appearance of a dying man leads to the obvious diagnosis.[163] Quickly

---

163 Hemorrhage is the cause of collapse rather than any other. Don't delay your actions to save him (LDR)

apply coagulant powders as we instructed in the chapter on wounds of the scalp.

Nature often restores the patient by delivering blood from the liver to re-fill the emptied veins, allowing the wound to continue to bleed heedlessly. Perhaps a contusion has been severe enough to continue to attract blood. And we see it can happen with a phlebotomy when the bleeding will resume after a delay while the restoration is in process. When there is no powder, no magic formula, no powerful stone (ie magnetite) that can arrest the hemorrhage, I advise, as did Master Hugh of Lucca, that you use a pressure bandage pulled tightly enough but not too tight. While you prepare the dressing, an associate should place his finger on the bleeding vessel to stop the flow. The finger should press parallel with the vessel, not just over the opening. The blood will thicken and clot. After the hemorrhage stops, treat the wound as you have learned.

When you take away the controlling finger, Master Hugh of Lucca advised always to spread this powder in the wound: Take two oz. of hepatic aloes, one-half oz. of bol d'armenico, one oz. of sandragon and three oz. of white and greasy frankincense. Grind the mixture to a powder. Put the powder in the wound and dust some wheat-flour over it, and lay on a compress moistened with egg-white and vinegar. Then elevate the limb.

Another method used by Master Hugh: While the finger pressure is in effect, irrigate the wound with cold water to cool the region and the blood. The longer you maintain the digital pressure the better will be the result. Continue the cool irrigation until the patient no longer feels heat in the wound and the blood does not boil.[164] Hugh also wrote that you may cool the wound by sprinkling wine and water, as we taught in the chapter on blood-clotting in wounds. [165]

As soon as the bleeding is controlled, remove the pressure pad and replace it with another, also wet with egg-white and vinegar. Replace it when it becomes warm, and repeat the action until the wound

---

164 Tabanelli explains 'boiling blood'. It was a misconception of the epoch that blood contained gas bubbles which were released and became clearly visible when a phlebotomist splashed blood from the arm into a basin and froth appeared on the surface (LDR).

165 Yperman cited Theodoric who wrote down what Hugh taught. Hugh did not write (LDR).

is no longer warm. When you replace the tampons, renew the under-lying powders and the spray of cold water and vinegar.

Some people misunderstand this and say, "cold warms and heat cools". They do not know what they are talking about. Really, cold cools the naturally warm blood, and warm water heats it. Remember that ' like attracts like'.

The barber-phlebotomist does not release cool blood nor does he warm it with cold water. When one bathes in cold water, his pores – the small openings in the skin through which the sweat emerges— are closed and his natural heat cannot escape. So one may say that cold acts to preserve heat.

And so it is that bathing in hot water during the winter makes one sensitive to cold for two or three days. Furthermore, if one strips down and bathes in cold water on a wintry morning, he shuts his pores and retains his heat and feels warm. And a cold bath in the summer months may leave one feeling warmer than before the bath, And if he pro-longs his immersion in the cold tub he will become hungry because the cold drives his natural heat inwards from the surface. That inter-nal heat will increase the rate of digestion of food in the stomach. If you have paid close attention to the foregoing, you will agree that it is true.

When the blood no longer froths, apply cold compresses wet with cold water and wine.[166] Afterwards, put the red powder in the wound and go on to treat the wound as you have learned. Later on, I will explain why we treat wounds differently according to where they are.

After the hemorrhage has stopped, as in the cases described above, provide food and give the patients beverages that promote the resto-ration of blood: capons, hens, geese, partridges and mutton with pars-ley. Add egg-yolks in all dishes. The patient should drink unwatered good wine; when he is well fed, he will recover by virtue of his own God-given vitality.

---

166 Yperman had no idea the bleeding patient's blood was 'watered' to maintain intravascular volume and sustain life and that thin blood lacked some of its frothing agents! (LDR).

Chapter 2 B. Fractures And Wounds Of The Clavicular Region[167]

Sharp weapons such as swords or sabers often wound the shoulder, and the clavicle or other bones may be broken. When a bone is divided or cut into, proceed at once to remove any bits bone from the wound and carefully assess the full depth of the cut. When you are satisfied, suture the wound with bites taken deep enough to approximate the full thickness of the wound, leaving no deep pockets in which pus can accumulate. Place the bites about a finger-breadth apart, spaced widely enough to admit your finger tip.

Insert a drain at the lowermost end of the opening; let it be of very clean old linen or of lint dipped in the red powder or Albucasis' powder, as we make it. Later, use black balsam (48).

Chapter 3 B. Stab-Wounds In The Chest

Stab wounds caused by knives, daggers, swords, picks, pitch-forks, javelins or by blows by clubs or wounds by arrows or darts—any wounds that can cause damage within the chest wall can penetrate the diaphragm or enter the pleural cavity wherein lie the heart the lungs, and can damage the esophagus that passes behind the trachea and carries what we swallow into the stomach, or cut the larynx (ie trachea) which carries air to the lungs. In such cases (ie penetrating wounds) look well to see if blood from the chest goes through the diaphragm. If so, try to evacuate the blood from the abdomen as I will explain below. Place a small drain in the front and a small one at the rear end of the wound to empty the chest cavity. Whatever you do not remove when the wound is fresh will be more difficult to remove later on. Soak the drains in warm oil of roses. You should have those materials ready at hand and be prepared to plug the wounds and prevent the escape of inspired air and to prevent the entry of ambient air. This caveat holds also when you make your own incisions (ie see

---

167 The title is misleading. The topic is all fractures of the shoulder region compounded by wounds by sharp-edged weapons (LDR)

below). If the trapped blood suppurates, you must irrigate the wound (ie the empyema cavity) with a tube and a clyster-nozzle attached to a pear-shaped bladder.

Insert the tube and inject the irrigant from the bladder and try to reach the entire cavity; while squirting, point the tube here and there and flush out all the accumulated matter from within. Use this irrigant: Take three oz. of rosamel which has been boiled with one-half oz. each of powdered myrrh, fenugreek and lupine flour. Add one lb. of sweet honey and two lbs. of water[168], and boil it down to two-thirds of the original volume. Strain it through a clean cloth and use it as above.

Afterwards, cover the wound with this plaster: Take four oz. of barley-meal and one oz. each of myrrh and powdered fenugreek, and gently bring it to a boil while stirring with a wood spatula. When the mixing is complete, add three oz. of previously filtered and purified terebinth. Mix all while it cools. While using the plaster be sure to keep the drains wet. Change them frequently until all the pus has been evacuated. You will know that the contents are no longer toxic when the patient says that he feels well, that his strength is returning, and that he breathes easily. When you see the last of the pus and the wound appears clean, shorten your drains and allow the wound to close.

If to the contrary the suppuration continues and you anticipate a lethal outcome, or if the toxicity persists in spite of less pus, and the patient cannot sleep and is anorectic, the prognosis is poor. There is little more you can do in such cases except to continue your cleansing and the use of the drains and plasters, trusting to God for the rest.

But if the wound resists and a bulge appears between the fifth and sixth ribs, [169] while it is still small, incise over the most prominent part of the mass and reach the pus and drain it. Treat the new wound as we recommended for the original one by cleansing, with drains etc, until it heals.

Indeed, when the blood and pus extends to the level of the diaphragm, it can no longer be drained through the primary wound. In such cases, a second incision is necessary. This new wound may be hard for the patient to accept, and he must be given to understand

---

168 In Part I of Book VII, the Ms uses 'pounds' as a measure of liquids, whereas in Part II the term is 'liters' (LDR).

169 A 'necessitating' empyema (LDR).

the risks of the inevitable dire outcome if it is not used. A posterior wound is more dangerous than an anterior one because the posterior part of the diaphragm is richer in nerves and is more fleshy.

If everything happens as I have described, the victim often will survive. But if you fail to treat properly, eventually the patient will cough up and expectorate pus.[170] He will cough ceaselessly and he will be struck down by the empyema. Sometimes he will cough up pieces of his lung with the pus.

When a chest wound does not enter the thoracic cavity, treat it as any other wound with plasters, black ointment etc.

CHAPTER 4 B. WOUNDS OF THE HEART

Because it is the primary organ of Man's body, which receives the Vital Spirit at birth and loses it at death, a wounded (ie penetrated) heart cannot be cured. It furnishes vitality to all the other organs through the vessels which belong to it, the veins and the pulsating arteries. The heart loses its blood through the wound, and its vital heat. Like a candle whose wick is deprived of its fuel, its flame is extinguished.

So it is with the heart that loses its blood. The Spirit of the body is extinguished. After it has lost its blood, the heart becomes dark (ie cyanotic) and the extremities—the hands , feet, nose etc. – become cold; the lips become pale and the entire body sweats. A wound on the left side of the chest or from behind or even from the opposite side may reach the heart.

CHAPTER 5 B. OTHER LETHAL WOUNDS

Other parts of the body may suffer fatal wounds. The victim of a wounded brain may suffer epilepsy and die. He is incontinent of urine and is agitated and he convulses. All of that occurs because the brain is the source of all the nerves. The spinal cord has the same two covering membranes as the brain, and a wound through the cord is equally lethal. The same is true for the lung, especially in the upper

---

170 A bronchopleural fistula or a lung abscess (LDR).

lobes. The wounded lower lobe may heal because it is less in motion than the upper. But if a lung is damaged by an effusion (ie an abscess or empyema) such that the medications cannot reach it, the patient will die of a phthisis. A wounded lung spills red blood within the chest. Breathing is rapid and the patient turns blue. If the wound of entry is small, enlarge it to enable you to instill this powder: Take mastic (juice or dry powder), frankincense, gum of tragacanth, gum arabic and fenugreek. Grind them to a fine powder. After applying the powder, provide the patient this potion: Take some water containing a sprinkle of wheat-flour and bring it to a boil. Filter it and add some sugar. Tell the patient to remain silent and to conserve his breath. Keep open the external wound to maintain access to the lung. When necessary you should clean it as I instructed in the chapter on the the thorax.

You cannot cure wounds of the liver unless they are very small. The small ones heal rapidly. On occasion some of the liver may herniate through a wound in the abdominal wall. The Four Salernitan Masters recommended applying this plaster over the extruded liver: Take equal amounts of a decoction of absinthe, sambuco (406), ebulus (165), honey, vinegar and wheat-flour . Boil all until the mixture is as thick as honey. Apply it at room temperature; it will help Nature. The patient's inherent powers will retract the liver. If the wound is too small (ie the extruded liver is trapped) you may enlarge it with a bistoury. The plaster will heal a wound on the surface of the swollen exposed liver.

A wound through the diaphragm also may be lethal when it is at the level of the floating ribs. The patient's breathing is rapid and labored and painful, and the breasts heave.

Galen said that a wound in the fleshy part of the diaphragm (ie not in the membranous parts) can be cured.

Wounds of the thinner bladder wall will not heal, because the tissue is nervous and categorically beyond cure. But wounds in the fleshier bladder-neck are curable, as we observe them heal after lithotomies to remove small stones in younger persons. In children even if there is a small leakage of urine, healing will ensue.

Wounds that enter the stomach may be lethal because ingested food and beverages are spilled. When treating the stomach, you may have to enlarge the abdominal wound for exposure. Sew the gastric wall with a fine waxed thread on a cutting needle. However, in the upper and fleshier part of the stomach, that is, the nervous part, do not suture, because it will be to no avail. After suturing use the red powder as we described it in the chapter on wounds.

Intestinal wounds, especially in the small intestine, are lethal because they spill feces. However, you may be able to save someone with a wounded colon. I will give instructions in the chapter devoted to that problem. For the present, know this: When the signs do not declare an impending death, give thanks to The Lord that all hope is not lost. Even so, you will have to attend during a long critical course before your cure succeeds.

Galen said that an abdominal wound that emits gas indicates a fatal outcome. The same holds for a wounded chest that blows air; the heart rate is rapid and the patient gasps for air.

Transverse wounds across the thigh within three inches of the knee, or a wound that divides the attachments of the leg muscles (ie below the knee), or a wound just above the wrist or across the middle of the arm, all of them must be judged to be lethal.[171] So said Galen and Almansor.[172] Muscles are only partly fleshy; the rest consists of nerves, tendons and ligaments; all together they are the contractile structures. Because they move, treating their wounds is difficult, and the healing process is defeated. Ligaments and nerves derive both from the brain and the heart. Wounds, such as those named above, transect muscles and do not lend themselves to treatment. In such cases (ie wounds in nerves and tendons) Avicenna recommend complete division of the partly divided structures, stating that it is better to save a life than to prevent paralysis.

Both Avicenna and Galen agreed that wounds which cut into richly nerve-bearing regions are to be dreaded. Often they are complicated by spasms, and disturbed speech (ie mania). We will discuss the particulars in the chapters devoted to the various wounds.[173]

---

171 The prognosis to be given before undertaking any treatments (LDR).

172 Almansor was not a person! It is the title of one of Rhazes' treatises (LDR).

173 Yperman's presentation in this confused and mish-mash of statement suffers when compared with the more elegant and better organized material that we read in the treatises by William of Saliceto, Lanfranchi, and, especially, Henri de Mondeville, all of whom preceded The Fleming (LDR).

Chapter 6 B. Wounds Of The Kidneys

Renal wounds usually are incurable and are lethal, because the tissues are soft and moist.[174] They digest blood from the liver after it arrives via veins called 'ilis' which lie against the vertebrae and connect the kidneys with the liver. The kidneys by Nature extract the watery part from the blood and send it as urine to the bladder. For that reason, a surgeon who treats renal wounds should insert fibrous drains wet with egg-white and prescribe this potion which is said to eliminate pus (ie infected urine): Take decoctions of polygonum (361), convolvulus (416), bryony (67), prunella (355) and caryophylla. The victim should drink as much of it as possible. Also give this potion made from the pharmacist's cold seeds (123a): Take equal amounts of melons (144a), cucumbers (144), bol d'armenie and white tragacanth. Boil the seeds in water until it is syrupy. The patient should drink it, hoping it will assist Nature where there is little to hope for and little else to do.

Chapter 7 B. Wounds Of Muscles And Nerves In The Upper Arm

When wounds at mid-arm or elsewhere cut across muscles, the prognosis is worse than if it completely amputated the arm. That is so because the retracted nerve is the source of the pain and of the spasm which forebode death. You know that a muscle is composed of nerve fibers, tendon and ligaments as well as of arteries and veins which come from the brain and the heart, as we have described them in our chapter on mortal wounds.

The Four Salernitan Masters said that you should apply a hot cautery to the ends of the cut nerve and avoid touching adjacent tissues. The cauterization will prevent the nerves from attracting more humors to the wound, an attraction mediated by the nerves for sensation. Galen wrote that humors always flow to painful places and that you should apply this paste to prevent it. Take decapitated and cleaned earthworms (499). Mash them with egg-white and apply it in the

---

174 As above, this is the prognosis rather than a declaration to do nothng (LDR).

wound. It will reach the hidden nerve-ends better than any other paste.[175] All the above is relevant for partly or completely transected nerves. However, when the nerves are incised in their long axes, cauterization is not indicated.

Avoid hot applications on nerves. That will provoke putrefaction (ie necrosis). Nerves are made from humors that are condensed by cold, everywhere in the body.

Now attend to an example given by Galen. A man pricked his finger with a needle. His tough skin closed over the tiny wound and it soon became inflamed, painful beyond the patient's tolerance. The surgeon used a heat-melted greasy paste (ie to relieve pain) and the finger became gangrenous. The patient then suffered convulsions and he died after seven days.[176] If instead the surgeon had used a corrosive paste to drain the pus, the patient would have survived. That is why the Masters have advised against hot or cold water [177] in wounds in regions that are rich in nerves, and so, too, for oil of roses that has been made with oil of green olives as its base in instead of oil made from ripe olives or with oil of nuts of Grenoble.[178] So when you encounter anyone with a needle-puncture in a nerve-bearing region, apply a cloth soaked in warm terebinth. It will relieve the pain. Then apply a paste of euphorbia and wax or the like.

Another for puncture wounds: Take armenian galbanum, serapinum (429) and opoponax (321). Mix and insert it in the wound with a needle or a nail or similar.

Those who are followers of Lanfranchi do this for trnasversewounds in the arm: When the muscle is cut or if nerves are divided, he sutured the cut ends of the nerves with a cutting needle.[179] Then he applied powdered quick-lime mixed with frankincense and sangdragan on the sutures, as I described in the chapter on sutures.

---

175 The burrowing propensiity of the earthworms is implied (LDR).

176 Tetanus (LDR).

177 The terms refer to more than the temperatures. Hot, cold, wet and dry also describe the character (ie the complexion) of substances and humors. Blood is warm and dry, phlegm is cool and moist, etc.see fn.181(LDR).

178 I cannot identify them. Perhaps it is a misreading of Granata, ie, pomegranates (LDR).

179 He did not suture the nerves themselves. Rather he roughly approximated the cut ends with mass sutures that closed the full depth of the wound (LDR).

When a coagulum[180] forms in the wound, he advised cutting the sutures and filling the wound with warm oil of roses mixed with egg-white. When fresh bleeding occurs, not an infrequent complication in a wound that has many nerves and blood vessels, one must exercise his best judgment. The bleeding may not be controllable except with the use of the cautery, and it may be difficult to cauterize the bleeding flesh without injuring the nerves and vessels, and you do not want to induce spasm, which is a threat whenever nerves are wounded. So you must anoint every part of the wound with an ointment that repels humors which could collect there, or at least to suppress them to a lesser degree. Use this: Take one-half oz. of bol d'armenia and two oz. each of oil of roses and vinegar and make an ointment as we did for the white ointment. We grind the clay finely in a metal mortar and add the oil and mix well before adding the vinegar. Make the paste very smooth (ie no lumps).

The foregoing applies to wounds of the mid-arm, the elbow, the hips, and the thighs, the lower legs and to all muscular regions where there are nerves and ligaments and blood vessels that supply them. Those are the motor nerves and do not transmit sensation. And the ligamentous tissues are not very sensitive.

When an open wound contains a broken bone, first set the fracture and lay the limb on a flat surface to maintain the reduction while you treat the wound. If you do not do so, the bones will not knit properly. Then carefully place the patient supine so that both he and his wound are comfortably at rest. Use warm wine as a dressing, first irrigate the wound with it, then dry it with lint or a linen cloth.

Chapter 8 B. Wounds At The Elbow And Other Joints

Wounds in the region of the elbow or near the wrist, especially the former, are very dangerous, because the vital synovial fluid is lost. Suture the wound as soon as you can and apply the red powder. Then dress the wound with a pad of lint moistened with egg-white in the summer and egg-yolk in the winter, and with both during the other seasons. The yolk is warm, more-so when alone than when it is mixed

---

180 A late hematoma (LDR).

with the white.[181] The proper combination, according to the season, will repel potentially harmful humors and blood from the wound.

CHAPTER 9 B. WOUNDS OF THE INTESTINES

When the abdomen is cut open by a knife or sword, the intestine may eviscerate. If they have not been sliced into or perforated, cover them with a sponge or a cloth wet with warm, milk, continued without interruption until the intestines can be replaced within the belly. If the wound is too small for an easy restoration, or if the extruded loop is inflated after its exposure to the outer air, or if they are filled with nutriments eaten before the wounding, you must enlarge the opening with a bistoury , exercising great care to avoid injury to the organs. If a strip of fat (ie omentum) has been extruded, cut it away

After a successful replacement, close the abdominal wound with two or three sutures to prevent a recurrence and apply a moist (ie egg-white) pad over which you place one or two dry pads bandaged in place for three days. Dress the wound on the third day and remove all the pads, but do not remove the sutures. Wash the area with warm water at each dressing, and blot it dry before applying the populeum ointment (365). Apply the black ointment (30) between the edges of the wound. Then lay some cabbage leaves on top (71). Drains are not necessary if you use the ointments and leaves and wound potions. [182] [183]

---

181 Yperman did not explain his use of the terms that describe his medications, as did his great predecessors. Warmth or coldness did not refer to the temperature, any more than did moist or dry refer to the actual wetness. All medicines and herbs as well as all humors and all parts of the body had natural qualities measured by degrees, usually on a scale from one to three. Phlegm was a cool moist humor. If the humor was unhealthy, one sought a cool medicine to ward it off with one of the same or nearly the same degree. The same held for melancholy, whereas blood was warm and dry, etc. (LDR).

182 Prof. Tabanelli reminds us that the substance of this and other chapters is an abbreviated version of what Lanfranchi had written in his *Chirurgia* Bk.II, Ch 7. et al.(T).

183 Whereas most Master Surgeons inserted a drain through a gap left at on end of the wound, Yperman said no. His use of greasy ointments and widely spaced sutures probably prevented the wounds from sealing before most of the bloody and serous ooze had escaped, thus avoiding suppuration (LDR).

CHAPTER 10 B. SUTURING THE INTESTINE

There are six parts to the intestine: jejunum, peritoneum, rectum, omentum, duodenum and ileum.[184] Three of them are not much at risks for wounds, while wounds in the other three can be treated by a surgeon.

An abdominal wound through which intestine has eviscerated is treated so. First examine it to determine if it has been damaged (entered). When the jejunum, the mirach (peritoneum) and especially the rectum have been incised or penetrated, the patient will suffer from hiccups and nausea and the wound may be fatal. Wounds of the omentum, duodenum and ileum may be treatable by a capable surgeon, even when they are completely divided.

First examine all of the extruded loop; often there is more than one wound, as many as three or four.[185] First cut away any damaged tissue or perforated intestine (ie including both ends of a transected loop), and prepare to suture a divided loop end-to-end. Have ready a tube of smooth elder-tree bark about the length of one finger. Insert it into the lumen and then suture the ends with sutures placed about a finger-breadth apart. Manipulate the tube within the intestine so it passes under the suture line and extends on both sides of it.

Apply an ointment over the sutures and replace the intestine through the open abdominal wound. You may have to enlarge it to reduce the evisceration without further damage. The abdominal wound must be kept open until you are certain that the intestinal wound has sealed. Dress it daily and medicate both the intestinal and the abdominal wounds. If the abdominal wound closes before the other, and the intestinal wound suppurates, the suture line will come apart and both the intestines and the abdomen will distend with toxic matter and gas.

That is a treacherous situation and you must recognize it at once and reopen it or the patient will die. It is said that the intestine will

---

184 It is difficult to explain the errors of Yperman's anatomy, especially since he had,Lanfranchi's more accurate descriptions. Here, too, as in so many places in Book VII, I must blame copyists and Van Leersum (LDR).

185 Here we observe an experienced 'trauma-surgeon' at work. However, Yperman did not explore the entire intestine; he limited his exploration to what had been exposed in the wound (LDR).

heal after about thirty days. Then you may remove whatever you had put in it. The sutures will come out by themselves and the abdominal wound will close. The bark tube will be passed per rectum.

CHAPTER 11B. HERNIAS WITH OR WITHOUT BLADDER STONES

The treatments differ even when the two ailments occur together.

When hernias appear suddenly in the lower abdomen, caused by shouting or climbing hills or by crying (in children), use a truss over the opening in the abdominal wall and push back the extruded viscera. If the patient is a baby with a recent hernia use a pad, with or without this medication: Take a fistful each of royal fern (181a), sedum (422a), comfrey (128), fennel and prunella. Soak the pile in wine. The dose of the winy decoction is one spoonful twice a day. With this potion and the truss the hernia will heal. Keep the truss snuggly in place until the herniated viscera remain within the belly. The opening will close, thanks to the treatments. It will take eight weeks.

When the treatment fails, you will have to operate. Follow the methods described in Roger's *Chirurgia,* a valuable source.

CHAPTER 12 B. OMENTOCOELE RESEMBLING HERNIA[186]

We encounter patients who are thought to have hernias but instead have a water-filled collection coming down from the flanks (ie into the scrotum). We evacuate the sac by a puncturing it with a needle or the point of a knife. Insert a wool thread to be left in place. Pull it back and forth daily to allow you to express all the water.[187] Then treat the small wounds.

---

186 Another confusion of terms. The chapter deals with hydrocoele, not omentocoele (LDR).

187 My interpretation of the text: The needle is armed with the wool thread and it penetrates the hydrocoele through-and-through. The thread is used as a seton. When a bistoury made the initial puncture, the threaded needle followed its lead! (LDR).

CHAPTER 13 B. BLADDER STONE THAT MOVES

Actor [188] said that bladder stones always are hardened humors, formed in the kidneys and concentrated in the bladder. They begin as gravel (sand) and can be treated at that stage with simple absorbents, or by using medicines that have the same degrees [189] of coldness as the gravel.

Take handfuls of the seeds of bugloss, (lithospermum, 69), parsley, fennel, apium (29), water cress (490b), cherry (104), peach and athamanta macedonia (? 29). Add two grains of geranium seeds (209) and one-twelfth the weight of the above of dried goat's blood or sangdragon. Grind all the dry substances. Then mix in the goat's blood (resin) until all of it is powdered. Then add sugar to sweeten it to taste. Moisten the powder with wine and take it daily, either as a powder or as a potion.

If that treatment fails, you will know that the gravel has already agglutinated and has formed a stone. More information on this subject can be found in Galen's *Universis Passionibus*, Book III. He tells us how the stone increases in size, how it arrived where it is and whatever more you wish to know. He gives more advice in his book *Liber Aureus*. He tells how to eliminate the sand with medications which rid the patient of the humors that are the cause of the malady. His advice was to do nothing more if the medications fail. The patient will have to live with his stone.

Roger's *Chirurgia* recommends cutting for stone, and he describes the operation.

CHAPTER 14 B. HEMORRHOIDS

Some hemorrhoids bleed excessively. But if you arrest that bleeding you may kill the victim. This is what happens. The contaminated blood from everywhere in the body tends to settle in the lower parts and it flows through the hemorrhoids freeing the vital organs of their

188 Tabanelli suggests that Actor may have been Atto or Acon, a physician for Empress Agnes, cited by Mesûe or Constantine Africanus. see fn 194 (LDR).
189 See fn. 181, Bk. VII, Part I, Ch. 8 (LDR).

bad matter.[190] When the blood in hemorrhoids coagulates, the bad blood now backs up and overcomes the internal organs, and may destroy the patient.[191]

Chapter 15 B. The Treatment Of Hemorrhoids

Before treating a patient you should determine what has caused them, their appearance and their size. After you examine him and his urine, feel his abdomen; is it hard and distended by the residues of digested foods which could not normally be evacuated, and serve to rid the organs of bad humors?[192] The patient's natural forces displace his contaminated blood to his lower belly whenever he feels he has to urinate. That (ie intra-abdominal) pressure (constipation and dysuria) impedes the flow through the five hemorrhoidal veins which are distended and appear large. Those five veins are called hemorrhoids.[193] They often seep blood and are painful.

To treat the suffering patient have him drink some of the previously described syrup of cassia. It will rid his body of the bad humors by defecating profusely. As a result, the contaminated organs will be clean and dry, and can attract the blood that had been misdirected toward the hemorrhoids. The latter may shrink and vanish, and the patient may be cured.

Then you may prescribe the three medicines described below to further dry the internal organs (ie and the internal hemorrhoids) and improve the patient's well-being.

Chapter 16 B. How To Use The Medicines For Internal Hemorrhoids

Three days after dosing the laxative syrup, give the patient a second medicine consisting of aloes, rhubarb, and scammony, or a mix-

---

190 Blood on its way to the colon for its final 'digestion' and elimination in feces. Some of the bad matter will be 'evacuated' in the blood that seeps from the hemorrhoids (LDR).

191 In other words, do not abruptly interrupt hemorrhoidal bleeding! (LDR).

192 Is he constipated? Does he strain at stool? (LDR).

193 Yperman emphasizes the etymology: 'hemo'=blood and 'rrhoid'= flow (LDR).

ture of equal amounts of all three, either as pills or as a powder to be drunk with water or warm beer.

The second medicine is given on the day it is made. Further dosage is given on the eighth day. However, if the patient shows signs of recovered vigor (ie after the strenuous laxation), you may give the added dose on the seventh day.

A third medicine, the esula cataputia (171), contains three parts of the milk of euphorbia and one part of esula. Another was described by Actor,[194] but it is difficult to obtain.

Whenever you can do so, treat without using the following medicines. But when you need them, use your common sense (ie about doses, etc.). For all patients with white urine (concentrated, milky or chalky), use this remedy: Pulverize one-half lb. of euphorbia and pass it through a fine sieve to make a powder as fine as wheat-flour. Grinding the seeds of cataputia esula in a mortar is not an easy task; the dose is twenty gr. Added to the milk.

Then take as much of the euphorbia mixture as fills the hollow of the palm of the hand as far as the base of the fifth finger. Add as much sugar as needed to make it palatable. Drink it down with warm wine or beer, or eat it as a paste wrapped in a crepe of dough. Do not dose it when the weather is too hot or too cold.

Chapter 17 B. When To Dose The Patient

Give the medicines at dawn after wrapping the patient's neck with a cold wet scarf that holds a pledget of linen wet with vinegar over his Adam's Apple. The patient keeps in hand an unripe (ie sour) apple to bite if he is nauseated.

Spray his face with cold water or slap it on by hand. Then return him to a warm place where he abstains from food and drink until evening. The room should be in the shade and protected from wind. He will have seven to ten evacuations during that day.

After the restoratives, let him eat hen's meat boiled in water with parsley and salvia, or fresh pork. He may drink a broth of wine and beer when the weather is very warm, and his urine feels equally warm.

194 I believe the name was Actuarius (d. 1283), a physician in the court of the Paleologi (probably John III or Michael. He wrote a well-accepted *Therapeutics*. see Baas p. 211(LDR).

He may eat bread and butter and all fresh foods, always in moderation. He should abstain from drinking liquids in excess of need and avoid stressing his internal organs.

CHAPTER 18 B. HEMORRHOIDS CAUSED BY DYSENTERY (BLOODY DIARRHEA)

Dysentery may cause hemorrhoids when the liquid discharge comes from an inflamed belly, giving rise to what is called 'morsicatura' (erosions). They attract the blood to the lower belly and congest the veins; they cannot resist distension and they dilate enormously and cause much distress.

You should prescribe medicines that eliminate the poisons in those veins. When that is accomplished, the dysentery will cease and the affected organs will return to normal.

The patient should eat foods that favor the growth of tissues (ie to fill the eroisions), such as roasted mutton and sour pears with waxy skins. They should drink only gascon wines until they are entirely well. After the body has been purged, apply constrictives (ie astringents) on the hemorrhoids, such as the populeum ointment (365) with equal amounts of zinc sulfate and sugar. Spread the ointment on a pad of oakum moistened with water. That will shrink them.

Another: Grind equal amounts of frankincense and alum in a mortar and add an equal amount by weight of salt and oakum. Add vinegar and egg-white while grinding until you have an ointment. Spread it on a pad of oakum.

Another: Incinerate equal amounts (ie by weight) of salt and oakum. Pulverize the residue, add honey and achieve a smooth paste to be spread on a thin cloth for application.

Another: Take equal amounts of celery, pastel (497), old rancid honey, mutton-fat and onions. Mix and grind them in a mortar to make a plaster to be applied as hot as is tolerable. While that is active, bleed the supine patient from a vein on his head. The hemorrhoids will disappear. Six days later you will need to decompress the feeder veins, using vesicants.[195]

---

195 This is unclear. Where does he apply cantharides or does he use cups? (LDR).

CHAPTER 19 B. THE THREE KINDS OF HEMORRHOIDS

The three kinds of hemorrhoids are: 1. The Internal, within the rectum, which impede defecation but do not cause much pain. 2. Those associated with fistulas that appear on one side of the anus.[196] 3. The external piles which are dilated masses which block the flow of blood. They cause much suffering.

If you attempt to treat with ointments, plaster etc. before purging the patient with laxative syrups et al. the patient may die.

CHAPTER 20 B. THE FIVE HEMORRHOIDAL VEINS

When the patient is constipated or has dysentery, his blood is carried below by the five veins that descend from the back. In degree determined by his innate vitality, the patient's blood accumulates painfully, causing the veins to enlarge suddenly and become hemorrhoids. Two are on the right side, two on the left and a fifth lies against the coccyx. That one may give rise to the most important (ie the commonest) fistula; it is the most difficult (ie of the three kinds of hemorrhoids) to treat. Often you treat it only with plasters, such as artemisia, absinthe and linseed oil, as the paste. Apply it as hot as can be tolerated.

CHAPTER 21 B. THE TREATMENT OF SWOLLEN HEMORRHOIDS [197]

Often the hemorrhoids are too swollen and bulky to lend themselves to treatment with medicines alone. Then you must incise them to make them bleed and obtain a rapid cure. Actor wrote that he knew many patients who were cured with incision alone.

Other surgeons advise ligating hemorrhoids with waxed threads. For those who first have been properly purged as described above, the treatment will be effective. However, if the ligation was not preceded by purgation the patient's life is put at risk. Indeed, the ligature causes suppuration and the hemorrhoid falls off. Then the blood

---

196 The Text says 'abdomen'. A scribe's error (LDR)
197 Type 3, the external piles (LDR).

which usually passes to the region has no means to escape and a fistula develops.[198]

In the absence of the escape route the bad blood backs up into them and does such harm to his organs that the patient may die. That is why I tell you to see the whole picture before you act.[199] Nature tells us that some bad matter may be lodged in some organ, no matter which, somewhere in the body and cause the faulty humors to emerge anywhere, from head to feet. Nature tells us to purge the body in order to restore health.

Some surgeons take a slim hot iron cautery, covered except for the tip (ie in a tube) and they burn a white spot on each hemorrhoid. That works well if it follows a purgation. But if there was no preliminary purge, the hot cautery touches a hemorrhoid already hot and distended with blood and lacerates it. The sudden hemorrhage may kill the patient.

I prescribe a refreshing syrup which will thin the blood and promote its evacuation. It dries the groins and cools the blood and makes the patient feel better as he recovers.

You may need to use emollients on the hemorrhoids, such as a plaster of linseed oil, fresh lard and white nettles, which you have ground until the leaves are saturated with the greases. That will soften and relieve the local discomforts, and help in the cure.

---

198 The Concept: The bad humors which cause the hemorrhoids come from the internal organs. The hemorrhoids then become the receptacles and the vents (ie by bleeding) that serve the organs, Therefore, unless you first purge the organs with laxatives, the preemptive removal of the hemorrhoids eliminates a necessary means for ridding the organs of their bad humors, which accumulate and threaten the patient's life (LDR).

199 The misconceptions in that era, carried over from earlier times and transmitted even until this century, included hygienic bleeds that were thought to cleanse the body's blood that had been tainted by bad humors, such that the kidneys and the intestines could not deal with all of it. After a bleed, the liver makes fresh blood to replenish the losses. Many Authorities believed that hemorrhoids in robust individuals that bled moderately were substitutes for phlebotomies and should not be treated except to relieve local discomforts (LDR).

Chapter 22 B. Knowing How To Treat Illnesses

Galen said that one should treat everything with great gentleness. No matter how minor the ailment may seem to you, it is painful enough for the sufferer. When you understand Man's innate Natural Force, there is nothing wrong in uttering wise saws, as are the following. 'Although you may have done wrong, you can make things right.' 'Often it is said that some persons do not end up well because they have been treated too long with gentle measures, up to the point where they were lost.' 'On the other hand, some persons are lost and die at the very beginning of a course of painful and difficult treatments.' 'So I advise those who are about to practice medicine that they do nothing to make an illness worse.'[200]

Chapter 23 B. Unnatural Treatments

The use of measures contrary to Nature for as long as two days may be enough to destroy your patient by bringing on a bad fever. Use your common sense and no one will die. Some persons have such noble natural qualities that we often can depend on their own powers for cures: those few who follow the rule of the four elements, the few who combat heat with cold, cold with heat, wet with dry and dry with wet.

When you apply hot remedies on an already hot body, you will oppress the patient; his own Nature already has heated him, and now you overheat him to a fever, and he may die of it. And if you add moisture to his own humidity, his natural force will be overcome by the 'flood'. Similarly, if you put a dry topical on a woman's breast [201] her forces will be depleted and she may perish.

When you try to relieve a patients suffering, always treat with contraries: hot combats cold, etc. That is how to obtain cures.

---

200 You may lose a patient after a long extended treatment, perhaps not intensive enough, but you have not made him suffer during the course. That is more acceptable than killing a patient with intensive and painful measures that he could not withstand. Yperman leans on Galen who quoted Hippocrates "First do no harm' (LDR).

201 I think that Yperman here refers to a woman's 'caked' lactating breast (LDR).

Chapter 24 B. Dislocation Of The Femur

A fall or a leap may cause the femur to luxate. If you fail to reduce the dislocation before the third day, the patient may be crippled for life.

One assistant holds the patient suspended over a padded beam set between his thighs. Another assistant lies beneath the patient and pulls on his leg as to straighten it while you are at his side and push your fist against the head of the femur and direct it into the joint. Then flex and extend the thigh to test the success of the reduction.

Have ready several bandages moistened with egg-white or the like, selected according to the season of the year, as we have taught. The bandages must be long enough to wrap around the body and bind the thighs together to prevent a re-luxation. The patient will lie supine for three days. Test the reduction again by flexing and extending the thigh.

Bathe and anoint the patient and replace the bandages for an additional fourteen days, changing the bandages every third day until he is cured. If he continues to have pain, prescribe baths and inunctions.

Chapter 25 B. The Head Of The Femur

The head of the bone that enters the hip joint is a round ball which narrows at its base. At its end there is a short ligament that fastens the ball to the hip-bone inside a cup-like concavity that accepts it. The ligament is stretched when the head of the femur is displaced. If the femur is not replaced within three days, blood (ie sanguinous humors) is attracted to the site.

That leads to further rotting of the nerves [202] and the patient may be left with a fistula, or else the accumulated blood may sprout proud flesh that can fill the joint so the head of the femur cannot go to full depth. Even when you empty the matter from the joint, the thigh—bone cannot be replaced; its natural site has been preempted by the

---

202 Another reminder: 'nerve' may mean tendon or ligament as well as nerve (LDR).

new tissue. Therefore, unless the dislocation is promptly reduced, the patient will always be lame and unable to continue at his former occupations.

Some surgeons recommend baths, inunctions and the application of a cireone.[203] However, those surgeons harm their patients. The nerves are naturally cool, and the baths and oils cause them to stretch. The same holds for the ligaments that bind the joints, and, as a result, the crippled patient's joint is looser than before.

CHAPTER 26 B. FRACTURE OF THE FEMUR

You will need two assistants to help you set a fractured femur. One of them grasps the thigh near the body and the other takes it above the knee. The surgeon stands alongside the thigh and instructs the assistants how and when to apply traction, and not to overdo it. He feels the femoral head [204] and can tell when the two fragments meet. He gently molds them together. He compares the two legs to see that they are alike in length. Then he applies the populeum ointment. The he wraps the thigh with ten long bandages, each half a hand-span wide and moistened with egg-white. Atop the bandages he surrounds the limb with a fluffy mat over which he lays seven splints. He holds them in place with three loosely tied cords, one at each end of the splints and one in the middle. Then he slips a tube of elder-tree bark under each cord and twists it (a tourniquet) until the binding is tight enough to secure the splints. The upper and the lower tubes are twisted counter-clockwise (ie to the west) and the middle one is twisted clockwise (ie to the east). Then he slips a wood or metal rod into each tube to fasten them in place. The whole apparatus must remain undisturbed with the patient supine in bed for nine to twelve days, longer if there are several fragments). Then remove everything, including the egg-white, and bathe the thigh with warm water. After

---

203 A waxy paste on a thin cloth. Tabanelli cites Paré who described the paste as thicker than an ointment and softer than a plaster. It adheres to the skin and acts as a very weak 'cast' to restrain motion (LDR).

204 I agree with Tabanelli that this chapter deals with fractures of the shaft of the femur, despite the statement about feeling the femoral head. Yperman meant the upper fragment of a two piece fracture, and Tabanelli is correct in stating that one cannot feel the ends of a fractured femoral neck (LDR).

the splints have been removed, the thigh is unrestrained and you must handle it very carefully lest you bend it or displace the fragments and have a life-long lame patient.

Wash the leg with a soft cloth and warm water and reapply the populeum ointment and repeat the entire application – bandages, pad, splints etc. Do it again after another seven days, and again at five.[205] After that he should be able to raise his leg from the supine, and to flex the thigh when arising from the bed.

He must resume activity with restraint. I recommend him to use crutches and not to bear full weight on the fractured leg, as he returns to his normal gait.

I advise baths, oils and cereoenos until the cure is complete, as The Lord may wish.

CHAPTER 27 B. DETAILS OF TREATING FRACTURES AT THE HEAD OF THE FEMUR

The femur is slightly bowed and is about the length of two hand-spans. One end is rounded based on narrow neck. That is where usually it is fractured, and that is where there are more muscles. Therefore, the repair involves the entire mass as well as just setting the bones in place, if you wish the patient to walk normally. The bandages must support the bone until the union is solid. However, the bandages should not exceed the length of two and one-half hand-spans, because the patient cannot tolerate multiple turns. When you go to place it, start above and crisscross as you proceed downwards, to hold the bones as healing is helped along by your topicals.[206] Avoid long bandages that have to be unwrapped every time you apply your medications, and risk displacing the bones, and end up with a permanently lame patient.

Actor was right when he recommended the use of short bandages.

On the twelfth day check to see if the fractured leg is straight and is equal in length to the other, and if the hip is tilted (ie the trochanter) or is higher or lower. Apply linen pads in an effort to restore

205 That is a total of 33 days: 12+9+7+5 (LDR.

206 The bandage does not encircle the patient's torso. It criss-crosses the fractured femoral neck obliquely, from side to side (LDR).

a normal status. Use the wax applications (ciroeni) and lay the pads over them. The bandages that are moistened with egg-white are removed after twelve days. Then use warm damp bandages.

Cover the ciroeno with a felt sheet and place splints, spaced a 'splint-width' apart to allow the thigh to be aerated. [207] If you do not leave spaces, and the felt completely covers the fracture, the thigh is at risk for inflammation. If that is not recognized when it first occurs, it can destroy the patient, or he can lose his leg.[208]

Do not move the patient during the (ie ? second) twelve-day period and cause him much pain, and interfere with a solid union at the fracture. When the patient thinks he is well enough to walk, test the union. The leg should hang free, allowing it to swing from side to side like a reaper's scythe.

CHAPTER 28 B. ON SPLINTING AND IMMOBILIZATION [209]

Whenever a bone is broken, you should use splints after verifying the fact, as we have instructed. After a positive diagnosis, reduce the fracture and apply a waxed film (ie ciroeno) and ointments until the cure is established. Some persons who are cured of fractures had good reductions and were restored to normal. Others (ie also with good reductions) believed they were cured but are lame because the limb had not been properly immobilized.

CHAPTER 29 B. DISLOCATIONS AT THE KNEE

A knee can be dislocated by a fall or a twist. The initial maneuver by the surgeon is to place his arm behind the knee while his assistant places his under the thigh. When they pull, the dislocation is reduced. A successful reduction allows the knee to flex and extend.

The kneecap also is easily dislocated. That makes normal movements difficult. In such a case, push back the kneecap into its normal

---

207 Yperman's timing is unclear. I assume that the splints, etc.came after the initial twelve days (LDR).

208 Yperman blames the ischemic gangrene of the leg on faulty aeration rather than on too tightly bound splints and dressings (LDR).

209 This is an epilogue for Chapters 26-28 (LDR).

place with your hand. Then set pads on both sides and wrap them with a bandage moistened with egg-white. Remove them after five days. Then apply the wax film, bathe the leg and use unguents until the repair is solid.

Chapter 30 B. Wounds At The Knee

When caused by contusions and or by lacerations, the knee cannot withstand some wounds at all and others may cause great damage. Hemorrhage may threaten survival if not treated at once, and a badly treated wound may become a fistula (ie osteomyelitis).

Arrest the hemorrhage with wet (ie egg-white) packs, bound as tightly as needed. Remove them after three days by wetting them with warm water. Replace them with tampons of linen cloth, or lint, or clumps of virgin wool, all saturated with olive oil, or a plaster made from cabbage leaves. Cover the surface around the wound, but not in it, with the populeum ointment. Then cover all with cabbage leaves. Dose the patient with a wound potion, and change the dressings at suitable intervals.

Chapter 31 B. Broken Legs

When you treat a patient with a broken leg, first palpate and locate the site of the fracture. While two seated or kneeling assistants apply counter-traction – one alongside the patient grasps the thigh, the other holds the foot, you, the kneeling surgeon, mold the fragments and set them, taking great care that a sharply pointed loose fragment does not perforate the overlying tissues; you push it back into place if you can. Then take a long (ie two arm-spans) bandage of medium width (one-half hand-span)[210], wet with egg-white, or mother's milk, or warm wine, or warm water, or black ointment or populeum ointment and apply about seven to ten turns. Then lay a felt sheet about eight inches long over the fracture site. Over that lay seven splints, each about one inch wide (ie one finger-breadth) and about

---

210 These measurements are approximately seven feet in length and four inches in width (LDR).

eight inches long. Bind them in –place with three cords, one of which is centered over the fracture and slip tubes of elder-tree bark under the cords and twist them to adjust the tension of the cords. Into each tube slip a rod to act as a stent.

Then compare the lengths of the legs to assure that they are equal.

Then place the legs in a trench made of three planks covered with soft cloth, to hold the leg flat and outstretched.

A good surgeon pays a daily visit to check on the splints and the tension of the cords. He applies the populeum ointment at the knee and the foot to reduce swelling. He wraps the knee and foot with cloths wet with vinegar to comfort the patient.

After twelve days undo the bindings and change the dressings. Wet the wrappings with warm water to make the removal easier, After washing and drying the leg, apply a ciroeno, a plaster of linen covered with equal amounts of wax, lard, white resin and soot, all melted together in flat pan. Dip the cloth in the pan, remove it and let it cool. When it is tepid, wrap it around the leg. Then roll on eight to ten layers of bandage and reapply the felt, the splints etc. That treatment is repeated during eight to ten weeks, until the leg regains its strength, a process abetted by good food. The patient must use crutches and not bear his full weight on the bad leg until the bony union is secure. I have seen a leg break again when these strictures were not observed. A misstep too soon after the fracture can lead to a lifetime of limping with a short leg.

Chapter 32 B. On Fractures Compounded From Within

When a pointed fragment of fractured bone thrusts its way through the soft tissues and produces an open wound, treat the leg as we did in the preceding chapter. If you cannot push back the exposed fragment, remove it with a forceps. You may have to enlarge the wound to permit you to gently lift it out. Then complete the treatment.

Chapter 33 B. The Methods of Other Surgeons

Here I shall describe different uses of the splints.

Some surgeons first lay on a cloth moistened with egg-white to cover the region and they wet the bandages with water. The first layer (ie by adhering to the skin) tends to hold the fragments as they were set, while the wet bandages temper the tightness of the inner layer. That is a good idea. When all the layers are moistened with egg-white, an unbearable tightness may follow as the egg-white dries. The discomfort will disturb the patient at night as well as during the day. The leg may be inflamed as the blood is forced into the foot, causing it to swell. The ensuing distress will last until the edema subsides. And that is not a good idea.

Chapter 34 B. Another Method

Some surgeons beat egg-white with water and use the foam to moisten their bandages before unrolling them on the leg. That is a harmful practice. If any at all, wet only the second layer (ie the first turn of the bandage atop the linen cloth) and use dry bandages for the other turns. That will prevent the bandages from shrinking and becoming too tight.

Chapter 35 B. Dislocations Of The Foot (ie Ankle)

To reduce a dislocated foot, you must stretch and pull as you set it right. Compare the result of the reduction with the normal foot. Apply one layer of egg-white-wet bandage and the others damp with warm water. Leave the dressings in place for five days. Remove them, oil the foot, apply a ciroeno and reapply a barely damp bandage. Repeat the treatment daily for an additional five days until the patient can bear his weight without pain. That will be the sign of a cure.

Chapter 36 B. A Sprained Ankle

A bad twist can injure the ankle and yet not cause a complete dislocation.

The condition may be neglected because the (ie untreated) patient can still hobble about.

Sometimes the blood that is attracted to the part is consumed (ie digested) locally and becomes pus.[211]

A fistula my evolve.[212] The poison lodged in the joint destroys the bone, nerves, vessels and the other tissues. Many draining openings appear near the malleoli and bits of bone are extruded—some tiny, some large.

Some surgeons think this is St. Louis' Disease.[213] Actor refutes that claim, saying that a patient who seeks good advice and treatment at the time of his injury he will not suffer this painful result of his own negligence.

Enlarge one of the openings with your knife, large enough to admit a finger to feel the diseased bone. Thread a cloth seton (ie using two opening) to keep it open for daily irrigations of vinegar and strong lye. After the drainage ceases, apply cabbage-leaves over the openings and use wound medications as you see fit. From time to time give the patient a spoonful of a wound-potion. Change the dressings daily. The setons should remain at least fourteen days before changing. All of the pus must be eliminated before you treat the external wound.

Chapter 37 B. Fractured Feet

Fractures occur in two places: at the middle (ie the metatarsals) and at the neck (ie below the malleoli). Set the fractures by traction and anoint them and apply a bandage moistened with egg-white. Cover the region with a sheet of felt and lay on four splints on the dorsum and four others on the sole of the foot. Knot the cords at one side. Tighten them with the tubes and stents, as we described earlier. The patient should avoid spoiled foods which can worsen his pain. He should position himself as is comfortable for sleep. There is no

211 The hematoma is absorbed but the edema persists. The edema-fluid is a kind of 'pus' (LDR).

212 How osteomyelitis occurs here is not explained. Was there an open wound? (LDR).

213 Scrofula, with draining sinuses, as treated by the Royal Touch (LDR).

need to repeat the treatments until the twelfth day. Re-apply them at intervals until a cure is obtained.

Chapter 38 B. Other Methods

Some surgeons use bandages moistened with wine when they treat fractures. That is acceptable because blood that is naturally warm and moist is attracted by the fracture A bandaged limb swells, but thanks to the wine, which is warm but dry, the blood is repelled to where it came from, and the patient is relieved.

Chapter 39 B. Other Surgeons

Some surgeons anoint the fractured leg with the populeum or the brown ointments, whichever they think is better suited. They wet their bandages with warm water or sugar-water, as the local condition indicates. They do well with good reason. Water and milk are naturally cool and the blood which normally is in the region of the fracture is warm and moist. That large amount of warm blood dries the tissues. The dressings (ie as above) moisten them. The snug bandage and splints, etc. repel the excess blood.

Chapter 40 B. (Untitled)
(A Miscelany That Includes Fractures And Head-Wounds)

Some surgeons use a ciroeno made of equal amounts of wax, lard, mutton-fat, resin and tar. They melt it in a flat pan and saturate a piece of linen cloth and wrap it over and around the fracture. It is harmful for the these reasons: The soft tissues have been stripped off the bone by the injury, and the bared bony fragments may over-ride each other, where they remain mal-aligned and cause permanent lameness. If they unite side-to-side, no one in the world can do anything about it, and when such a union occurs, the patient will be lame. Actor recommended the application of egg-white (ie on bandages) directly over the fracture (after a proper end-on-end reduction). The warmer the bones, and the drier the action of the egg-white, the better they will hold the fragments and insure a good recovery.

Although different authors do more or less the same things, they criticize each other about certain details. Yet all do well.

Some use the ciroeno from day one and leave it until the twelfth to eighteenth day. Actor forbade that, but he agreed that all the other things were used correctly.

But when the bone is not broken and only has been bruised, the use of the ciroeno is approved; the healing is internal.[214] But when a fracture exists, the treatment must be external, using a properly applied apparatus, to remain in place for twelve to eighteen days, until the union (ie by callus) is secure. Later on, bathe the part, dry it, anoint it with the populeum. Then use the ciroeno, felt, splints, cords et al. The status of the reduction must be checked from time to time as the healing proceeds.

Master Ancel of Genoa (? Geneva) treated all-head-wounds with an ointment without anise and he received many plaudits in his home city. He insisted that his patients drink only the strongest wine that they could obtain and that they should eat more meat, all of which is contrary to the methods recommended by the medical and surgical authorities, as you find them described in our chapters on diets and beverages. Also, you will find there our lists of forbidden foods and beverages.

Here is Ancel's Ointment; I make no claim for its worth.[215] He took one lb. of white resin, five dr. of oil of roses, three dr. of white wax and he melted them in a lead-lined ceramic pan. When it was sufficiently liquid he poured in some white wine and brought all to a boil. Then he soaked a cloth in which he had poked many holes, and using a forceps, he put it on the head. Over it he placed a lint pad moistened with warm wine and over that a dry lint pad. Then he wrapped the entire head to hold fast the dressings, When the wound

214 With potions, purges and other measures prescribed by the physicians (LDR).
215 Tabanelli notes that some (Van Leersum and Haeser) claim that Yperman disdained Ancel as an ignorant lay practitioner who prescribed unorthodox diets and medications. Despite that, Yperman cited him. Ancel of Genoa, also was called Ancel de Genes. In the more complete citation found in the London Ms, he was named as one of the lay practitioners that had the support of the ignorant populace despite his failures and limitations (T).

was large, he closed it with sutures. In that way he avoided anise! And those who died were buried; there were more who died than those who survived. Nevertheless, he received more praises for his work than did the surgeons who followed the more accepted practices. He was not among the surgeons who try to act rationally and who value a good reputation above the acquisition of a profitable trade, as do the ignorant lay practitioners.

We have another here, a native of Flanders, William of Zieriksee in Zeeland. He prepares his ciroeni as follows: He melts ram's and hog's fats and mixes them with wax and some verdarain (481). After straining it through a cloth, he saturates a piece of linen and cuts off a strip just the size of the wound. When it is fouled, he wipes off the pus and replaces it with the fresh face down. He never closes the wound with sutures but he washes it with warm wine before he replaces the ciroeno. For this treatment he has garnered a great reputation, acquired without just cause.

There is another at Poperingen, a woman named Lisa Pauwelins, who treats all wounds with potions. In the wound itself she places a small amount of lint atop which she lays a red cabbage leaf. She treats many patients and many of them die. Nonetheless, she receives much more praise than is given an able surgeon. I will tell all of you, including the surgeons-in-training, who aim to be Masters not to be surprised (ie disappointed). The successes of the ignorant lay practitioners come through sheer luck, not by their setting goals and achieving them.[216]

HERE ENDS BOOK VII AS TAKEN FROM THE CODEX OF
BRUSSELS

---

[216] These concluding critical remarks reflect the bitterness expressed through the centuries by members of the 'righteous establishment', angered by the aspects of wealth and fame of the usurpers. Yperman's criticisms seem petty when compared with the brilliant vituperations written 250 years later by the surgeon of Queen Elizabeth I. The Reader will reward himself with great amusement by spending an hour with the treasury of antiquackery put into the words of rich invective that he will find in *The Selected Writngs of William Clowes,* ed. by DNL Poynter, London, Harvey and Blythe, Ltd., 1948 (LDR).

PART II
FIFTY-ONE CHAPTERS FROM THE CAMBRIDGE CODEX[217]

CHAPTER 1C. EXCEMA AND SCABIES

Here I will discuss scabies and explain its true nature. Patients who suffer with it often are referred to surgeons for treatment as well as to physicians. Therefore, I will describe the treatments for scabies which I have taken from Galen, Hippocrates et al.

First of all, know that the eruptions of scabies and excema appear (ie on the surface of the body) because the sick person's internal vitality is not potent enough to deal with the faulty humors within the body; the weakness may simply be due to old age. [218] Therefore, we recognize the fact that the eruption is the riddance of a serious malady, and it lends itself to a perfect cure. Another type of rugosity[219] appears in persons who consume rotten foods and bad wine. Some eruptions occur because a person cannot expel corrupted foods except with strenuous efforts (ie constipation) and the matter remains in the body as a source of putrefaction.

This is how I treat it. First of all evacuate the bad matter. After a proper laxative syrup has done its job, mix some of it with an extract of fumitory or the like as suited to the patient's age; that will make a laxative that can purge the humors, as described in our antidotary. After the evacuations, in the evening smear this anti-scabies ointment on the nude patient while he is standing near an open hearth to provide warmth; cover the wrists, elbows and buttocks.

---

217 These chapters appear only in the Cambridge Codex, in the edition of E.C. Van Leersum. The chapters will be numbered 1 C, 2 C etc. (LDR).

218 The concept here is that an exanthem represents the attempt of the body to discharge the faulty humors through the skin, having failed to eliminate them by digesting them and evacuating the residues in feces, urine, sweat, emesis or blood (phlebotomy). Scabies was thought to be a systemic malady, not an infestation by the sarcoptes mite! The extensive treatments reflect the concerns for more than the skin (LDR).

219 The rough skin, considered of itself to be an exanthem, is the chapping induced by constant scratching of the scabetic 'itch'. The dorsum of the hands, the interdigital webs, the soles of the feet etc. were favorite places for the mites to burrow and afflict (LDR).

The ointment: Take quick lime, aloes, olive oil and make an ointment. Ponatur in Pixide Cerate.[220]

Another: Take one oz. of aloes and mix it with vinegar to apply on the wrists, elbows and buttocks.

Another: Take two oz. of walnut oil and one oz. of wine vinegar and add one oz. each of powdered litharge and gold. Boil and stir well with care to avoid charring it after it has been inspissated. Keep it in your storage bin until you use it.

Another: Avicenna said we should anoint the wrists, the elbows and the buttocks with this ointment after he bathes in a heated tub: Take powdered litharge and gold, live sulfur, and powdered alum. Boil with vinegar while stirring with a spatula until it is as thick as an ointment. Put it on the itching regions. Keep it in a clean container.

Another: Take two oz. of walnut oil, one oz. of scabious and two oz. of a good vinegar. Boil them while stirring without pause and avoid charring. When the watery part is gone, PPC. This ointment also is effective against tinea, impetigo and spots on the face as well as scabies anywhere on the body.

Another: Steep some pitch in water (352) and filter one oz. through a fine cloth. Add to the filtrate two oz. of walnut oil and two oz. of powdered sal nitri (402). PPC.

Another, used as above by Master Gilbert [221]: Take garlic cloves and split them open. Mash them and add pork-lard to make an ointment. PPC.

Another recommended by Galen to be used three times to mature (ie digest) the humors and to eliminate them through the urine: Take two drams each of sulfurous wine, black hellebore (164) and mercury (288); and one-half dr. of staphisagre. Grind them fine and add pork-lard. Mix them while heating. PPC. Anoint the mixture. Avicenna used this ointment to treat carious bone (ie osteomyelitis).

Another: Take three oz each of the juice of bryony (489)[222] and

---

220 This is an apothecary's instruction for storage, "Let the compound be kept in a wax-coated (lined) container (box)". Henceforth I will abbreviate 'ponatur pixide cerate' as PPC (LDR).

221 Gilbertus Anglicus. See Appendix II. (LDR).

222 I think that Tabanelli's 'vitellini' is a misprint. for 'viticelle', white bryony (LDR).

radishes, three oz. each of vinegar and walnut oil and one-half oz. of aloes, amd mix. PPC.

Another, cited by Pliny : Wash the region containing decayed bone with water in which lay a drowned man (492b). The abscess was cured by the water.

Another: A twice daily bath in this is good treatment for infected bone and purulent eruptions: Take one-half lb. of minced fresh bryony roots (67). Boil them in fresh water until it foams. Strain it through cloth and use the clear liquid as a lotion.

Experimentator [223] says that the roots of garlic (porrum, 365a.) laid on the ganglia that serve decayed bone cure it. The recipe: Two oz. of walnut-oil, one oz. of wax, one oz. of garlic juice, all mixed over a flame. PPC. It is a valuable ointment.

William of Medicke [224] was the first to offer the following for scabies: Why was he the first? That is strange, because the benefits and the actions of mercury are so good and so certain and have been so well-tested. The recipe: Take two oz. of mercury, three dr. of gold litharge, two dr. each of euphorbia and staphisagre, one-half lb. of salt-free fresh lard. Mix over a flame. PPC. Use this from the elbows to the feet. During the summer, apply it after the midday meal while he (ie undressed) is exposed to warm sunlight. During the winter anoint him in a room near an open hearth. If he has not been cured by the fifth day, wash his belly with warm wine containing rosemary (387). Cover the cleaned belly with a piece of old cloth saturated with the ointment, protecting the rest of the body from contact with it. I, myself, have cured many patients with scabies everywhere in the body. In its distribution over the body, scabies resembles leprosy.

Hugh of Lucca often used the following with success, by applying it to the palms, the wrists and the soles of the feet he completely

---

223 Tabanelli says that the name is apocryphal. Sarton says that it was the name of a lost treatise, not a person, that was cited by the Flemish Dominican encyclopedist, Thomas of Brabant (Cantipratanus) fl. circa 1250. The lost work probably was contemporary with Thomas. see Sarton, Vol. II, p. 593 (LDR).

224 Not identified by Tabanelli. I think the mispelled name was William of Moerbeke, 1215-1286, another Flemish Dominican (like Thomas above, easily accessible to a neighbor at Ypres !). William of Moerbeke translated Greek sources. see Sarton, Vol.II, p.829 (LDR).

eliminated the rough skin and the scabetic lesions in less than one day. I have had similar successes. Hugh bled the patients from an hepatic vein (ie dorsum of the hand) after the applications. The recipe: Three oz. of oil of laurel, one oz. of powdered olibanum, eight oz. of common salt, equal amounts of the juices of plantain and fumitory and one-half lb. of pork lard. Heat the liquids gently while stirring. After they have cooled, add the powdered olibanum. PPC. Set it aside for use when desired.

Many people prepare it this way: Take three oz. of laurel oil, one-half oz. each of powdered aloes, powdered arsenic (34), enula (168a) and radishes. Cook to make an ointment. Then add one oz. of mercury tempered with saliva. PPC.

Hugh of Lucca also used this ointment against scabies and rough skin: Take one oz. each of the juices of chelidonium, fumitory, scabious, lapathum (236), powdered gold, powdered ceruse, black and white hellebore and one-half lb. of laurel oil. Mix to make an ointment. PPC. Use it on the soles and palms. If the eruption appears elsewhere , anoint the wrists and buttocks.

A respected colleague gave me this recipe which he used to treat his own itch. He mashed hedera (120) to obtain its juice. Wherever he had to scratch he first wet his finger nails with it and was cured. When his legs itched, he applied the leaves of hedera with success.

Another recipe, from the book of gold:[225] Three oz. of oil of roses, and enough wax to make an ointment. Then add one oz. of mercury temperted with saliva. PPC

Another by William of Congenis, to be applied at the wrists:[226] Take three oz. of oil of laurel, two oz. of lard from an old pig, one oz. of mercury tempered with common salt, three oz. each of the juices of plantains and fumitory. Heat while mixing to boil off some of the fluid and observe it carefully to avoid stringiness (ie as of kneaded dough). Cool it before adding the mercury. PPC.

Avicenna said that the juice of wild celery (29) is good for rough dry skin and to relieve the itch. He said that we should split the stem

225 Probably Nicolaus Myrepsos of Alexandria, the so-called Alexandrian Gold (LDR).

226 Fl. mid-century 13. Probably southern France and Montpellier. Copied Roger Frugard (LDR).

in half and wrap it in cloth and heat it with salt. Use it to rub the patient when he is bathing.

Sulfur-water is an astringent that promotes healing, as does incinerated abrotonin (35). The last-named also softens the skin and dislodges scales. The same is true for goat and bear-grease (206).

Another: Take four oz. of burnt lead (253) finely ground and mixed with honey. PPC.

Another: Scoria of silver (419) is useful for chapped skin.

Another: Powdered safron mixed with vinegar. Also, very hot water will get rid of rough skin by washing away flaked pus.

Another: Chelidonium applied during an evacuation (ie phlebotomy) will help purify the body.

Another: Powder incinerated frog meat (129) and mix it with vinegar to treat excema.

Another: Fresh calamint applied with massage when the patient is in the bath.

Another: Oil of wild mustard (297) is good for chapped skin. Apply it in sunlight or near an open hearth.

Another: Take two oz. each of coriander (132) and dill (26) and wine lees (175). Heat in an oven until a dry powder remains. Mix it into oil of eruca (171) for application on rough or itching skin. It is a well-tested recipe.

Another: Mix acorns with rue and wine vinegar. Boil and mash the pulp to use as an ointment. PPC,

Another: Take two oz. of olive oil, two oz. of the juice of calamint and add wax. It is very effective against severe excema when used as above (ie on a bathing patient).

Another:: The juice of coriander is very good to eliminate rugosity. Avicenna used it. Garlic is good for dry excema, and so is mustard. And old urine will calm an itch, as will droplets of boiled-down wine.

Avicenna said that burning torches near the legs can eliminate purulent itching crusts.[227]

Chapter 2 C. Warts

Warts derive from a superabundance of melancholic humors.

---
[227] Probably fueled with pine-pitch (LDR).

Avicenna gave us a sure cure for them. Take green acorns (203) and grind them with chicken-fat. Cook them well and sieve them through a fine cloth. Apply it on the warts and it will destroy them.

Another good remedy used by many Master Surgeons: Rub on some rich soil taken from nearby graves.

Another: Apply minced galbanum over the base of recently snipped off warts. The galbanum can cause the eyes of a partridge to disappear.[228]

Another: Take crushed cashew nuts (25) mixed with onion juice. PPC. Use it on and around the wart.

Another: Take the juice of (or powdered dry) round aristolochium mashed with onion juice. It is an astringent that will shed crusts and yield soft skin. The roots of parsley are equally good.

Another: Experimentator said to roast chicken legs on charcoals until the skin comes loose. Rub it on the warts three or four times a day until they fall off.

Another: (also by Experimentator) for treating internal warts: Drink the juice of pimpinella (349). When the warts have smooth surfaces, drink the juice as well as make a plaster. Avicenna said that minced portulacca (366) spread over the warts will kill them. He also said that the feces of an eagle rubbed on a wart will kill it.

Another by Gilbertus Anglicus: Wash the warts with water in which a drowned man had rotted (492b). The same benefits are obtained with rostrum porcinum (392).

Constantine the African offered this: Crush flowers of salex to obtain the juice. Apply it and destroy the warts. Another from Constantine and other sages: Take chick peas (112) and rub them on the warts. Then wrap those peas in a bit of cloth and toss it over your shouilder, and Presto!, the warts will disappear. Some wise men think that is a hoax.

Peter Lucrator[229] offers these: Apply the milky sap of fig trees, or use orpiment with vinegar.

Another from Gilbert: Snip off the wart and apply the juice of titimalle (173) – the plant or its milk.

---

228 I cannot interpret the phrase. Perhaps the eye of a partridge describes a
    kind of a wart (LDR).
229 Not identified (LDR).

Another that is a strong corrosive: Take lye made from wood-ashes and add potash. Let it set for three days. Then add a cupful of quick-lime until it all has the consistency of honey. Put it on the wart after it has aged a while, apply it up to twenty or thirty times a day, until the wart falls away with a gentle brushing. Or you may tie a string around the base and lift it off.

If the patient tends to form new warts, purge the bad humors with goat's milk whey (286).

CHAPTER 3 C. SMALLPOX AND MEASLES[230]

Here we shall discuss smallpox, a pustular eruption in people of all ages. The malady strikes with great fever and pustules form. The victim suffers backache, an itching nose and has nightmares in his sleep. When you encounter such a patient, know that the signs indicate smallpox. Most patients also present with itching backs and noses. Your treatments should begin with the earliest signs.

First perform phlebotomy, only if the pustules have not yet developed. After they are present, eschew phlebotomy. Prescribe boiled figs that may favor the fading of nascent pustules. Or, have the patient drink this hot potion three times a day: Ten dr. each of dry figs and lupin-flour, five dr. of gum tragacanth, four lbs. of spring water. Boil it all down to 6 (ie error)) liters. Filter it through a linen cloth and add dr. of powdered saffron before drinking. The potion should be taken until all the pustules are dry.

Another: All green clothing can act against pustules. Avoid all things that cool the body from within, because they will cool the blood and dry it and favor clotting. When the pox appear, you mature them (ie cause to suppurate) by exposing them to steam. Then open them. If some foul stuff persists in the patient's eyes, instill drops of rose water and follow with the juice of meadow –rue. Use it when red spots appear on the whites of the eyes, when the eyes itch and when tiny white spots appear in the red ones. When none of that is noted and

---

230 This is another jumbled chapter, quite typical of Book VII C. The confusion of terms and the disordered descriptions of clinical signs, diagnoses and treatments certainly labels it a product of a careless scribe trying to make his way through Yperman's Flemish Ms. Yperman himself should not be blamed entirely for what we read here (LDR).

the pustules are small, use only the general measures. But when the itching persists or increases or becomes prickly and painful, use drops of egg-white and whey. Do not to use steam fumigations too often when treating the eyes. That warning is more important when treating measles, because that disease derives from black bile and is under the influence of the moon. It is not easy to clear it from the eyes. In those cases prescribe pomegranates, barley-water, cucumbers (144) and melons, and add a mucilage of psillium (353).

When the patient continues to suffer and faints with anxiety, have him drink a decoction of fumitory, and massage his body with soft towels until the redness (ie here it is measles) fades . Then go to other measures. Save the urine for inspection.

You will know that the patient has a terribly bad case of the disease, a malignant form capable of great harm, when you examine the whole body and you see blood seeping from the newest red spots.[231] Then seat the patient close to a steam bath.

The pustules of variola are small, yellow and hard and do not fade on pressure. After a phase of deep red color accompanied by much general malaise, the patient is left with a pitted face. The pustules are malignant and can be lethal. When you diagnose variola, have the patient gargle rose-water to relieve his sore throat. Irrigate the eyes from time to time with his face upward, using rose-water mixed with vinegar. That will temper the eruption of pox in the eyes. Have him breathe through his mouth rather than his nose so to rid himself of most of the pox (ie in the nose and throat) and relieve his discomforts. The palms and the soles of the feet can be relieved by frequent massage with a cloth wet with very hot water. It will hasten desqammation.

Do not press food on patients with either of the two maladies. Let them eat in moderation until they lose their bad breaths and foul catarrh, which are symptoms of measles. Frequent bathing after the crusts have fallen away will sweeten and purify the bodies of the victims of the pox, and much of the scarring and pitting will fade.

---

231 Here I think the author meant small pox. The text often does not indicate which disease the author was intending and, of course, it does not distinguish rubeola from morbilli (LDR)

Use this ointment (ie pomade) to improve the scars: Take two oz. of powdered litharge and boil; them in oil of roses; three oz. of millet seeds and rice-flour; one and one-half oz. of powdered dry bones. Mix all with barley-water and spread it on the involved surfaces. In more difficult cases, have the patient drink white wine after he bathes and use steam baths in which you have added such active substances as incinerated ceruse. However, when the pock-marks are as small as seeds of lupin, brush on soothing substances made from dates as follows: Take the soft meat of dates mashed to the consistency of an ointment and smooth it on until it adheres. Or use this: Take three oz. each of plump figs, apples with seeds and flax-seed mucilage. Mix them with bean-flour. PPC. Anoint it alternately with hot hen or rooster fat.

Chapter 4 C. Leprosy

Leprosy is a filthy disease appearing in four types. One derives from putrid phlegm and is called tyria, named after the tyrian (ie from Tyre) serpent encountered at Jericho. The serpent molts its skin as it ages; a new skin appears just as the old one finally is shed. One can see it happen when the reptile slithers between two fallen branches and strips off what remains of the old skin. In Latin the shed skin is called spolium, which becomes a useful part of many medicines.

Now that we know its name,[232] let us describe its manifestations: the matter (ie pus etc.) and the appearance of the leper's body and eyes.

Tyria is caused by the abuse of certain foods. When a person with a phlegmatic complexion eats too much of soft fish that have phlegmatic humors, such as fat eels, carp and barbels, that get their own food in the bottoms of streams; when he drinks too much sweet wine and eats too much of fat geese and swans, be not surprised that such a person who lives on those birds [233] become leprous.

---

232 Tyrian because the leper also sheds his epidermis in flakes and shreds (LDR).
233 Birds that 'laze' about in ponds rather than fly (LDR).

Chapter 5 C. The Signs Of (Tyrian) Leprosy

The eyebrows are sheds and do not grow back. The eyelids thicken and the eyes are teary. The nostrils are half shut and are filled with matter, which makes breathing difficult. The lips and gums are purulent and bleed easily. The chests are sunken and the voices are hoarse. When you wash a leper with water you make him worse off.

The medicines (ie to be described in the following chapters) are effective only if used promptly, at the very onset.

Chapter 6 C. Leprosy Called Alopecia Or Fox

This second type of leprosy is called alopecia or fox;[234] it derives from tainted sanguine humors which are caused by eating rotted foods which cause plethora. Bleed those patients early. They can be recognized by these signs: Their faces are puffy and flushed, the color of leprous flesh. They shun sexual activity. The eyes are puffy and tearful. The veins around the eyes and on the face are congested (ie telangiectasia). The nostrils are collapsed. The gums bleed when touched. Their chests are sunken and spots appear everywhere on their bodies, which blanch when pressed and then reappear. Their urine is red and thick, and so is the blood taken from their veins. It turns brown when standing and thickens as it cools. One can feel many lumps (ie in the subcutaneous tissues) and there are many wens. The flesh (ie muscles) are soft and scrawny; the skin is pale, sweaty and loose. The patient infects many cohabitants; those who have direct contact with his body may putrefy to the same degree.

This second type of leprosy closely resembles the first type since they both derive from moist humors.

Chapter 7 C. Leonine Leprosy

A third type of leprosy is called leonine, lion-like [235] and choleric. It is hot, dry and fetid, similar to people with choleric complexions

234 Alopix is Greek for Fox, which sheds its hair annually. This leper loses his hair (LDR).

235 The leper's face is wrinkled, thrown into thick folds, especially the forehead, resembling a male lion (LDR).

who prefer spicy and salty foods and who drink strong wines, and add pepper and garlic. They corrupt their own bile.

CHAPTER 8 C. THE SIGNS OF LEONINE LEPROSY

The skin of the eyebrows sags; the facial skin yellows, but that of the body reddens. The eyes itch and burn and the eyelids are wide open; the irises are dilated and they stare fixedly straight ahead (ie at eye-level). The nostrils are narrowed and are blocked; the gums recede from the teeth; the lips adhere to the teeth; the chest is sunken; the belly is constipated; the urine is red; here and there body will itch. The blood that is released at a phlebotomy is yellowish when it first spills forth and it flows easily, and it dissolves quickly when dripped in water.

This leonine species of leprosy is common. Even when it first appears the patient is noticeably restless and disturbed.

CHAPTER 9 C. ELEPHANTINE LEPROSY

This fourth type of leprosy derives from melancholic humors. The name describes the thick and horny skin and the long period of incubation before the diagnosis is clear.

The signs are: a dark pallid face and body. The eyebrows sag; the eyes are round; the nose changes colors; the tongue is covered with small swellings that resemble warts; the web between the thumb and index finger is wasted. This is their course: They exhibit the signs of the fox and the serpent (ie other types of leprosy); their urine is scanty and ashen gray in color. When bled, their blood clots rapidly and when you place a coagulum in water it becomes more dense. When the clot is left alone it does not become pale. You can see thread-like formations in the clots, like tiny vessels or nerve-fibers. When he is struck by the illness (ie after the long incubation) it happens all at once. It seems that the entire body is involved at a clap of the hands; the eyebrows and many sites in the body are involved all at once.

SOME INFALLIBLE TESTS FOR ALL KINDS OF LEPROSY

First noted are twinges of pain, often transient and soon to recur. The thighs, feet and hands lose sensibility such that the patient does not jump away when he is pricked with a needle or some sharp instrument, in the buttocks or elsewhere. He favors cool fresh air where he can seat himself. The loss of sensibility is the result of the corruption of his humors.

Another test: Add three gr. of salt to some of blood obtained at a phlebotomy. The salt will dissolve at once, whereas it will not dissolve in healthy blood.

Another test: Smear some of the patient's blood clot on your palm to note if it feels greasy. That is a sign of putrefied humors. Note also that the skin is thin and shiny at the forehead and nose, as if it had been oiled.

When treated for scabies, a common malady among lepers [236], it recurs and forms tiny pimples that resemble wens, even after they had been eliminated by the surgeon. After bathing in water, the leper's body dries quickly, as if he sheds water from oily skin.

The voice has a nasal quality because nasal breathing is difficult. The breath is foul, sometimes coming up from the stomach, sometimes coming out from the brain. His sweat stinks. When touched by a flame he may react little or none at all. The elephantine types lose their hair.[237]

Avicenna said that leprosy can be recognized anywhere in the body. The patients turn away their eyes and look no one straight in the face, because they are very distrustful and as if they wished to spread their leprosy to everyone. They are irritable and utter foul imprecations. They are only slightly feverish if at all. When a fever does appear on the fourth day, it soon goes away or is easily treated.

A touch by a lepers hands can make a healthy person sick. That accounts for the fear of lepers among the populace which shuns them, as is advised in both the New and the Old Testaments.

Avicenna said that whatever good blood remains in a leper is

236 The reference is to crusted and itching skin, not only to true sarcoptic scabies (LDR)

237 This is probably is an error. See fn.234 (LDR).

contained in his stomach. Robert (?) attests to the fact that even though she is tainted every where, a leprous woman may bear a child. Part of the similar advice Avicenna gives to lepers who want to prolong their lives is to abstain from sexual activity, so that at least for the rest of their lives, their lower bodies will remain free of the disease.

If you wish, you may offer the following treatments to bolster a leper. If prescribed, they should be conducted only by an experienced physician.

CHAPTER 10 C. VENEREAL LEPROSY

When leprosy is the result of sexual contacts with a leprous woman, you must learn whether she was a hot or a cold leper as well as her symptoms, because that will determine the treatment you will use.

When Leprosy is contracted from a phlegmatic or melancholic woman you will know it by her ugly face. After the reported contact, when you look for the signs to first appear, those who are affected by blood or bile will be worse off than the others, and their treatments will be prolonged.

If the source is a leprous woman of the warm type, the signs will appear more rapidly. You will know she is of the biliary type if her natural heat is directed inward and her skin is taught (ie and cool). She reacts to a prick sometimes as if from a burn and at other times as if touched by ice that makes her shiver. Often she will flush and then turn pale.

The patient's natural vital force brings the bad leprous matter to the surface, under the skin, over the underlying fleshy tissues of the face, making fine wrinkles like the tracks of lines of ants. That sometimes causes 'tics' (prickling). The face already is ruddy and congested by heat and by twinges of pain, and the expression is one of terror.

If the faulty humors are cool, the face is puffy and the skin everywhere else is heavy (ie edematous) and the patient does not want to bestir herself from her seat. One can feel the coolness through her skin, especially on her face and forehead. [238]

---

[238] Where other than here has my reader seen mention of an action performed by earnest mothers everywhere: touching her child's forehead to detect a fever ? (LDR)

Here is how we treat a leper who is overly agitated. Immediately bleed from both arms and cause the blood to clot with this potion: Take two oz of ozzysaccara (330). three oz. of syrup of fumitory, four oz. of a decoction of fumitory, two oz. each of scabious and borrago (63a). Mix and make a julep, one hot mouthful to be drunk in the morning and evening. Then fast for two hours. Then administer this laxative: Take two dr. of ozzisaccara and hierarufinum (219d). On the third day wash the patient with cool plants. After that administer two parts of rubea trosciscata (393) and one part of greater theriac (462) with the juice of fumitory. This is to taken when warm. Repeat after three days. On the fourth day, bleed again, this time from an hepatic vein. The following day bleed from a capital vein in amounts tolerated by the patient. Allow three days for the patient be kept warm near a stove, and then prescribe opium. Repeat the bleeding after three months.

Scarify the legs and apply cups under the chin and produce a blister (80) on the legs at the same time as above. In the morning dose him with diaprunum (355) and dianthus (155a) or with rosamel. Then give him more syrup of fumitory. Twice weekly mix a yellow ointment with oil of roses and apply it on the face and cover it with leaves of plantain. Leave it overnight and remove it in the morning.

This is how we medicate the lepers whose disease was caused by cool phlegm and melancholy. Bring the bad matter to head with this potion: Take two oz. of oximel diuretic, one oz. of syrup of fumitory, four oz. each of decoctions of borrago and fumitory and dose in the morning and evening. Follow this with a laxative purge: Take two dr. of ieralogodon (219b) one dr. of ierarufin. Keep it warm on the stove for two days, adding water and leaves of sambuco, ebulus, scabious, fumitory and some lapis lazuli. After a steam bath, dose the patient with Galen's theriac and warm syrup of fumitory. On the third day bleed from an hepatic or capital vein and scarify and apply cups under the chin. To improve the dark skin, apply green wine in which you have macerated some powdered rhubarb. Apply it twice a week to moisten the face.

Chapter 11 C. Valuable Preventive Treatments For Leprosy

Take some gold filings (249a) and make a fine powder and mix them with the juice of borrage (63a). Another: Take a small amount of bone, called deer's horn (62), and make a fine powder to mix with the juice of scabious. Use it as a potion. Another from Theodoric: Take a serpent that lives on a desert mountain and keep it in a dry cage. When ready, cut off its head and let it thrash about and bleed until it dies and lies still. Remove its skin ,[239] eviscerate its body and boil the flesh (273a). Have the patient eat some of it, not knowing what he is eating lest he reject it. And he should drink the water in which the snake was boiled. Continue until the patient is distended and begins to shed his own skin. Then sit him near a stove (ie now he is unclothed as well as desquammated) and anoint him with oil in which you have boiled some of the serpent. Repeat the treatment until the patient's own skin and deeper tissues are renewed. This is a well-tested method.

Avicenna and other surgeons used this: Bury a decapitated and tailless serpent until it is covered with maggots. Then let it dry (ie exposed to sunlight). Then boil it in wine and add honey before the patient drinks it. Another by Avicenna: He frequently bathed the patient's beard with the water in which a snake had been boiled. Another: Macerate some maize[240] in the boiled serpent-water and feed it to chickens who also will drink the water. After they shed their feathers, cleanse them and boil them (ie the chickens) and feed their meat and the broth to the leper. Use the broth to wet the patient's face and hands. Bleed him four days afterwards. Another of a similar type: Place a snake in a tightly stoppered small cask of wine and wait until the flesh is completely macerated. Use the wine. Another: Desiccate salted snake-meat in a casserole and make a powder of the residue. The patient should add some of the powder to all his foods.

239 The loss of skin betokens the remedy against leprosy (LDR).

240 An anachronism. Maize (indian corn) was not introduced into Europe before the return of Christopher Columbus after 1492. The generic term 'corn' was used for all food-grains, especially wheat. I assume that is what Yperman-Tabanelli intended here. In the USA the word 'corn' has replaced the word 'maize' and refers to no other grain (LDR)

Or use the powder to make a potion which is effective against leprosy and other foul diseases. Also useful are mixtures containing almonds, borrago, calamint, dipsaccus, tragacanth, radish, scabious, tartar (456), ierarufinum and Galen's great theriac.

CHAPTER 12 C. ANTIDOTES FOR INGESTED POISONS

The immediate remedy is a drink of hot water and oil to produce three or four emeses. Some people vomit better after drinking milk with oil and butter .

Observe the patient's symptoms: If he is feverish and has a flushed face and yellowed eyes and a foul breath, have him drink cool things to calm him and cool him. But if he has a headache and is sweaty, give him stimulants such as asafoetida (37) etc. If anyone is uncertain whether or not he has ingested a poison, have him drink fig juice with oil of walnuts and take morning doses of Galen's theriac with terra sigillata (460). Another for suspected ingestion of poison: Repeat the above treatment after the patient has been given an emetic and he has vomited.

If the patient collapses, that is a sign that the poison acts contrary to the complexion of his heart. When the treatments are not effective, prescribe some balsamodendron (48) as an antidote. I have seen it work against aconite which is a very potent poison. A potion of musk (291a) or cinnamon or cumin or Galen's theriac will help.

CHAPTER 13 C. TREATMENT OF POISONING BY CANTHARIDES (80) [241]

Use these antidotes to counteract poisoning by cantharides. The signs are bloody and dark urine, which you can cure by drinking almond oil. Also, have the patient drink celery-juice, asafoetida and Galen's theriac. When the patient is nauseated give him milk to drink and prescribe two doses of vinegar containing one oz. each of asafoetida and juice of calamint with added sugar.

---

241 I have re-ordered the sentences and phrases here in an attempt to make some sense. The ancient copyist's jumble has been faithfully repeated by Tabanelli, and it remains hardly comprehensible (LDR).

Another: A decoction of psyllium as a potion. It also is effective against poisoning by coriander, which can be detected on the patient's breath.

When anyone eats too much hot roasted meat directly from the oven or the spit, before it has cooled, he should take nettles stripped of their 'hairs' and drink juices of styptic plants, and go to bed. On arising he should bathe.

If someone eats tainted fish, older than one or two days, he should drink a potion of undiluted wine contained ground pepper, and he should eat hazel nuts.

If a patient has fits (ie after eating bad food), give him sweet fruit juices and electuaries of diateron (341). Give him undiluted wine and apply oil of nard on his belly at bedtime and cover it with a warm cloth.[242]

Chapter 14 C. Snake Bites

When a person has been bitten by serpent, apply myrobalans (298). If bitten by an unidentified animal (ie while he is asleep) apply cups over the bite to suck strongly at the openings, Then smear on some wild polycaria inula (360a) and place directly over it the head of a crayfish (138a) and the sandy contents of its abdomen. When the fang—marks begin to fill and swell and become hot, you will know that it is the bite of a very venomous beast. When the bite putrefies and blackens, you will know that the poison is still active in the body. However, that does not mean that it will destroy the whole body. When a bite is near the heart it is more threatening, or near an important artery that can carry the venom to the heart. Be well aware that the great theriac of Galen is a good remedy against serpent bites, as are the mithridaticon (288b), asafoetida and hermodactyl (219) The victim should drink only undiluted wine.

---

[242] And even now, seven hundred years later, many mothers and grandmothers apply a square of flannel cloth wet with some greasy substance on the aching bellies of children. Not all of them emit the sweet odors of nard! (LDR)

Chapter 15 C. Scorpion Stings

When a man is bitten or stung by a scorpion, immediately dose him with Galen's theriac followed by undiluted wine. Then let him eat pomegranate fruit. Suck out the venom and place the leaves of chicory (taraxicum, 113), alkanna (15) and screpellacio (gentian) over the sting.

Chapter 16 C. Bee Stings

After a bee sting, bathe the region or the whole body, or cover the region with sand or roll the person in sand, or apply warm ashes.

Another remedy: Take a handful of senecio (426a) and half as much of wild celery (97). Mix and grind to a powder. Use it on bee and wasp stings. You may apply this ointment on and around the sting: Take one oz of wine vinegar, one-half oz. of oil of violets and mix and make an ointment.[243] When the stinger remains in the skin, rub it out with the oil of violets. Then rub some ashes over the region and apply the oil. Then wipe it clean to inspect and make sure that the stinger is gone.

Chapter 17 C. Bites By A Rabid Dog, The Worst Bites Of All

When you know that the animal is really rabid, treat the victim. The signs are described by Bernard of Gordon in his *Lily of Medicine*. [244] First apply a cup over the bite to extract the venom [245] Then apply a medication made of eruca (171), camphor and salt-free butter. The victim should drink a potion to prevent suppuration, such as a decoction of caprifolium (84) and the like. Limit his diet.

---

243 The phrase 'to make an ointment' usually meant to add enough white wax or thick oil to achieve the consistency of honey or thicker (LDR)

244 Bernard of Gordon's *De morborum prope omnium curatione*, 1322 (LDR).

245 The viral cause for rabies was not known until the 19thC. All authors believed it to be an envenomation (LDR).

Chapter 18 C. Remedies For Poisons

These are poor-man's remedies which succeed if used immediately. Take the juice of agrimony (13) and drink it with white wine. It works well against venomous snake bites, dog bites and human bites, and it is useful in treating venomous abscesses.

Another equally good remedy: Take one oz. each of the roots of tansy (454) and tormentilla (465). Grind them fine and drink one dr, in white wine. It has been proven to completely rid one of poisons.

Another: Take roots of asphodels and make a powder to be drunk (ie with wine). It will save the drinker from poisons, and from spoiled food and beverages.

Others to use against poisons and venomous bites: asphodel, asafoetida, garlic, bdellium, bedegar (53c), centaurea (100), balsam, draguntum (161), mint (288a), carrot (152, dipsaccus (159), gentian, iris-roots, lily, honey, opoponax, pitch (352), horseradish (373), rue, spikenard (437), tussilago (470), squills (443), salt, sambucus (406), chicory, terra sigillata, zedoaria (503).

I use the following electuaries, all called opiates: esdra, littontripon, Galen's ierologodon (the strongest kind), mithridaticon, the great theriac.

Chapter 19 C. Nodules (Ganglia) Called Scrofules

These lumps are called scrofules because like a sow's (scrofa) litter, they come in clusters. The nodules are firm, consisting of matter (ie suppurated) and melancholy. They appear in the neck near the throat and under the jaw, and in the axillae. When they suppurate in the neck, they erode and become ulcers. In that event they are called the King's Evil by some authors, who believe that the King of France can cure it simply by touching it with his hand. Also, it may be possible to find a cure as an act of faith, because faith comforts the body and a healthy morale triumphs over a disease. That can happen when the suppuration is not extensive. However, Nature's resistance cannot overcome a chronic and very difficult case.

Another method has been tried by some surgeons who make use

of certain beliefs. They lay the patient on the ground near a swiftly flowing stream during the night of St. John in mid-summer. While there, they bleed him in such a way that his blood falls into the water. They claim many successful cures. But, see it this way: After a long series of set-backs, people will try alternative methods to obtain a cure, applying themselves as required of them.

In truth, these nodules appear in persons who are difficult to dry (ie edematous), in those who are viscous and over-filled with humors, and in those who eat and drink more than their bodies can digest. Therefore, the superfluous undigested matter inflates the nodules which may become abscesses. The excess dilates the nodules, and the abscesses end up as draining fistulas or hemorrhoids [246], etc. The undigested residues of food and drink accumulate in the ulcerated nodules and that is why these patients often suffer from hunger, and why abstention is an important part of the treatments. Those who do not wish to understand its importance and will not follow the dietary regimen are difficult to cure.

First of all, instruct the patient not to bend his head forward and to avoid laughing, crying and vomiting.[247] Try to clean away the pus by prescribing electuaries of turbith (469). The nodules derive from phlegm and melancholy and the electuaries purge those humors. Prescribe this for the same actions: Take three dr. of turbith-gum, one-half oz. of white sugar. Grind them to a fine powder and dose the patient with two dr. but use only one dr. if the patient is not robust. Give it at midnight so the patient can sleep until the laxative begins to act. The patient should not drink water and he should not eat any cold foods. Cupping is good as an additional evacuant.

Some surgeons question the value of cupping. However, after neutralizing the bad matter, you should try cups to eliminate it before it erupts and becomes a chronic ulcer no longer suitable for internal absorbtion (ie and elimination by purges and bleeds). But, when the lesions already are draining, use this plaster before the lesion becomes a chronic ulcer (ie a fistula): Take red snails (249) and cook

246 If the scrofules are in the groins (LDR)

247 Activities which move the neck and disturb the scrofules. Remember Galen's and Avicenna's caveat that a wound cannot heal if it is in motion. Here, al;so, Yperman hints that moving the head will attract the scrofule-causing humors to the head and neck (LDR).

them with lard from hogs and birds and some wine. Make a plaster to place on the mass.

Another: Take some goat turds mixed with honey and vinegar. Cook it and apply the paste while it is warm.

Another used by Avicenna who declared that it is effective: Take lily bulbs, flax-seeds, and pigeon droppings. Mix and boil with wine. When the gland and nodules have cool complexions, add more of the excrements. If the patients are children or women use only one-fourth the amount.

Another good plaster for glands before they erupt: Take two oz. of flax-seeds, two and one-half oz. of sulfur, one oz. of honey. Mix and boil. Apply it warm.

Another: Take three oz. each of the roots of bryony and pigeon droppings and cook them with hog lard. It will absorb the nodules and retract them.

Another from Dioscorides [248]: Take the roots of burdoch (433) and boil them in wine. Apply when warm.

Another from Macer[249]: Take equal amounts of live sulfur, pigeon droppings, flax-seeds and seeds of nigella (307). Grind and mix with warm wine, and then bring to a boil. Apply as a warm plaster, and it will make the nodules vanish.

Another from Gilbert: Take one fried egg, some anabula – euphorbia (173) and add wine. Drink some in the morning and evening of three consecutive days and take little else to drink or eat. Many have attested to its effectiveness..

Another recommended by me after many successes: Take equal amounts of very dry pigeon droppings, deer and cow turds, litharge, the roots of the cold-seed plants, apium, galbanum and bitter almonds. Mix and add some olive oil and old hog lard and some milk. When applied it will destroy the scrofules, but first you must purge the patient with laxative pills of turbith.

Another: Take mustard-seeds ground with hog lard and milk. Apply it after purging with turbith. It works well.

Another: Take common plantain leaves, rub with salt and apply.

248 Greek botanist-herbalist (c. 50 AD) whose great pharmacvopeia was a major source during the ensuing 1500 years (LDR)

249 Tabanelli says this refers to Macer Floridius. However, that name refers to an herbal of great renown written by Odo of Meung ca 1075 (LDR).

Another from Avicenna: Grind bean-flour and apply it.

Another from Gilbert: The blood of snails.

Another: Take equal amounts of the juices of rue and abrotonin. Use it on ulcerated lesions.

Another, praised by many surgeons: A plaster of diachylon (153).

Another: Take one lb. each of mucilages made from fenugreek, flax-seeds and althea (18); one lb. of litharge; two lbs. of olive oil. Make a plaster.

I often prepare this plaster, which I prefer as better than all the others: Take: one lb. of all the plants listed below and make a muci-lage, of which take one lb. Then take one and a half lb., of litharge finely ground, two lbs. of olive oil and one-half lb. of wax. Mix all to make a plaster.

The following is a watery solution[250] that dissolves scrofules, nodes and fragments bladder-stones. It softens hard livers and kidneys as well as of metal (?) in less than three days. The plants are chelidonium, hyoscyamus (217), titimals (173), cicuta, (115), wild rue, asphodel and malum terrae. Grind them in a mortar (ie to obtain their juices) and sublimate (ie distill) them three times in an alembic. Label it to warn others that it is poisonous .

CHAPTER 20 C. MALODOROUS ARMPITS

We call this disorder 'hyrcus'. To get rid of it do this: First shave the hair and rub the axillary skin with a good wine with added rose-water and a decoction of cassia (94) or ambergris. [251] Use it in the evening before retiring.

To treat a swollen face due to a dental abscess, boil cinnamon and powdered dry figs in wine and make a plaster to apply warm.[252]

---

250 The solution alone is a potent topical distilled from the juices of the plants and must not be taken by mouth (LDR)

251 I cannot identify ambergris as a medieval surgical medicine. I assume the author meant ambrosia, a type of artemisia (35) (LDR).

252 There is no explanation why the copyist placed this malady in the chapter dealing with malodorous armpits (LDR).

Chapter 21 C. Buboes [253]

These abscesses are called buboes after the owl that hides in trees, barns, churches etc., because the bubo escapes detection, hidden in the neck (beneath the ears and the jaw), in the axillas and in the groins. You should not use cool plasters as treatments [254] because the swelling in the neck allows the brain to rid itself of its superfluous humors through the erupted bubo which releases a flow of pus as from a streamlet.

For axillary buboes purge[255] the heart, lungs and the chest. For inguinal buboes cleanse the abdominal organs – the liver, spleen, kidneys and intestines. Since we cannot directly use topicals on those internal organs, we treat them with cool medicines (ie potions, not topicals) to dispel their bad matter toward the neck, axillae and groins so it can be eliminated via the suppurated buboes. The internal accumulation of the bad matter puts the patient at risk for aposthems, dysentery, deafness and many other ailments of the organs. Therefore, we use our treatment to bring the buboes to a head, to ripen them and cause them to erupt and to cleanse themselves. To do that we first apply this emollient: Take two oz. each of mucilages of flaxseeds, fenugreek, mauve-roots and bismalve and add enough porklard. Mix, heat and apply when warm in the morning and evening until the bubo is soft. Before every reapplication, wash with warm water. When you see that it is 'ripe', open it by incising in its long axis. Empty it and insert a cloth drain that was prepared in advance. Atop that, apply the brown ointment as a paste. Leave it until the next day before removing it and washing the abscess with warm water, Dry it with a cloth. Then insert a drain dipped in ta detergent, and put brown ointment over it. The detergent is made so: Take three oz. of celery juice, one and a half oz. of wheaten flour. Mix and bring to a

---

253 Suppurating lymphadenitis, not plague (LDR).

254 Which suppress suppuration. Instead, use warm applications on the buboes as described (LDR).

255 The physician prescribed laxatives that were specific for every organ, season, phase of the moon, side of the body etc. The surgeon acceded to this product of the clerical ascendancy. Yperman never exhibited disgruntlement, as did Henri Mondeville, who knew much of it was foolish domineering humbuggery (LDR)

boil. Immerse the drain. This is more than a good detergent because it also stimulates the re-growth of normal flesh.

Avicenna used this ointment when there were multiple draining suppurating buboes: Take one-half lb. of white resin, five oz. of wax, two oz. of wine vinegar. Boil off the wine and keep it in a proper container. That ointment is useful in treating all draining wounds.

CHAPTER 22.C FISTULAS

A fistula is an open lesion extending from outside to the inside. Surgeons describe many kinds of fistulas, but the ancient Masters said that the true fistula is a firm tube from its onset, and, according to Avicenna, that is how it got its name (ie a musician's whistle).

The source of a fistula is either internal or external, be it an abscess, an ulcer, a maltreated wound or an excess of a humor that corrodes and forces its way through its confines or is attracted toward a cancer that cannot repel it. When we come to treat it, we must know the type of humor that is its cause so we may purify the patient with the correct medicines. That is to say, we begin with medicines that will mature the humors; by prescribing the correct laxative pills, dosed for one or two days. You can find several of them in our Antidotary (ie the Compendium Pharmacopeia).

When the offending humor is sanguine and there is a plethora, bleed from a vein that is suited for the region of the fistula. When necessary, you may bleed with cups rather than by phlebotomy, or when the fistula has developed in a fleshy region where there are many nerves, or in the nerves themselves, or in the necrotic shaft of a diseased bone.

In that last case, you must scrape and cleanse away the necrotic bone. Use the proper instruments which have angled ends. Remove the diseased bone and leave behind the healthy, as Hippocrates taught. True[256] Surgeons know that a fistula cannot be cured if one leaves

---

[256] Yperman uses the term 'Master' when he refers to a formally trained Surgeon, the product of the Scholia. Roger Frugard was the first to use the term 'Doctor' when referring to Physicians, whereas the common term before him was 'Master'. The term 'Ancient' did not alone describe someone from a much earlier epoch; rather it could refer to someone immediately preceding the writer, including his own teacher (LDR).

behind a shred of diseased bone. Do this: Dilate the outer opening of the fistula with the pulpy core of an elder-tree twig, increasing the diameter of the twig as the wound enlarges until you can gain admission for your powders and lotions made from wine and honey or other equally gentle substances. In time you will abate the purulent discharge and eliminate the vile tissues. Here is one recipe: Take quick-lime, atrament, bronze flower (186b) and alum. Grind them to a fine powder which you put on a strip of cloth previously moistened with egg-white. Or use verdigris instead of the other powder. Or use a drain covered with soap and dipped in vinegar.

Another: use powdered verdigris (481) and white alum mixed with honey.

Another: take incinerated salt and verdigris in equal amounts and make a powder.

Another: fill an empty egg-shell with orpiment and vitriol (490) and an equal amount of human feces. Incinerate them and pulverize the residue. Cover a drain with it and insert it to cure a fistula.

Another uses powdered euphorbia.

Another: take a live toad, some lumpy fibers of cannabis, some juices of rue and beans. Put them in an earthenware jug with some horse-manure and clay (32). Mix well and incinerate in an oven. Do not open the jug until it is cool. Pulverize the contents and insert it into the fistula. Use all the powders cited in this chapter until the drainage ceases.

Another: Constantine (ie Africanus) said that the ashes of an incinerated dog's head will cure a fistula.

Another: The Four Salernitan Masters recommended this: Take one ounce each of agrimony, saxifrage (413), arnaglossus (27a), centrum galli (196), tartar, and tartar with verdarain (481). Clean the area around the opening and insert a drain covered with the powder.

Another: When the fistula has several openings and your treatments cannot dry all of them, apply some warmed pellets of deer—feces ground with honey. The ensuing inflammation will induce suppuration, leading to a cure of fistulous cancers[257] and other infections.

---

257 Any type of necrotic ulcer (LDR).

Another for the same purpose: Take two oz. of powdered charred desiccated human feces (179) and one-half oz. of pulverized long peppers. Mix and apply.

Another, for fistulas with external openings:[258] Mince dove's foot geranium (160b) and crush it. Introduce the juice into the fistula. But if the opening is internal (ie not accessible), have the patient drink the juice.

Another, for fistulous cancers: [259] Boil the juice of titimal with sow-milk and add some myrrh. Wet a drain with it and insert it. It will dry the fistula, as I have observed many times.

Another: Cook euphorbia in white wine. It will dry the fistula and kill any worms that may appear, according to Master Gilles.[260]

Another: Take pigeon droppings and heat them with goat's milk. Use it to clean the fistula.

Another Take the juice of tassus barbatus (457) and boil it with honey until the juice boils off. Add powdered pomegranate peel and yellow myrobalans. Grind them and apply the paste.

Another: Grind sagapenum (399) with salt and apply it.

Another from Gilles: Desiccate the roots of titimal in an oven. Pulverize the residue and put it on a drain to be inserted.

Another: Apply ground orpiment, live sulfur and honey. Use it three or four times.

Another: Grind and apply a mixture of white pepper, dry figs and roots of parsley.

Another from Gilbert: Introduce the blood of snails.

Another: Introduce a fine powder of olibanum mixed with wine.

Another: A marvelous potion to be drunk when you cannot see an internal opening. I have seen it destroy fistulas and discharge the sequestra of necroitic bone: Take one-eighth maniple[261] each of

258 The surgeons and physicians believed that most fistulas began as chronic external ulcers that burrowed inward to reach an internal terminus. Occasionally, as expressed here, the source was internal, such as osteomyelitis (LDR).

259 Again be reminded that the author means any necrotic, undermining, excavating chronic ulcerating lesion, be it a phagedenic ulcer, a gangrenous or infarcted patch or a basal cell or epidermoid carcinoma (LDR).

260 Gilles of Corbeille. A 13thC Salernitan physician to King Philip Augustus. He wrote a book on urine, largely about urinoscopy, mostly taken from a book by Isaac Judaeus the Elder (c. 900 at Tunis).

261 Maniple: more than a pinch, less than a fistful (LDR).

arnaglossus (ie here it is strawberry, 446d) cannabis, seeds of lapathum, tormentilla, scabious and centaurea; two mpls of tansy. Mix all and cook them in two liters of white wine until it is reduced by half. Then add foamed honey. Dose two spoonfuls twice a day.

Another: Take one mpl each of red cabbage, abrotonin, fragaria (strawberry), cubebs (143), herb Robert (6), apium, and cannabis. Boil all in two liters of white wine with foamed honey until reduced by half. Filter and dose as above.

Another: Take one mpl each of the juices of betony (56), agrimony, artemisia, rue and marrubium. Mix with wine. Dose as above.

Another: Take one mpl each of cannabis (seeds or roots), strawberry, agrimony, arnaglossus, tansy, caryophylata (93), asparagus (39), herb Robert, blackbnerry (58a); one and one-half mpl of garance (197). Boil all in two liters of white wine, while adding foamed honey. Reduce by half. Filter before drinking. Dose as above.

Another: Take some wild salvia and mash it wine. Apply the plant on the fistula. It will work if you persist with it.

Another: Some authors say that you can obtain a cure by drinking the juice of nettles (305).

Another, recommended by Albert The Great[262]: Dose round aristolochium in white wine as mouthfuls of the liquid or as pills, three times a day, to empty and cure the fistula.

Another: Saint Benedict's herb (115) in wine. Drink four doses a day, and lay the macerate plant on the fistula.

Another: Take the juices of germander (200), herb benedict, agrimony (13) and add wine. Dose as above. Agrimony is known as one of the best remedies.

CHAPTER 23 C. THE APOSTHEM CALLED BILIOUS FIRE

Some authors call this abscess erysipelas because it is more fiery and dry. It meets no resistance as it enlarges and it turns black . The inflammation and the burning heat derive from bile which is concentrated in the lesion. The local heat chars and blackens and produces a metallic sheen. It does not come to a head and erupt and empty

---

262 The polymath Sainted Albertus Magnus, 1193-1280 (LDR).

itself of pus leaving an exposed cavity in which you can introduce medications.[263] It begins with redness and heat and induration.

The region ripens and rapidly erodes in the hottest spot, but it discharges very little. The opening soon ulcerates. The ignorant lay practitioner, not recognizing what it is, nor knowing what to do about it, not having studied the problem, and fearful in face of it, comes forth with some foolish ad hoc suggestions. He says that the abscess is due to a failure to light a candle at Arras, and that the victim should correct that deficiency by undertaking a pilgrimage to that shrine.[264] With that deceit the practitioner is freed of his patient, or the victim consults an ignorant physician who pretends to what really he does not know, and he advises the fellow to exhaust what is left of his native energies by wandering off to find some 'holy man' with a staff or a candle, to pray for help. When that 'saint' doesn't respond to the plea and the Natural forces have been expended, the victim dies. Everyone knows well when a person does not eat, The Lord cannot feed him, and in spite of his prayers and great penance, he will die of starvation. And so it happens, when the illness is serious and Nature alone cannot overcome it, you must use medicines to prevent the death of your patient. If the faulty humors are not potent, Nature alone may win, and can protect the patient. Therefore, before you do anything, pray to our all-powerful Lord, and bow to Saints Cosmas and Damien, [265] and then we may help Nature with our treatments. When a patient is at the point when he cannot eat or drink, we must relinquish him to God, yet try to help him as best we can.

The bilious mass that we call erysipelas is surrounded by a zone of heat and redness caused by the seething bile that brings inflammation to the surface from within. When it is ripe, the abscess softens as do most abscesses. [266] At times the inflammation spreads in the sur-

263 This is an open lesion, not the usual abscess, and cannot be treated as such (LDR).

264 Henri de Mondeville provided this comment: "In France it is called St. Mary's Disease; in Burgundy it is St. Anthony's and in Normandy it is St. Laurent's fire, And there are many more names."(See Henri de Mondeville's *Chirurgia*, op. cit. Tr. II, Doct. II, Ch. 1). St. Anthony's Fire also was the name for Ergotism (LDR).

265 Roman surgeons martyred in the 3rdC, later to become the patron saints of Surgery. St. Cosmas name became the title of the Parisian Society of Surgeons in the mid 13thC. (LDR).

266 Edema of the overlying skin (LDR).

rounding region, as a measure of its own virulence; at times it remains unchanged. When there is not much pus; at times it subsides
on its own. At times an abscess will erupt and discharge some dark
pus and bits of black tissue, as if the heat of the erysipelas had charred
them. The latter events often are the result of the poor surgical technique of someone who does not understand what can happen when,
for example, one wraps a bandage or binds splints too tightly when he
treats a wound or a fracture. That happens more often in young patients who bleed more vigorously, in whom the wounded region swells
to a greater degree, or when the medicated dressings are piled on in
excess of the need for compression. The tissues undergo necrosis
and turn as black as coal, as also happens when a horseman in cold
and wet weather rides in cold water and then tries to re-warm his
numb (ie frost-bitten) feet, not aware of the heat of the flaming hearth.
They may burn black and die.

Now let us go on to the treatments. When you are called to attend
a patient with erysipelas and the zone surrounding the lesion already
is red, he has waited to long. When the redness is intense, the heat is
great and the region is puffy and has suppurated[267] apply this repercussive: Take two oz. of bol d'armenie, one-half oz. of sangdragon, one
oz of terra sigillata and four oz. each of oil of roses and a good vinegar.
Mix by grinding in a mortar and apply it on and around the lesion.
Some surgeons use cool plasters hoping to reduce the heat, which
instead should be allowed to escape rather than be driven inward.
They believe that they will help destroy the abscess with cold, whereas
they simply increase the heat. Consider this analogy. An uncapped
jug that is boiling allows its hot steam to escape. And consider a person who bathes in cold water or has fallen into a cold pool or who
washes his hands in cold water on a cold wintry day or a ragamuffin
who owns very items of clothing. All those people retain heat because
their pores close. When we go to the public baths or sit by our stoves,
we open our pores and our heat escapes as if the door to a hot room is
opened wide,. and when our heat is lost, our nutriments are poorly
digested. Hippocrates said that bathing when your belly is full can
cause a fever. The food remains undigested in the stomach because

---

267 Obviously not a flood of laudable pus! Yperman describes the foul thin
    liquifaction of necrotic tissue (LDR).

the heat needed for digestion has escaped the body. Perhaps that explains why some people digest better than others during the winter than in the summer; the ambient cold causes (ie the pores to close) the body's heat to be retained.[268]

Use topicals to moderate the local heat and calm the inflammation and yet allow the heat to escape. The very wet plasters and their vapors act to reduce the bad matter, lessen the stiffness and gently relax the patient. The following is a good calmant to apply on the place where the abscess is pointing: Take bread-crumbs (65) and wine and make a plaster and some bread-soup. Apply it warm.

Another. Boil barley-flour, wine and butter to make a warm plaster. Then bleed from the nearest vein. That will shrink the lesion. Never apply a cup over the 'point'.

Chapter 24 C. Burns By Fire Or Hot Liquids How To Treat Burns Of All Kinds

Take finely minced pili lepre (345) and lay it thick on the burn.

Another for burns by flames: Split the roots of salex and mince the halves and mash them to a sort of ointment to apply directly.

Another, by Experimentator: Apply an emulsified egg-yolk with a feather-brush. That will suppress infectiion (ie inflammation).

Another by the same author: Make a fine powder of atrament. Mix it with egg-white and oil of roses until it is a medium-thick paste and spread it on the burn. The inflammation will subside as the burn heals.

Another: Lay a very thin sheet of lead on the burn.

Another: Incinerate some snail shells and pulverize the residue. Mix it with oil and wine and anoint the burn.

Another: Experimentator advised an immediate application of warm wine and warmed bovine feces and an emulsion of egg-yolk.

Another: Boil portulacca in water and apply the leaves.

---

268 This bit of reverse physiology, as completely wrong as it is, nevertheless represented an effort to explain what was observed in an epoch before there were thermometers. The fact that such a conjecture reflects the kind of science that was awakened by the likes of Roger Bacon, William of Okham and Robert Grosseteste in Medieval Europe. Wrong as it was, it was more than just an ignorant acceptance (LDR)

Another (a salve to keep in mind): Take the soles of old shoes (242a), some wax and oil of roses and cook them until the leather is gummy. When applied, it will ease the pain and heal the burns and other areas that have lost skin.

Another by Experimentator: Mix two egg-yolks with olive oil and apply.

Another: Beat olive oil and rape plants (377) in water until the leaves are saturated. Apply the oil with a feather-brush and cover the area with a thin cloth.

Another from Galen: Chop the rind of fresh limes (250) and boil them in water for a long time. Remove the soggy pieces and apply the decoction with a feather-brush.

Another recommended by The Four Masters: Distemper quick-lime nine times to weaken it. Then grind it with oil of roses and egg-whites. Then whip it into a medium-thick ointment. Apply it with a brush.

Another: Boil lime-peels in water for a long time. Mash the strips with the oil of the feet of oxen [269] (204) and oil of camphor. Warm it before brushing it on with a feather.

Chapter 25 C. Phlegmon Caused By A Sanguinous Humor[270]

This abscess is infiltrated with greasy blood. It is reddish but not deep red as is erysipelas, and it is not inflamed (ie hot) because it contains more of the serous element of blood mixed with the red matter. It enlarges and bulges, appearing like a loaf of bread. When it points and drains it discharges both blood and white (ie watery fluid) pus. It does not empty easily; rather, many small openings appear. Some call it 'four eyes'.

Treat it first by phlebotomy from a vein that is a tributary directed toward the affected part. If you want it to erupt, apply mitigatives and treat it as we do erysipelas.

---

269 Probably the collagen rather than an oil (LDR).

270 This aposthem probably is an edematous bruise with hematoma. The 'watery' leakage through many openings probably describes lymph emerging through pores (LDR).

Chapter 26 C. The Cool Swelling Called Zimia (Edema)

Zimia is a cool swelling derived from phlegm in joints or as encountered at the base of a limb, especially in a person who is cool and phlegmatic. Sometimes it is inflamed (ie firm); then it may redden. If that occurs, it seldom becomes hot except briefly. Occasionally it is discolored by bile (ie the yellow of a fading hematoma). This swelling never suppurates and erupts because it always matures inward (ie is absorbed). If it grows it promotes the formation of pustules by corrupting the veins and the arteries. If you want it to 'ripen' you must use warm medications to counteract the cool matter. Do not apply viscous topicals because they will promote the internal drift of the pus (ie the lymph) and discharge it inside. That will transform the humors and provoke abscesses in the lungs and fistulas.[271] The following are viscous and sticky medications and should not be applied on the cool phlegmatic masses: flax-seeds, malva, bismalve, lily-bulbs, psyllium, fenugreek and others like them.

On the other hand, use warm and dry medicines which include lyes (254) made from the ashes of grape-vines and oak wood. Soak a cloth pad, folded twelve times. in the lye and apply it warm for a good result. Then you may incise the swelling with a bistoury and introduce a drain of lint wet with warm wine. The next day, repeat the treatment after washing the wound with warm water or wine. Blot it dry and apply this detergent: Two oz. of the juice of wild celery, one oz. each of honey and wheat-flour and bring them to a gentle boil. Remove the pot and save the contents in a container. Use the medication on drains. Then cover the wound with a plaster made with the black ointment. The recipe is in our antidotary.[272]

It is the most useful of all the ointments. My recipe is as follows: Take one and one-half lbs. of olive oil, one oz. each of galbanum, mastic, frankincense and terebinth; four oz. of wax, two oz of colophony, three oz. of purified naval tar, one oz. of an ointment of sagapenum.

---

271 I can conceive the case of a 'milk-leg' or 'phlegmasia cerulea dolens' with iliofemoral venous thrombosis, massive edema, congested veins, pulmonary embolism and infarction leading to lung abscess, empyema and bronchopleural fistula! The 'pustules' on the leg are patches of ischemic necrosis (LDR)

272 This another version of Yperman's Black Ointment, the famous Ointment of the Apostles with its twelve ingredients. See Book I, Ch. 7 and 8, footnotes 18 and 19 (LDR)

Heat the oil and wax and let it settle before adding the colophony and naval pitch. Again let it stand. Then add the ointment of sagapenum and the terebinth. When the mixture is uniformly smooth, take it from the flame and allow it to cool until it is tepid before adding the finely ground mastic and frankincense. Continue to mix until it is cool. Keep it in a container.[273] This ointment warms and dries, and there are many uses for it in surgery. Many apothecaries stock it in their shops where it can be purchased.

CHAPTER 27 C. YPERMAN INTRODUCES THE FOLLOWING CHAPTERS ON WOUNDS

I, Jehan Yperman, now will deal with wounds of the veretebral column. When a wound enters the spinal canal and injures the spinal cord (ie marrow) high up where it meets the wide part below the brain, death is near, after much suffering. The same lethal outcome may ensue when the nerves emerging from the marrow are divided even though the marrow itself is intact; and the same holds for wounds that damage the 'tongue' of the cerebellum or that divide the ligamentum flavum alongside the spinal column. When the spinal cord is transected the result is lethal because the brain will empty itself through the cut end of the marrow. The treatments for all these wounds are the same, for the marrow, the bones, and the nerves. I will deal with them in special chapters.

CHAPTER 28 AND 29 C. WOUNDS OF THE LIVER

A wound that enters the core of the liver itself is always fatal. The victim loses his strength, as his blood is corrupted. But if the wound involves only the periphery, it can be treated as we do other wounds through the abdominal wall.

If some liver bulges through the wound in the abdomen wall, apply this decongestant; Take equal amounts of the juices of absinthe, the small sambuco, honey, vinegar and wheat-flour. Cook them all until the mix thickens to the consistency of honey. Make a plaster and

---

273 Probably PPC. See Chapter 1C, footnote 220 (LDR).

apply it. If that does not succeed, enlarge the wound and push back the eviscerated liver. Then treat the wound.

CHAPTER 30 C. WOUNDS OF THE KIDNEY

There are no curative treatments for wounded kidneys, because their tissues are firm, dry and too friable to hold sutures. The wound continues to discharge the urine which it removes from the blood reaching the kidneys from the liver. Nevertheless, as mortal as it may be, provide treatments for the external wound, using techniques and medications familiar to all Master Surgeons.

CHAPTER 31 C. WOUNDS OF THE URINARY BLADDER

When the membranous bladder-wall is penetrated, attempts to cure it will be to no avail. However, wounds in the bladder neck, the fleshier tissues, can be cured. In those cases, lay the patient supine[274] and limit the intake of fluids. Apply this powder in the wound: Take one oz. of bol d'armenie, two oz. of sangdragon, one and one-half oz. of hepatic aloes, one-half oz. each of frankincense (tus) and mastic. Pulverize all and apply it. Over it lay the constrictive plaster that we described in the chapter on wounds of the ear and the nose.

CHAPTER 32 C. WOUNDS OF THE INTESTINES

Here I will repeat what I have learned from the *Chirurgia* of Roland of Parma. Wounds of the small (ie narrow) intestine will leak liquid feces and are incurable. They always are mortal. That is not the case for wounds of the large and fleshier intestine. Sometimes a small wound can be successfully treated with wound potions alone. You can find prescriptions for them in the chapter on removing projectiles.

Larger intestinal wounds should be closed with sutures, allowing the long ends of the threads to dangle out the abdominal wound after you have replaced the wounded gut within the belly. Keep open the abdominal wall until the intestinal wound has sealed.

---

274 The wound is in the anterior suprapubic region. The supine position does not favor leakage (LDR).

At your first encounter with a patient with an abdominal wound (ie when the intestine is intact), reduce an eviscerated loop. If, as a result of prolonged exposure to cool air, the loop is distended, re-warm it with applications of warm wine or other liquids. If the open-ing is too small for an easy replacement of the eviscerated structures, enlarge the wound with your bistoury. Then treat the wound as we have taught.

Chapter 33 C. Treating Hernias Without Incisions

Not infrequently hernias appear with little discomfort. In such cases the surgeon can call them ruptures of the peritoneum only, and if they are fresh they can be treated with potions by mouth and appli-cations of plasters and pressure pads. I have been successful in many such cases at Ypres, but only for recently acquired hernias. If you can feel a firm margin of a hernia ring you must use the knife rather than medicines, and I advise all surgeons not to use non-operative treat-ments for ruptures that are old and have scarred margins; they are incurable except by cutting.

After a non-operative treatment, remand the patient to bed for six weeks and feed him a diet of flesh-forming foods which include warm milk, eggs, dates and butter, some veal, pork and mutton, and cooked buttered potatoes. He may eat small cooked patties of green veg-etables and butter.

My successes included the use of this potion: Take one mpl each of roots of royal ferns (181a), consolida, self-heal (424a), bruscus (66a), bugia (68). Grind them in a mortar and boil them in two liters of slightly pink white wine until reduced by half. Filter it through a cloth and dose a small swig three times daily until the hernia closes.

On the surface of the bulge snugly bandage a small plaster to keep it in place, the so-called hernia plaster.

Another potion: Mince and boil one oz. each of scabious, centau-rea, royal fern, European sanicula (424a) and herb Robert in two l. of wine and reduce by half. Filter and dose as above.

A woman who lives just outside the walls of Ypres had a two-year-old child with a scrotal hernia containing intestines. She reduced the hernia and put the child to bed and fed him small doses of minced herb Robert in wine. She cured him in one month without the use of a pad or a truss. That was possible because the hernia was fresh and the patient was a child.

I used another remedy to cure a forty-year old man in less than fifteen days. I took four mpl each of leaves and flowers of scabious (jacea) and caprifolia (84). I minced them and brought them to gentle boil in one l. of sweet wine and reduced it by one half. After filtering it I dosed him five spoonfuls twice a day. At the same time I gave him a thimbleful of this powder mixed into the potion: One dr. each of cinnamon, galanga, cipress nuts (149) and caryophyla and valerian, all pulverized. Also, I applied this plaster for treating hernias without incisions: One lb. each of colophony and wax, one dr. each of bol d'armenie, frankincense, mastic and the ashes of incinerated paper (107), three dr. of terebinth. Make a paste to be spread as a plaster; apply it when the patient lies supine and wrap a bandage to hold it snugly over the defect.

Roger (Frugard) described another plaster: Take one lb. each of naval pitch and resin, one-half oz. each of sangdragon, and human blood, three oz. each of terebinth and milk. Make a plaster and apply it on the hernia.

Another from Galen, which he used with his potion, with many successes in the city of Milan.[275] It works well for all kinds of rupture: Take three oz. each of naval tar, lard, wax and colophony; one oz. each of litharge, ammoniacum, galbanum, opopopnax, sumac, bdellium, serapinum, mastic, roots of consolida (both kinds), gum arabic and hare's beard (burnt); six oz. of mistletoe (211). Mix all with four oz. of a decoction of lambskin and viscous psyllium. Apply the plaster with a snug bandage and dose two spoonfuls of this potion twice daily. Take one mpl each of Blessed Mary's seal (361) and Solomion's seal (361), and the roots and leaves of plum tree and fennel. Boil in a lot of rain-water and make a decoction. Add sugar. Galen (Lanfranchi) cured many people at Milan with that combination of potion and plaster.

---

275 Certainly a copyist's error. The surgeon was Lanfranchi of Milan (LDR).

CHAPTER 34 C. APOSTHEMS OF THE PENIS THAT ARE CAUSED BY GAS

Some swellings of the penis derive from hot gasses. They inflate the bladder and then distend the penis. Sometimes penile swellings are soft, but they are different from the inflated and can be distinguished as follows. When you handle it remains erect and you can feel three caverns (ie the corpora cavernosa and spongiosum). That is a sign that it is inflated with gas. [276]

Treat that swelling (ie aposthem) which is quite common in children, as follows: First deflate all the gas. Then carefully anoint the penis and the scrotum with this: Three oz of oil of roses, one oz. of wax, melted together. Pour it into a mortar and grind them while they are warm. Pour in some cold water. Repeat the heating and dowsing with small amounts of water until the wax mixture can take up no more. Save it in a jar. and anoint the penis and scrotum as above. You may apply cloths soaked with a warm decoction of water lilies (491).

THE TREATMENT OF SOFT APOSTHEMS OF THE PENIS

These yield to digital pressure which produces a persisting indentation.

Formulate this medicine: Take thirty grape leaves, one dr. each of powdered frankincense and ceruse and enough rose-water to make a mild and soothing pomade. Apply it twice a day after first washing the part with warm water. Occasionally, when the penis is inflated, urination is painful and difficult to initiate. In that case, immerse the patient in a tub of warm water and allow the patient to urinate therein. Then bathe the penis and apply repercussive ointments to the entire region. Prepare them as follows: Mix one and one-half oz. of oil of roses with some rose-water, one oz. of wine vinegar, two oz. of bol d'armenie and one-half oz. of sangdragon.

Another: A tub bath of warm water containing simple invigorating

---

276 This concept of the nature of priapism comes from Galen (see *De Usu Partium*, Transl. by MT May, Ithaca, Cornell Univ. Press, 1968. Vol. II, p.656). The rapidity of erection and detumescence was explained by gaseous inflation and deflation. Humors cannot not move that quickly! (LDR).

agents such as violets, morel, chelidonium (mentelicum) et al.

Another: Some surgeons prescribe tub baths in warm sugared milk.

Another: When the erection is hard and pale, apply a plaster containing the ointment of absinthe described in the chapter on swollen testicles. Always wrap a clean bandage about one finger-breadth wide, beginning tightly at the tip and decreasing the tension as you approach the abdomen. That will disperse the humors and blood in the swollen organ towards the body. When you have concern for heat and inflammation, bleed from an hepatic vein behind the malleolus at the ankle to favor the evacuation from the penis and the re-absorption by the body of the flatulence that could be the source of the erection.

Another ointment: Boil four oz. each of the juice of solathrum, joubarbe (229) and two oz. of oil of roses. Add barley-meal to reach the consistency of honey. Keep it in a box. Use it twice daily after bathing the organ. The ointment calms and decongests.

Another for use in the winter when you cannot find morel (290a): Grind white bread-crumbs with rosamel and oil of roses. Heat while stirring until it is very smooth. Then add water to cool it. Apply it as warm plaster.

Another: Cook flax-seeds with malva to make a mucilage. Add oil of roses and apply as a warm paste.

CHAPTER 35 C. ULCERS ON THE PENIS

Treat open sores with detergents and desiccants. When the pain is caused by both internal and external lesions, first bathe the organ with warm water alone or with water that had been boiled with morel and leaves of violets. Then insert a strip of silken cloth to clean the inside of the urethra. Then use this cleansing powder as a soap in open ulcers: Take two oz. of finely powdered round aristolochium which you keep in a box.

Another powder that I have used to treat painful open penile sores: Desiccate common nettles in an oven and finely grind the residual cake. Use it as a powder. Over it apply this ointment: Take one-quarter lb. of ceruse, one-half oz. of litharge, one oz. of burnt lead (354). Add some oil of roses and wax and combine them by grinding in a mortar until the solids are inspissated. Save it in a box. When the glans is ulcerated, peel back the prepuce to expose it and apply the ointment on the ulcers. It abets the powder.

Another for an inflamed but not ulcerated glans (ie balanitis) requiring peeling back the adherent prepuce: Use a decoction of violets and mentelicum to bathe the organ twice daily. Then use a syringe designed for this purpose to inject some clean warm water in which you have boiled some mentelicum into the urethra. Irrigate as well as you can with three injections. As a fourth injection use a decoction of water-plantains (490b) and common plantains. Use it twice daily.

When the prepuce itself is ulcerated, apply the powders and the ointment as above.

Here is Hugh of Lucca's Treatment

When the penis is swollen and is covered with sores and the prepuce cannot be retracted, first bathe it with warm water. Then insert the small tip of a sound between the prepuce and the glans and gently work it all the way around. Then cover the tip of the sound with a bit of medicated cloth to clean the crevasse. After three such moves, dip the sound in oil of roses and repeat the action. Then wrap the glans with a strip of cloth wet with oil of roses to trap some of the oil under the prepuce. If there are sores on the shaft of the penis, apply our powder and then a plaster of the Rhazes' white ointment or this ointment : One oz. of fresh wax, three oz. of juice of morel and one oz. of juice of mentelicum. Cook until the juice begins to evaporate. Remove from the flame and PPC. I have used this to treat horrible lesions. It comforts. I inject some of it (thinned) into the urethra and the patients have recovered rapidly.

Another recipe given to me by a physician: Take a decoction of common plantain and inject it with a syringe and irrigate as well as you can. Then milk out the pus from the urethra. Scoop up a bit of the ointment on the tip of a sound and insert it between the prepuce and the glans, using three or four aliquots, or until the space is very clean. Then dip the sound in oil of roses and gently insert a strip of cloth wet with the oil, and allow it to remain. Then cover the part with a plaster made with Rhazes' Ointment: Use two oz of ceruse, one and one-half oz. of oil of roses, one oz. of white wax, one dr. each of powdered frankincense and myrrh. PPC. Apply it twice daily.

CHAPTER 36 C. ERYSIPELAS OF THE PENIS[277]

When first you encounter such a case, cut a pomegranate in halves and cook them in vinegar. Mash them in a mortar and apply the warm paste as a plaster. Then use the following repercussive around the lesion to prevent its spread to the abdomen: Take three oz. of bol d'armenie, one-half oz of terra sigillata, two dr. of sangdragon, four oz. of oil of roses, one oz. of wine vinegar and one-half oz. of rose-water. Mix and use as a defensive. PPC.

Another as a substitute defensive: Mix the juice of portulacca with a small amount of powdered camphor. Keep it in a jug, to be applied to the entire organ. If it is not effective and the erysipelas involves the glans which turns black, apply this ointment over the entire region until the necrotic parts become purulent: Take one oz. of a mucilage of fenugreek, one-half oz. of honey, one oz. of unsalted butter or fresh lard, one and one-half oz. of oil of violets and make an ointment to use as a plaster. This will cause the bad tissue to be demarcated from the good.

Another plaster: Mix and boil together three dr. of wheaten flour, two oz. each of egg-yolk and oil of roses, two oz. of the head ends of joubarbes, one oz. of vinegar to make a warm plaster. Keep it in place until the inflammation (ie heat) subsides and the necrotic proud flesh has demarcated. Then gently moisten and dry the organ, using warm wine. Then sprinkle this powder on it: Pulverize one-half oz. each of hepatic aloes, mastic and myrrh. Keep it in a container.

Another used by Roland (of Parma): When necrotic slough has come away, take two parts of rose-water to one part vinegar and wash the organ. He also said to wash the organ frequently with this decoction: one-quarter lb. of wine, one oz. of alum, one-half oz. of verdigris. Bring all to a boil and drip it on the exposed drain and cloth already in place. That will help to evacuate the pus..

277 See fn. 263 in Ch. 23 C (LDR).

Another (anonymous source): Use this irrigant: Take one lb. of rose-water and one-half lb. of wine vinegar and add this powder to the mixture: four oz. of ceruse, ten oz. of litharge, one oz. each of burnt lead (354), mastic and frankincense. Pulverize finely before adding some rose-water. Keep it for use, then warm it to clean the organ.

Another, for use when there is too much granulation tissue – a matter for the surgeon to judge: Apply this potent powder: Take equal parts of tartar, quick-lime and daffodils. Mix the powder with a lye made from bean juice. Use it only to erode all the granulation tissue. Another powder may serve as well: One-half lb. of finely powdered alum placed on a slate in an oven to incinerate it. When the powder has caked and is white, take it from the stone and grind it in a mortar. Put it on the proud flesh. It will eat it away and dry it. I have often used this powder of alum and I prefer it as better than that made from quick-lime, which is dangerous to use near blood vessels. You know that is the case with the penis. If you corrode into a vessel it will bleed.

After the eschar has separated, use the powder and the ointment that I prefer.

At times, some of the glans or the prepuce may hang loose. Cut it away and stem the bleeding with Lanfranchi's powder, described in the chapter on the head.

Chapter 37 C. Foods and Beverages

Warn the patient to avoid spoiled foods and beverages, and spicy foods such as garlic, onions, peppers, strong wine and cheeses, herrings and raw meat.

The sick man should drink sparingly and avoid salted foods. He should take only small amounts of beer, some teas and a small amount of still white wine. He may eat some eggs, butter, and every few days he may eat salted mutton or beef that is salted when it is raw (ie corned beef). He may eat small fish with white scales, such as carp, silver fish, pike and perch when they are freshly caught. He should add very little salt to his food to reduce his thirst. He should shun foods that heat the blood.

The sick man should be kept free of pain, limit his ambulatory activities and restrict his unhealthy emotions. His penis should be carried in a sack suspended from his waist.

Chapter 38 C. Cancer Of The Penis [278]

When the potions that we have described in the preceding chapters are not effective against the necrotic ulcer, you will know that it is a cancer of the penis. A cure can be obtained only by burning it away with a hot cautery.

Be near a hot fire (red charcoals) when you need to heat and apply a cautery. After that, apply unsalted butter or lard twice a day to calm the inflammation and to cleanse the burnt lesion.

Another cleansing and desiccating medicine to use after the eschar comes loose: Take one oz. each of arsenic (34) and alum and incinerate them in an earthenware dish. Then take four oz. each of human feces and dark blue cloth and incinerate them. Add some pomegranate peels to the ashes and pulverize all in a mortar. Apply the powder to the lesion and it will destroy the cancer. Then you will see clean red granulation tissue.

Follow with this powder: Take three oz. each of hepatic aloes, mastic and olibanum; one oz. of sangdragon, one-half oz. each of burnt lead (ashes) and ceruse. Pulverize and store in a box. Apply it twice daily. Make a plaster of the white ointment as follows: Take two oz. of ceruse, one and a half of oil of roses, one oz. of wax, one oz. each of powdered frankincense and myrrh. Make an ointment. PPC. Use it as a plaster. You can find an ointment for your purposes among the many listed in the previous chapters on ulcers of the penis.

Chapter 39 C. How To Arrest Bleeding From A Penile Ulcer

I have often seen bleeding from sores on the penis that has been so profuse as to enfeeble the patient before I was called to attend him. Once, at Ypres, I treated a poor peddler who suffered from a deep penile ulcer. It involved the dorsum about a finger-breadth proximal to the glans, and was full of foul matter. He had been treated

278 Any necrotic ulcerating lesion (LDR).

by an ignorant practitioner who had introduced a potent corrosive that had eroded a vein. It began to bleed furiously about midnight and continued until 10:A.M. The stupid surgeon did not know how to stop it, and they called me. I found him moribund, unconscious, seated on a cushion. Immediately, I placed him supine and pressed my thumb on the open vein, and held it a long while, while the peddler regained consciousness. Then I took some of the famous red powder and applied it to plug the opening in the vein. Atop it I placed some Indian maize-flour (granturco)[279]. and over that I set a piece of clean linen cloth folded in four plies, wet with the proper medication (ie see below). Before I left him, he had fully recovered his senses. When I returned to dress him the following morning, I used warm water to clean around the bleeding zone and I wet the compress to enable me to remove it without disturbing what was beneath it. Then I wiped the ulcer dry before I refilled it with the red powder. This time I covered it with a tampon wet with a decoction of plantains. Then I applied the 'proper medicine', Master Hugo's powder, made so: Take equal amounts of the whitest and most viscous frankincense (ie tus), hepatic aloes, sangdragon and bol d'armenie and made a powder, and PPC. This powder arrests bleeding and regenerates flesh to fill the defect. At every dressing I washed the wound with warm water and then with wine. I dried the wound and replaced the medicines. Then I anointed the abdomen down to the ulcer with this repercussive: Mix in a mortar three oz. of oil of roses, two oz. of bol d'armenie, one oz. of terra sigillata, one-half oz. of vinegar and three oz of rose water. I keep it in a jar to use as a defensive.

Another remedy used by Hugo; he often placed this plaster over the powder: Three oz. of oil of roses, one oz. of white wax, two oz. each of terra sigillata, burnt lead and litharge, to make a pomade which he stored in a jar.

Lanfranchi use this powder to control hemorrhage: Grind three oz. of oily white frankincense, one oz. of hepatic aloes and two oz of myrr. PPC. He made a paste of the powder by adding some of it and

---

[279] An anachronism. Indian maize was introduced into Europe by the Columbian voyagers 175 years after Yperman Granturco is a modern Italian word, it may not be the correct translation of the Flemish original or van Leersum's word for another coarsely ground cereal grain. (LDR).

some linen lint to the white ointment, and he spread it on a cloth moistened with a decoction of plantains.

CHAPTER 40 C. ABSCESSES AND SWELLINGS OF THE SCROTUM

These are caused by wounds, by overheating[280] or by congestion with the blood produced by it. These are the diagnostic signs: Redness; palpable heat; much inflammation (ie a tender mass) and severe pain. Treat them as follows: First bleed from basilic vein on the affected side. Then apply simple coolants, such as violets, hedera (215b) and solathrum. Boil them in water and let them drip almost dry before grinding them with whole-wheat grains. Then reheat with small amounts of wine and water and oil of roses. Apply as a warm plaster, twice a day. Before laying it on, wet the region with some of the water used to cook the medicines. Also, you may use a sitz bath based in the same water.

Another: Soak some compresses in wine vinegar and rose-water and apply them warm, twice daily, and then apply a cooling ointment described in our shapter on aposthems.

Another: When the foregoing are not effective, use this plaster: Take four oz. each of mucilages of flax-seed, psyllium and fenugreek; four oz. each of the gums of bdellium and ammoniacum; five oz. of wheat dust (177). Grind all and then boil. Apply as a very hot plaster. As always, wet the scrotum before applying any plaster.

CHAPTER 41 C. SCROTAL SWELLINGS CAUSED BY COOL MATTER

You recognize these by their pallor, hardness of the testes and by their terrible radiating pain. When the testes are firm and heavy use this plaster: Mix soft absinthe, deer-feces, mud from cow-pastures and pigeon droppings and heat them while continually stirring in wine. Make a plaster and apply it hot, after bathing the scrotum, with this lotion: which may also be used as a fumigant: Take two mpl of bismalve (18), one mpl of malva (273) and boil them for a long time in about six liters of water. Remove the greens and use the water to fumigate the scrotum. Then use it as a lotion before the plaster.

---

280 A euphemism for sexual hyperactivity (LDR).

Another: Take one mpl each of fresh absinthe, water cress, abrotonin, betonica and sambuco. Mash them and cook them in a wine of the Poitou. Make a warm plaster.

Another for swollen and inflamed testes: Take four oz. each of the juices of Herb Robert (cicuta), three oz. of vinegar; some fine bean-powder. Cook until just before they burn. Apply it as a very hot plaster. It will dispel the inflammation.

Another against cool humors:[281] Take equal amounts of beans, fenugreek, flax-seeds, anie, coriander and camomille flowers. Pulverize all and cook them in wine from the Poitou. A hot plaster will discharge the cool humors, as Master Louis von Mache claimed (ie unidentified).

Chapter 42 C. Scrotal Hernia

There are two kinds of testicular (ie scrotal) hernias: one is the hernia carnosa (omentocoele) called vlasch carnouffel in Flemish;[282] the other is the gaseous, or vind carnouffel.

The only cure for fleshy hernias is careful excision. Incise the skin at the groin and strip away the covering membranes, and free them from the canal (ie the spermatic cord and hernial sac) that suspends the testis. Transfix the isolated 'canal' with a threaded needle in two directions near the ring as we do for the other (ie not scrotal) hernias and we tie the threads amd excise the isolated structures. Then cauterize the cut end of the ligated mass to seal it and prevent a recurrence. Let the ends of the threads dangle out the wound until they come loose by themselves. Keep the patient flat in bed and treat the wound.

Chapter 43 C. Hydrocoele and Hernia Ventosa

A hydrocoele collects in the scrotum and appears as a tumefaction in the sac near the epididymus which is attached to the testis. Here is how you examine it and get rid of the fluid.

Some ignorant practitioners treat it by excising the testis as we do

---

281 Cool melancholy was the humoral cause of most 'cancers' (LDR).
282 Either a neoplasm of the testis or orchitis (LDR).

for hernias, and that is all wrong. They know not what to do. This is the correct way: Take a long curved cutting-edged (ie triangular) threaded needle and puncture near the bottom of the scrotum and enter the didymus and exit the opposite side of the scrotum followed by the thread. The fluid will escape. Leave in the seton for seven days; then you treat the small puncture wounds.

Some surgeons treat gaseous omentocoeles (ie hernias ventosa) in the same way, with a seton.[283] Others excise it with a bistoury and get rid of the gas and the swelling.

Chapter 44 C. Another Cure For Hernias

In a preceding chapter we taught how to treat hernias with potions and plasters, and trusses, without operations. Only recent hernias can be treated so. Now we will deal with hernias that are not cured in that way, using a method that does not sacrifice a testis and does not cause much pain. Prepare this medication: Pulverize two parts of quick-lime and one part of atrement. Grind the powder with some black soap to the consistency of bread-dough to use as a corrosive cataplasm. Lay a piece of leather with a hole set directly over the hernia defect in the groin, over the pubic bone. Put the caustic paste in the opening in the leather and leave it for an entire day. Then apply butter or lard until the eschar separates and comes away. That will expose the canal (ie the spermatic cord and processus vaginalis) that suspends the testis. Incise the 'canal' in its long axis. Follow the cut with a red hot cautery and burn right down to the bone; anything less will be to no avail. Then anoint the char with unsalted lard until that eschar also is discharged. Fresh granulation tissue will fill the defect and the scar will prevent further herniation from within the belly. Then treat the wound as usual.

During the course of the treatment the patient must spend forty days on his back, avoiding straining, sexual activity and eating fattening and gas-forming foods. That regimen begins three or four days before the operation and includes a light diet that keeps the body

283 This outrageous claim for successful treatments of 'gas hernias' by punctures
   or excision makes Yperman suspect for lack of personal experience with the
   terrible consequences of puncturing a gas-filled loop of intestine, which
   indeed is the wind-containing part of the hernia (LDR).

healthy and the belly flat. Before you apply the corrosive paste, carefully reduce the herniated intestine; it must remain within the abdomen where it is not at risk for damage by the caustic mixture.

Some surgeons do not use the caustic; they burn through skin (ie with the actual cautery) and all else down to the bone. Then they follow the measures described above. When properly performed, the treatment is secure and it spares the testis, although it makes great demands on the patient to endure the cautery. That is why many patients do not accept it and many surgeons do not use it. I myself never use the cautery alone because it is too dangerous.

CHAPTER 45 C. UMBILICAL HERNIAS IN CHILDREN

The navel may be very large in some children, and it may continue to enlarge and be very difficult to close by cicatrization. When it can be cured without an operation you first empty it by grasping it between your thumb and fingers and pressing the contents back into the abdomen; be certain that is complete. When some of the contents cannot be reduced (ie in cases of incarcerated hernias) the baby resists your efforts strongly and cries, indicating that there is pus and that you should not proceed further.[284]

When the color of the umbilicus is the same as the surrounding skin and you have reduced all of its contents, apply a previously prepared truss with a small pad at the center of a broad bandage which you set directly over the hernia. Knot the bandage over the pad. The pad covers a glob of this ointment: Mix equal parts of the ashes of lupin and linen cloth with vinegar and bits of lint. Change the paste and pad every day.

Another plaster for the same use: Take four oz. of black pitch, one-half oz. each of powdered mastic, frankincense and bol d'armenie. Melt the tar alone and remove it from the stove before adding the powders. Spread it on some hempen cloth.

When the treatment fails, do this: Grasp the umbilical skin with a forceps and completely reduce its contents. Then close the clamp at the base to keep the intestines within the belly. Ask the patient to suck in his abdomen if he can. Thrust two needles threaded with

---
284 Yperman describes a strangulated hernia with infarcted tissues (LDR.

strong threads through the skin at right angles. Encircle the sac and knot the threads and firmly close it. Then cut off the sac beyond the threads and remove the clamp.

The threads will remain until the infarcted tissue falls off. Then apply a desiccative paste. Continue with the pad and truss and watch the defect closely until it has healed.

CHAPTER 46 C. HEMORRHOIDS AT THE FUNDAMENT

Hemorrhoids are excrescences at the anus which at times are inflated by humors that collect there, especially blood that is oily.[285] They may burst open or leak blood. The symptoms of chronic hemorrhage are pallor of the face which may be yellow [286], the belly and the flanks may be distended with gas and the legs feel heavy.

There are four types of hemorrhoids. Some are long and broad, like mammary nipples; they are the worst. Others resemble mulberries and are the commonest. Still others are small, like grape seeds, and they are the least troublesome.[287] Some of them appear in front of the anus near the scrotum, others are further back at the sides of the anus. Some protrude and ooze, others are internal. The ooze usually as bloody but may be black like bile; it rarely is yellow bile, and even less often is phlegm.

The hemorrhoids that leak black bile are the worst type (ie teat-like). The mulberry types ooze pink blood. Those that leak phlegm (ie mucus) usually do so when the weather is warm and humid, especially in countries that have that climate. When the phlegmatic stuff is like egg-white, the belly may rumble.

When the hemorrhoids bleed, touch the bases with a hot cautery.[288] Galen taught that we should leave an opening in hemorrhoids that have oozed moderately for a long time, an opening through which the patient can continue to discharge faulty humors. Avicenna said that when you completely obstruct the hemorrhoids which are vents,

285 Contains small slippery clots (LDR).

286 We may guess that the cause of the hemorrhoids here is portal venous hypertension in a patient with cirrhosis of the liver, with jaundice, ascites and hydrops (LDR).

287 The fourth type probably are internal (LDR).

288 The bold advice is very different from the cautionary recommendations in Chapter 21 B (LDR).

you impose risks for hydrops, phthisis and mania, because Nature cannot purge the body as it had done by long habit. That is why you bleed from an hepatic vein in the right arm (ie as a preliminary measure). After such a purge and an evacuation by laxatives, you may treat the hemorrhoids externally with simple measures to dry them. Here are some remedies:

Pulverize equal amounts of the ashes of burnt lead and incinerated iron filings. Apply the powder frequently.

Another: Pulverize three oz. of acacia and two oz. each of ceruse and adracanth. Mix the fine powder with the juice of arnaglossus (93) and make an ointment. PPC. Apply it twice daily.

Another: Pulverize desiccated tassus barbatus. Apply it twice daily, PPC.

Another described by Roger: Pulverize pomegranate peelings (psidia –364) and grind them with vinegar. Apply on the hemorrhoids to dry them. If they are inside the rectum, insert drains covered with the ointment.

Another by Isaac (see Appendix II): Boil some beans and place them on lint as an application on swollen and inflamed hemorrhoids that are not bleeding.

Another: Chop roots of spica (celtic valerian) and cook them. Mix with wax and pitch. PPC. After using the paste for three days, bleed from an hepatic vein apply cups as near the anus as feasible.[289]

Another: Boil apium in wine and apply it on hemorrhoids and abscesses (ie fistula in ano)

Another: Apply walnut oil repeatedly.

Another: Mashed celery (root) with honey for use on bleeding piles.

Another: Powdered nettles and aromatic dill mixed with honey.

Another for use on Type I hemorrhoids: Mix powdered deer-antlers with wine cooked with honey honey, or with diasenna.

Another for use in cases caused by disordered brains:[290] Pulverize red and white coral, tragacanth and barley-meal. Put some of the

---

289 To cause the piles to extrude and be accessible for treatment (LDR).

290 The term remains unexplained. Perhaps the Author refers to the constipation, hemorrhoids and other afflictions of the inmates of the 'mad-houses' that existed in most cities (LDR).

powder under the tongue and let it melt before swallowing it. If it causes nausea, drink the powder in the juice of plantains.

CHAPTER 47 C. FISTULA-IN-ANO

Some fistulas are seen at the anus, other within the rectum, and some perforate.[291] You recognize it by its discharges of matter and gas. Other fistulas simply are pockets of pus that do not leak gas or feces. Perforating fistulas cannot be cured by drying medications; a surgical operation is necessary. Either use a seton or cut it open with a curved knife (ie shaped as a scythe). Then treat the open wound with the basilicon ointment to generate new tissue. After the fistula has been laid open with the knife, the patient is incontinent and there is no way to deal with it inasmuch as you cannot obstruct it.

However, you may be able to treat a very low (ie subcutaneous) fistula with potent topicals which I have listed in the chapter on fistulas. You can find many powerful detergents useful for cleansing them. One good ointment for cleansing and regenerating tissue is this: Take four lbs. of old lard, one oz. of verdigris, one-half oz. of sagimen and mix them. PPC. The ointment suppresses the drainage and eats out bad tissue (ie the indurated scar lining the tract).

CHAPTER 48 C PROLAPSED RECTUM

The rectum is the fundament and it may prolapse as a result of a swelling of nerves in the rectum and vulva. Treat it so: First have the patient sit in a hip-deep tub of water containing a decoction of equal amounts of balaustium, galls, oak-bark, pomegranate peels, acorns, and hypocystus (224).

Another: Take roots of serpentaria (35a) and wheat-flour. Bake it as bread in an oven. Have the patient eat some of it after heating it in a sauce pan.

When the rectum prolapses, wash your hands in warm water in which you have boiled and macerated psyllium (ie as a gel). Then push back the prolapsed part of the rectum.

291 The surgeon conceived the fistula beginning as an ulcer at the surface, which eats its way into the rectum (LDR).

If the extruded portion has cooled after a long exposure, bath it with warm red wine and sprinkle it with this powder before pushing it in: Take two oz. each of balaustium and cypress nuts, three oz.of mastic-tree bark and one oz. of ceruse.

Here is a suppository for the rectum: Grind and make suppositories with four oz. each of galls and cinnamon. Or fill two small sacks with the powder and dip them in rain water. Warm them before before inserting, one at a time, alternating them when they cool. Repeat the cycle many times.

Another method: Incinerate some grape vine shoots and serpentaria. Macerate the ashes with red wine and make a lye which you introduce as a clyster. Or use it in a sitz bath and its vapors will penetrate. It is a good remedy.

Another: Boil minced galls, acorns, balaustia, hypocystis, sumac and psidia with pomegranate honey and the peeled skins of medlars (274) in a basin. While it steams seat the patient over it and let it fumigate his fundament. Then give him a laxative of jacea (228b) or costus (135).

CHAPTER 49 C. TREATMENTS FOR LESIONS ON THE LEGS

Here I shall deal with the ulcers of the legs that surgeons call 'male morto', which are putrid.[292] When that appears behind the knee it is called 'mormael' (ie Flemish) or an abscess in bone. These lesions may be large or merely pustules with scabs. They may drain pus through several openings, pus which derives from melancholy.

To initiate your treatments, prescribe twice daily doses of this potion to hasten suppuration (ie to mature) in the offending matter: Take four oz of oxymel and two oz each of spring-water, white wine and a decoction of fumitory. Mix. Dose four small spoonfuls. After all of the potion has been consumed, purge with hierapicra (219d), as found in the pharmacopeia, The patient should abstain from foods that generate black bile, and he should take foods that are active against leprosy and cancer.

Bleed the patient from a splenic vein on the left arm. Do not wash the feet, but you must deterge all the pustules and ulcers to remove

292 Probably fetid chronic stasis ulcers (LDR).

the pus and to dry them. This is a good ointment for the purpose: Take two oz. of litharge, one oz. of ceruse, three oz. of oil of roses, three oz. of wine vinegar and one-half oz. of wax. PPC. Use it to make plasters. Always swab out the ulcers before you apply the plaster. Use this oil of the wood of the fraxinus tree for that purpose: Set two basins, one over the other, as we do for making the oil of juniper berries (479), a method called Ebe Mesûe. This oil of fraxinus is the best for use against scabies, excema and herpes zoster, as is described elswhere in this treatise.

Here is a pomade to relieve itching: Take one lb. of lard from nursing pigs, one lb. of ceruse and one lb. of salty mayonnaise. Grind them together until it is uniform and make a plaster. When applied warm, on a cloth, the mayonnaise alone relieves itching around wounds and ulcers.

CHAPTER 50 C. ABSCESSES ON THE LEGS

The aposthems of the legs, from knees to feet, that are fixed to bone and erode through the overlying skin are incurable. Even at the onset, if the inflammation makes the knee or the feet swell, the treatment is difficult. The color of the skin is a clue to the cause; it is due to blood destroying from within.[293] Begin your treatments with decongestive maneuvers and a limited diet that avoids foods that corrupt the blood.

The patient should take three oz. of 'triferamino'[294], one-half oz of thus and ginger. Drink some of the mixture twice a day. Apply this ointment over the bulges: Take one oz. each of powdered aloes, myrrh and acacia. Mix them with styptic wine and a decoction of cypress leaves or cyclamen. In hot weather anoint the affected region with a hot pogram (?) When the abscess threatens to erupt or leak, open it at once and treat it as we described in the preceding chapter.

---

293 Here Yperman refers to the 'blue' skin overlying bunches of distended varicose saphenous veins (LDR).

294 An unidentified plant. One that bears flowers three times a year (LDR).

CHAPTER 51 C. CANCER IN THE LEG

Crusted tumors are cancers, usually caused by salt-phlegm or altered black bile. They are very difficult to treat. The phlegmatic source is revealed by these signs: itching, abundant scabs and desquamation. There may or may not be an ulcer. Treat it so: Dose the patient at night when his stomach is empty. Give two and one-half oz of Mesûe's fetid pills (264), or use this: Take one oz. of black hellebore, one-half oz. of scammony, two oz. each of turbith and opium and make pills by moistening them with wine in which you have boiled some fumitory. Make the pills the size of chick-peas and always dose an odd number of them.

Give one or two oz. and then bleed from a dorsal vein on the hand between the fourth and fifth fingers. That vein attracts blood from the entire body, ridding the blood of its black bile. The vein is situated in the same region as the vein used in the chapter on mal mort (Ch. 49).

The sick man must avoid foods that form black bile in the blood, and we should follow this course of treatment (for cancers due to melancholy): First expose all the lesions (ie remove scabs, etc.) and apply this paste which the authorities claim will cure : Take one oz. each of ceruse and sulfur, one-half oz. of mercury and make an ointment. Then add the whites of two eggs and a small amount of vinegar. PPC.

When the ulcer stinks, it is a cancer, and one uses the Venus ointment, prepared so: Take two lbs. of olive oil in the winter and three oz. in the summer; one lb. of mutton-fat; five oz. of wax, six oz of naval tar, some gum ammoniacum, opoponax and galbanum. Pulverize the gums and grind them with the others and add hot vinegar. PPC. Follow that with a consolidative.. In these patients we use purges and bleed from a basilic vein on the foot.

Another detergent to remove crusts and smooth out irregularities: Take a strong wine vinegar, heat it and wash the sores every day. Then apply this plaster: Take one-half lb. of honey, four egg-yolks and beat them together while adding barley-meal until it is well saturated. This will cleanse and regenerate.

HERE ENDS THE CAMBRIDGE CODEX

PART III
ELEVEN CHAPTERS TAKEN FROM THE GHENT CODEX[1]

Chapter 1 G. On Dislocations

A wound or a contusion or a fall or a leap or a yawn may include a dislocated joint. All of them may a require a surgeon's attention.

Chapter 2 G. Dislocated Mandible

One person holds the patients head and the surgeon inserts a finger or thumb in the mouth and reduces the dislocation.

Chapter 3 G. Fractured Mandible

Set the fracture by traction on the loose fragment. Then wrap a bandage as we described it in the chapter on fractures. Add a second bandage to hold a pad in place over the fracture-site. Treat the patient as for other fractures.

Chapter 4 G. Dislocated Necks

An assistant inserts a strip of wood cut as thin as a bread crust between the victim's teeth to maintain an airway. Place pads over the shoulders and allow other assistants to support the body and pull the arms in the axis of the body, while the surgeon (ie with feet against the shoulders) distracts the head by the hair or hands under the chin and reduces the luxation.

---

1 These eleven chapters are fragments remaining in the Ghent Codex in the text of Van Leersum. They will be numbered 1 G, 2 G. etc. (LDR).

CHAPTER 5 G. DISLOCATED SHOULDER

One assistant holds the body while a second pulls the arm and the surgeon pushes from beneath the axilla and directs the humerus into the joint.

CHAPTER 6 G. DISLOCATED ELBOW

One assistant pulls the humerus while the surgeon flexes the forearm and uses his thumbs to press the dislocated bones into the joint.

CHAPTER 7 G. DISLOCATED HAND (IE WRIST)

While an assitant steadies the arm, the surgeon pulls the hand and molds the bones at the wrist.

CHAPTER 8 G. DISLOCATED FINGERS

An assitant holds the hand while the surgeon pulls the finger.

CHAPTER 9 G FRACTURED HUMERUS AND FOREARM

A single curved bone occupies the upper arm, whereas two straight bones are in the forearm, where one or both may be fractured, with or without open wounds. A fracture of one forearm bone is less serious than a simultaneous fracture of both bones, and a compound fracture is the most serious.

When the single bone (ie the humerus) is broken you will need two assistants, each to hold a fragment and apply traction so the surgeon can place them on end, and feel crepitus as a sign of success. Then apply pads and bandages.

When an open wound exists, lay pads of four plies of linen about a hand-span in length alongside the wound and thick enough to push the wound edges together when they are bandaged. Wrap them with four narrow bandages no closer than a finger length or farther than a half hand-span from the edges of the wound.

When there is no wound, use eight bandages and three pads, folded in four. Wrap them thickest where the skin is thinnest directly over the fracture, and decrease the tension as you approach the ends of the dressings. Wet the bandages under water and squeeze out all the air. Then dip them in egg-white. In that way you will distribute the medications the length of the arm, with more of it at the middle (ie the fracture-site).

When there is only a small wound, cover it with a medicated pad and two compression pads, each of them two finger-breadths long. Wet the bandages with egg-white and squeeze out the excess. Cover one bandage with the red powder and be careful not to bend the arm while you wrap all the bandages, one atop the other. The pads alongside the wound should lie in the axis of the arm to allow you to expose and treat the wound. Lay thin wood splints over all. They should be shorter than the arm and not touch the skin beyond the bandages. Use as many splints as are necessary, spacing them to allow free aeration and to avoid gangrene or overheating, which can be harmful. By the application of two many splints and by binding them too tightly a bad surgeon will cause erysipelas and much suffering.

Cover the intact surfaces away from the wound with some linen cloth, a sheet of felt or of very closely shorn sheep-skin, no longer or wider than the medicated arm. Over all tie three cords, one at the center and two at the ends, to enclose four or five splints, leaving gaps for aeration etc. Tie the cords loosely enough to let you slip under them three tubes, about the length of a finger, made of silver, bronze or elder-tree bark. The tubes should be well oiled inside and out. The will be twisted (ie tourniquets) to adjust the tension. Turn the center tube clockwise and the end tubes counterclockwise. When the proper tension is reached the tubes should meet end-on, This type of binding and splinting also is used for treating fractured legs.

The splinted flexed arm then is held to the chest by a scarf. The splinted leg is held extended and slightly elevated in a tub or suspended between two straw pads, each as thick as an arm.

When you remove the bandages to treat wounds, be sure to maintain the immobilization of the fracture until the fracture is united.

Chapter 10 G. Fractured Clavicle

When the fragments are displaced (ie over-ride), the surgeon uses traction to separate and to reposition the ends. Then lay a large pad over the fracture and place a round cushion in the axilla. When the fracture is real but not displaced hold the flexed arm in a sling until the fragments are united (ie by firm callus).

Make a paste of lint moistened with egg-white and some other medicine in water (ie a decoction) Use a very long and wide bandage that passes over the shoulder to hold the pads. The medicated plaster over the clavicle is held by criss-crossing over both shoulders and under the opposite arm. Use seven or eight turns and sew the bandages in place, and leave them as long as necessary.[295] The followup treatments are those we used for fractured legs.

Chapter 11 G. Fractured Ribs

When you treat fractured ribs, cover your hands with a thick honey or resin. Place cups over the fracture and replace them as soon as they need re-heating. Then jerk them off quickly. Repeat the maneuvers frequently until the depressed fracture is drawn into a normal alignment. Then apply the apostolicon spread on a piece of leather. We use no pads; simply bandage the medication in place.

HERE ENDS THE GHENT CODEX

---

295 The wrap is like the modern Velpeaux dressing. By holding the elbow against the chest, the cushion in the axilla is a fulcrum over which the lateral fragment of the fractured clavicle is distracted (LDR).

APPENDIX I A SURGICAL PHARMACOPEIA

A LIST OF SIMPLES AND COMPOUNDS
THE FORMAT

This long list of medications is compiled from the English editions of the eight treatises by Roger Frugard, Roland of Parma, Bruno of Longoburgo, Theodoric (by Campbell and Colton), William of Saliceto, Lanfranchi of Milan, Henri de Mondeville and our Author here. In the treatises of William of Saliceto, Lanfranchi of Milan and Jehan Yperman the substances are numbered so to more easily identify them in the pharmacopeias which I have appended to all seven of the works translated by me.

The numbered medications are the major element in the list, and they include most of the items used by the authors in whose Englished texts numbers are not used. In other words, most of the medieval surgeons used the same medications in common with their surgical and medical contemporaries and predecessors. A few items that are not numbered in the alphabetized list denote medications used only by one or two of the group.

Therefore, most of the un-unumbered items are common names for popular herbs and medicinal substances, variant spellings and some terms that may lead the Reader to what she or he seeks among the numbered items.

Following each entry there are synonyms, one or more common names and variant spellings, and the names which modern translators have used in the Italian and Anglo-Norman French editions of Roger and Roland (**R** for both of them), the Italian of Bruno (**B**), The English of Theodoric (**T**), the French of William (**W**), Henri (**H**), and Yperman (**Y**) and the Middle-English of Lanfranchi (**L**). The initials in bold-face type placed at the end of most of the entries indicate the authors who mentioned the substances which I have culled from the texts that were available to me. Many of the items are followed by "see" which refer the reader to numbered items for additional information.

Wherever I can do so, I identify the plants by botanical terms in an *Italic font*. I cannot claim accuracy in many cases, especially where the 19thC and 20thC botanists and herbalists have themselves confused me with variant nomenclatures. I have used Professor Saint-Lager's terminology in Henri de Mondeville's text and Mrs. Grieve's book as well as dictionaries and encyclopedias for assistance in those matters. The Alphita has helped in some cases.

As stated in my General Introduction, I believe that there are only a few items missing from the list, and I apologize for any such deficiencies. The list probably is a nearly complete *surgical* pharmacopeia for the century-and-half during which the major works were written.

A PREFACE FOR THE LIST OF MEDICATIONS

A Medieval Surgeon's materia medica for the most part were Topicals. The List that follows here names the substances used by the surgeons as Simple Medicaments or as combined in various forms of Compounds, nearly all of them for external applications, that is, as Topicals. Many of the same substances, indeed many more than appear here, were used by the non-surgical Physicians who prescribed them as medicines to be taken by mouth or administered as clysters, etc. Aside from the very few of them that the surgeons were permitted to use, the laxatives, for example, and some potions, they are not in our list.

WEIGHTS AND MEASURES FOR MEDICINALS

The standards changed from epoch to epoch and from place to place, and the modern equivalents are approximations.

Baas (cf. p.263) cites The Antidotarium of Ncolaus Praepositus of

Salerno (1140):

1 scruple (scrupula)	20 grains (grana)
1 dram (drachma)	22 scruples
1 hexagium	1 1/2 dram
1 ounce (uncia)	6 hexagia
1 pound (libra)	12 ounces
1 sextarius	2 1/2 pounds

Hunt (cf p. 59) states that the Salernitan system was based on the grain (grana)

1 siliqua	1 grain of wheat
1 obol	3 grains
1 scruple	2 obols
1 dram	3 scruple
1 ounce	6 drams
1 pound	12 ounces

Other measures are stated in the texts. For examples:

A maniple in Yperman: Somewhere between a large pinch and a small handful.

A liter in Yperman: A liquid amount somehow equivalent to a pound.

THE LIST

1.	Absinthe	oil of wormwood, avrotonin, aloisne. *Artemisia (sev.species).* **R B W L H Y**
1a .	Abrotonin	aurone, southern-wood. see 35. **Y**
2.	Acacia	sap of *Acacia arabica,* Gum Arabic.sometimes dry prunella (368b) see 212. **B T W L H Y**
3.	Acanthus	Bear's breech. see 64. *Acanthus mollis.* **L**
4.	Ache	apium. see 29, 97. *Apium graveolum..* **R W L Y**
	Acedula	rumex, acetosa. see 395. **R**
4a.	Acetum	vinegar. see 484
5.	Acoris	sweet sedge. see 74, 75, 422, 434, 444. **W L**
	Acorns	glans quercus. see 203, 309a. **Y**
6.	Acus muscata	Robert's herb, crispula, geranium, Gratia Dei. see 209, 366.*Geranium Robertianum.* **H Y**

7. Adiantum   delicate ferns, maiden hair, venus hair. see 362, 363, 476. *Adiantum capillus veneris.* **T W Y**

Adeps   beef lard. see 206. **Y**

8. Adracanth   tragacanth, diagradon. see 466. **H Y**

9. Adustum   ashes. see 38. **L Y**

10. Aes   chalcanthum, ios, bronze. see 65a, 482. **W L H**

Affodil   garlic. see 43,198 and sometimes daffodil 301. **R**

11. Agaric   a mushroom. *Polyporus igniarius.* **R T W H**

11a Agnus castus   goat-weed. see 22, 205. also chaste-tree, *Vitex trifolia.* **T**

12. Agresta   sour-grape (uva acerba) juice, verjus; (also memitte, a poppy). see 245a, 335, 478. *Vitri vinifera.* **T L H**

13. Agrimony   the herb. see 172. *Agrimonia eupatorium.* **T H Y**

Ailes   allium. see 16a, 43.

14. Airaine   'flower' of bronze, areim, ereim, eneim. see 481. **R W L H**

Alabaster   calcium carbonate, resembling gypsum. see 214. **Y**

Albugasse   donkey's milk. see 286. **W**

Alexander's Ivy   lovage. see 247, 256, 430. **T**

15. Alkanna   henna *Lawsonia inermis.* **T W H Y**

15a. Alkitron   cedar resin. See 96b. **H**

16. Alleluia   a clover, weed sorrel, oxalis, paniscuculi. see 395 et al.. **R L H**

16a. Allium   garlic. see 43, 198. **H Y**

17. Almonds   bitter or sweet. see 309. *Amygdalis communis.* **W H Y**

18. Althea   guimauve, geumalve, marsh mallow, bismalve. see 273. **R B T W L H Y**

19. Aloes   aloe vera, picra, pigré. Horse aloes are unpurified. *Aloe socotrina.* **R B T W L H Y**

20. Alum   (alun) from wine lees (potassium tartrate) or from crystals. Alun de roche is sugar-alum (aluminum sulfate), alumen de pluma (feather

alum) is halotrichite (iron-aluminum sulfate) etc. **R B T W L H**

20a. Amber   see 85. **T W H Y**

20b. Ambergris   from whales. here more likely ambrosia. see 35. **Y**

21.   Amidum   flour of various grains, amylum, usually wheat, froment. see 177, 187, 395a, 436, 494. **T W L H Y**

22.   Ammi   goat (or gout) weed, seeds. see 11a, 205. *Ammi visnaga or majus.* **W**

23.   Ammoniacum   hore-hound. resin of *Dorema ammoniacum.* or *Bubon gummifer.* **B W L H Y**

24.   Amome   ginger family. see 201. **W**

24a. Amorantus   almarus, amens. see 42 *Amaranthus hypochondria and blitus.* **T H**

24b. Anabulle   euphorbia. see 173. **H Y**

25.   Anacardus   cashew nut, elephant-foot tree. *Semicarpus anacordium.* **T W L H Y**

      Anagallis   pimpernel. see 292, 348. **Y**

25a. Andronium   a primrose. *Primula vulgare.* **T**

25b. Anemone   wind-flower and herb. *Anemone pulsatella.* **T**

26.   Aneth   dill, or sweet anise. see 158. *Anethum graveolens.* **R W L H Y**

26a. Angelica   emperor's herb. see 167. *Angelica archangelica.* **W H**

27.   Anise   leaves and seeds. see 349. *Pimpinelle anisum.* **R W H Y**

27a. A(r)naglossa   arnaglossus, plantain. see 93, 202, 353. **Y**

      Anthera   from roses. see 389. **H**

28.   Antimony   stibium, metal filings. **T W L H Y**

28a. Ants   insects and eggs. **T L H**

28b. Apis   honey bee. **H**

29.   Apium   many species. ache, batrachium, patalupi, wild celery, persil, wild parsley, petroselinum. see 4, 97, 344. *Apium graveolens.* **T W L H Y**

30.   Apostolicon   Apostles'Ointment from twelve ingredients:

23, 33, 53, 188, 194, 253, 299, 312, 321, 379, 482, 493 also called Black Ointment and Venus ointments. **R B T W L H Y**

30a. Apricot — see 33a. *Prunus armenica.* **T**

Apple — poma. see 363a.

30b. Aqua forte — nitric acid. **W**

31. Araignee — spider web. **R H**

31a. Argentum Vivum — mercury. see 283. **W H Y**

31b. Arancium — orange. see 119, 322. **W L H**

32. Argilla — terra sigillata. clay. see 59, 119a, 460. **W L H Y**

33. Aristolochium — snake-root, malum terrae, polyrrhyzon, clematis, birth-wort, serpentaria, see 58, 120, 142, 376. *Aristolochium rotunda.* **R T W L H Y**

33a. Armoniacum — armenian apricots (not ammoniacum). Sal armoniacus see, 30a, 424. *Prunus armeniacus.* **R T W**

34. Arsenic — auripigmentum, orpiment, sublimate of arsenic sulfate or oxide. see 43c, 327 (not 424). **R B T W L H Y**

35. Artemisia — abrotonon, citronella, mugwort, armoise, aurone, ambrosia St. John's plant, absinthe. see 1a, 20b. *Artemisia vulgare.* **R W L H Y**

35a. Arum — dracuntium minus, cuckoo-pint, dracunculus, calf's-foot. see 500. *Arum maculatum, Dracunculus vulgaris.* **T H Y**

35b. Arundo — marsh-reeds. see 386. **W**

36. Asa Dulcis — laser, benzoin, tapsii. see 41, 447, 461. *Styrax benzoin.* **T W H**

37. Asafoetida — assa *Ferula foetida.* **B T W L H Y**

38. Ashes — see 9, 60, 99, 111, 117. **R B T W H Y**

38a. Ash tree — tamarix. see 189, 264, 453. **R H**

Aspen — tree poplar. see 364a.

39. Asparagus — asperge, asparagus roots or stems. *Asparagus officinalis.* **T W H Y**

40. Asphodel — albutum, anthericon, centum capitum, porrago. roots of *Asphodelus albus.* **W L H**

41. Assefan   styrax. see 36, 447. **W**
41a. Assius lapis   a stone from Assa (the Troad). **W**
     Atrement   atrament. vitriol based. see 490 et al. **W Y**
42. Atriplex   hortense orache, arroche, pes locustae, straw-
                        berry spinach, blite. see 24a *Atriplex hortensis*. **T
                        W H**
43. Aulx   ailes, garlic, allium, elinnium, affodile (wild),
                        ramsome, porrum. see 16a, 43, 365a. *Allium
                        sativum*. **R T W L**
43a. Aunée   scabwort, inula. spikenard. see 437 et al. *Inula
                        helenium*. **T W**
43b. Aurea   aurum. a decoction of gold particles in water
                        or vinegar. **T**
43c. Auripigmentum.   orpiment. see 34, 327. **R T W L H**
     Avellana   hazel-nut. see 309.
     Avena   oats, haveron. see 310. **T H**
     Avrotonin   abrotinin. see 1a, 35. **T W L Y**
44. Axonge   lard, lardon, oint, sui, axungia. see 206 et al. **R
                        L H Y**
45. Bacca populi   poplar berries, bourgeon. see 364a. **W**
46. Baccar asarum,   asarabacca. *Asarum europaeum*. **W**
47. Balaustium   wild pomegranate flowers. see 364. **R B W L H
                        Y**
48. Balsamdendron   balm of gilead, xylobalsamum. see 53, 90, 299.
                        Balsamodendron opobalsamum. **T W H Y**
49. Balsameta   St. Mary's herb, costmary, mace. see 454
                        Tanacetum balsamita. **H Y**
49a. Barba hircina   salsify, goat's
49b. Bardana   sorrel. see 236 and 395 ety al. (also Burdock).
                        R H
50. Barecha   melon. see 144a 280, 369. **W**
     Barley   see 323
50a. Basilicon Oint.   53, 206, 312, 360, 379, 493. see 314. **H Y**
51. Basilium   basilicon, herb basil, wall-thyme. *Ocymum
                        basilicum*. **T W H**
     Battitura   chalcanthum. see 106 et al. **T**

52.	Baucia	pastinaca. parsnip or carrot. see 152. **L H**
53.	Bdellium	procerion. a balsamic resin. see 48. *Balsamodendron africanum.* **T W L H Y**
	Beans	fava. see 178.
	Bedegar	wild roses, eglantiere. see 53c.**R H**
53a	Bees	**H Y**
	Beeswax	mu. see 176, 293, 329a, 397 329a.
	Belladonna	henbane. see 217 et al. **Y**
53aa.	Belliculus	blata bysantia, belliculli marini. purple and white marine snails, source of royal purple dye. **T W**
	Belsegensina	coriander. see 132.
53b.	Ben been.	*Moringa aptera* .**W**
53c.	Bendegard	bedegar. gall from stem of eglantine rose. see 389. **W Y**
53d.	Bennett	Herb Bennett. see 115, 116. **Y**
54.	Beta	Bleta , betta, beets. *Chenopodiacia.* **W H**
55.	Berberis	bartberry, cortex bugia. see 68. *Berberis vulgaris.* **L H Y**
55a.	Berula	an herb, a variety of apium. *Berula angustifolia.* **T H**
56.	Betonica	betony, scrofularia, figwort, vetony,. citonia. see 109, 155a, 185a *Betonica officinalis.* **R T H Y**
57.	Bile	melanchiron, fiel, fellis. see 183. **B T W L H Y**
	Bindweed	scammony. see 416. **H Y**
58.	Birthwort	asirinum, aristolochium, snake root. see 33 et al. **T Y**
	Black Ointment	see 30. **Y**
58a.	Blackberry	sometimes mulberry.see 294, 393. **H Y**
	Blood	see 409.
58b.	Blueberry	whortleberry, airelle. *Vaccinium* var. **H**
59.	Bol d'armenie	a clay containing iron oxide, various clays— German, Bohemian, etc.—sometimes fuller's earth, cimoleam. **R B T W L H Y**
60.	Bombacyna	ashes. see 107, 333. etc. **T W**
61.	Bone-marrow	medulla, midolle, meule. see 275. **T W H**

62.	Bones	of geese, hens, deer. etc. hooves, ivory, horns, antlers, squid etc., all burned and powdered. see 133. **T W L H Y**
63.	Borax	borax, sodium borate; see sal de nitre, also sagimen nitri, nitrum, boracis, bourach. see 402. **R W L H Y**
63a.	Borrago	borrage. *Borago officianalis.* see 69. **R T L H** y
	Bouillon	see oat, wheat.
63b.	Boxwood	dogwood, ammon's horn. *Cornus amonum and floridum.* **T H**
63c.	Bran	sou. see 21. **T H**
63d	Brandy	of any fruit. Eau de vie is from grapes **H**
64.	Branca Ursina	acanthus, brama, bear's brush. see 3. *Acanthus mollis or Heraclium spondylum.* **T L H Y**
64a.	Brassica	generic term. see 71, 377 et al.
65.	Bread	crumbs are mica panis, see 285. **T W L Y.** Panata is bread soup. **W Y** Opirus is whole-wheat bread. **T**
	Bresillet	caesalpina sappan (later called the Brazil tree) **H**
65a.	Bronze	aes. see 14, 481. **H**
66.	Broom	planta genesta. *Cytisus scoparius.* **H**
	Brown Ointment	a regenerative mentioned only by referrence to Nicholas.
66a.	Bruscus	butcher's broom. see 221, 226a. *Ruscus aculatis.* **T W Y**
67.	Bryonia	brionee, viticelle, root of bryony, also sicadis, labrusca. see 120, 144 182, 489. *Bryonia dioecia.* (White bryony, a poison, is *Momordica elaterum,* really a cucumber). **R T W L H Y**
68.	Bugia	root-bark of barberry bush, cortex bugia. see 55. **W H Y**
69.	Bugloss	borrago, blue weed, lingua bovis, lithospermum. see 63a. *Echium vulgare, Borrago officianalis or Anchusa officianalis.* **R T W L H Y**
	Bulbus	onions. see 319, 415.

	Burdock	sorrel. see 236 and 395. **R Y**
	Burith	soap. see 412, 430. **R**
70.	Butter	from cows, also sweet butter, May butter, bure de mai. **B T W L H**
71.	Cabbage	choux, chaux, caulis, cholet. *Brassica oleracea.* **R T W L H Y**
	Cacumia	climie. see 121.
71a	Cadmia	cadmium sulfate, sory, climie. see 96a et al.
72.	Calamint	thyme. see 278. *Melissa calaminthus.* **T W H Y**
73.	Calamite	styrax. see 447. **T W**
74.	Calamus	aromaticus, squinanthus, sweet sedge, sweet flag. see 5, 75,422, 444. **B T W L Y**
	Calf's foot	arum. see 35a et al.
74a.	Calx viva	quick-lime. see 251. **L H Y**
	Camedreos	germander. see 200.
75.	Camel grass	calamus. see 74, 416a, 422, 444. *Andropogon schoenanthus.* **H**
76.	Camomille	chamomile (several varieties) cotula. *Anthemis nobilis and A. pyrethrum.* **B T W L H Y**
76a.	Campanula	rampion. *Campanula indicas.* **T**
77.	Camphor	champhore, caphura. *Laurus camphora.* **R T W L H Y**
78.	Cannabis	hemp seeds or leaves, chévenis. *Cannabis sativa.* **H Y**
	Canne	reeds. see 378a and 386.
79.	Cannelle	cinnamon. see 94, 117a *Laurus cinnamomum.* **R W H Y**
80.	Cantharides	spanish fly. Eloe vesicatorum. **B T W L H Y**
81.	Capers	capparis. fruits, shells, bark, oil. lonacera, a honeysuckle. *Capparis spinosa.* **R T W H**
	Capillus	veneris venus hair. see 7.
82.	Capital Powder	19, 33,188 228, 299, 325, 329, 408, 410. For head-wounds. **T H Y**
83.	Capitellum	capiteils, potash lye, lessive. see 254. **R L H Y**
	Capreoli reeds.	see 208.
84.	Caprifolium	caprifici, chevrefoile, honeysuckle, licium. a

fig. see 260. *Lonicera caprifolium.* **R H Y**

84a Caputpurge head-purge. a mega-compound laxative containing marjoram, chelidonium, nasturtium, pyrethrum, staphisagre, nutmeg, long peppr, euphorbia, scammony and rose water. **H**

85. Carabe amber, possibly containing a scarab beetle. see 20a. **W H**

86. Cardamom amomie, granum paradisis, granum solis. *Amimum cardamomum.* **T W L H Y**

Cardo see 102. **H Y**

87. Carmingella an aromatic herb, unidentified **W**

88. Carnis serpentum snake meat. see 129. **H**

89. Carolus dry-rot wood of fallen trees. **W**

90. Carpobalsama mace. see 49. **W H**

Carrot see 52, 152. **T Y**

91. Carthame safflowers and seeds. see 397a. *Carthamus tinctorius.* **R W**

92 Carvum caraway seeds. *Carum carvi.* **T W**

93. Caryophyla garyophyla, giroflé, sanamunda, herb-benedict, cloves, eugenia, arnagallus, carnations, chickweed, stellaria, ipia, horse-foot. see 122, 202, 279. *Caryophylus aromaticus or Geum urbanum.* **B T W L H Y**

Cashew see 25.

94. Cassia 'bastard' cinnamon. and many others. see 79, 427 *Laurus cassia.* **T W L H Y**

Cassilago henbane. see 217. **R H**

95. Castor bean ricinus, cataputia, cocconidium. Diacastor is a laxative electuary. *Ricinus communis.* **B T W H Y**

96. Castoreum beaver musk. **B H Y**

96a Cathimia cadmia, lapis calaminaris. see 71a, 121, 439. **T H**

Cauda equina horse-tail, hippuris. see 170. **W H**

Caul cabbage. see 71. **W H**

96b. Cedar tree of Lebanon.see 15a. *Cedrus libani.*

97. Celery (wild) see 4, 29. **R T W L Y**

98. Celandine   chelidoine (probably the 'lesser'), figwort;. see
                      56, 109. **T W H**

99. Cendre de chêne ashes of Turkish oak (Quercus cerris) lexivium,
                      see 117, 254. **W**

100 Centauria   jacea, narce, thistle, teazle. see 458. **T W L H Y**
    Centinervia   rib-wort. see 428.

101. Cepa   oignun, ascalonia. onion. see 319. **W L H**

101a. Ceratonus   any of four legumes including carob. **W**
     Ceratum   beeswax. see 176, 329a

102. Cerdone   cardo, chardun, calendula, thistle, senecio. see
                      100, 458. *Centauria centaurium or Cardo benedictus.*
                      R H Y

103. Cerebrum galli chicken brain. **H**

104. Cerisier cerice, cherry tree, bark, sap. *Prunus avium.* **R L Y**

105. Ceruse white lead, psimythion, minium. see 242, 253. **R T W L H**
                      Y
     Ceterach   see 69, 417.

106. Chalcanthum   copper sulfate and other metallic salts, battitura
                      see 481, 482. **T W L H Y**
     Chalmedrys   kamedrys, germander. see 200.

107. Charte de soit   bombacyna, papyrus. ashes of paper made from
                      silk. see 38,60,117 333. **T W**
     Chaux   lime, calx. see 251 et al.

108. Chebules   kebulus (from Kabul). see 298 (unripe). **T W**
                      L H Y

109. Chelidonium   celidoine salvage, celandine, mentelicum. see
                      98, 155a.. *Chelidonium majus or Ficaria*
                      ranunculoidis. **W L H Y**

109a. Chenopodium   pigweed, dog-foot. *Chenopodium alba and rubra.*
                      H
     Cherry   see 104. **Y**

110. Chestnut   nux castanearum, chastaine. see 309. *Castanea*
                      sativa. **R T L**

111. Cheveux   humaine ashes from human hair, capillae
                      humani. see 38 et al., 117. **T**

112. Chick peas   cicer. *Cicer arietinum.* **T W L H Y**

Chick-weed   stellaria. see 445a.

113. Chicory leaves. endives, scariola, groin du porc.*Cichorium intybus.* **W L Y**

China root   galingale. see 193.

113a. Cicada   incinerated insect. **T**

Cicer   chick-pea. see 112. **H**

114. Ciclamen   pome de terre, malum terrae, sowbread, cyclamen, earth-nut, panis porcinus. see 262. *Conopodium majus or Cyclamen hederifolium.* **L H Y**

115. Cicuta   cowbane, water hemlock, cicuta virosa, benedicta. see 116.*Conium maculatum.* **R L H Y**

116. Ciguë   hemlock seeds, herb bennett, beneite. see 115.*Conium maculatum.* **R W H Y**

116a. Cimolea   chimolea, cymolia, terra cimolea. mud containing metallic and stoney bits accumulated under whet-stones. see 289. **H**

117. Cinis   ashes.various woods, bones, crabs, mouse, rabbit, scorpion, sponge, hair, grapevine, oyster shell, sea-shells, seashell, hair, paper, etc. see 38 et al., 111. **T W L H Y**

Cinnabar   mercuric sulfidesee 283. **W**

117a. Cinnamon   see 79, 94, 117. **T W H Y**

Cinq-foil   tormentilla. see 465.**T H**

118. Cissus   cissus, hedera, Virginia creeper. *Vitis hederacea.* **H**

Cistus   ladanum. see 234

Citonia   and oil. see 56

119. Citrons   various citrus fruits and melons. Venarum citrinum is citrus fruit pulp, citron pips were used alone. see 31b, 250. **B W H Y**

Citrullus   gourds, melons. see 125, 280

119a. Clay.   all types. see 32, 59, 460.

120. Clematis   the flower, ground-ivy, liere, viticella, vitis petit vigne, hedera, flammula, aristolochium. see

33, 215b, 376. *Clematis vitalis and Hedera helix, etc.* **R T L H Y**

121. Climie argenti metallic oxides, especially silver, gold and zinc. also cacumia, cathimia, spode, tuthie, iron, couperose. see 253,441. **T W L H Y**

122. Clove see 93, 202.

122a Clover various trifoils. see 277, 344a. *Trifolium pratensa.* **T**

Cochia a laxative compound pill, hierarufinum. see 125, 219d. **T**

122b. Coctana dwarf figs. see 185. **W**

123. Coing quince. citonium, diacydomite. see 372. **W**

123a. Cold Seeds 'cold-weather seeds'. The Greater are 137, 144, 191, 280. The Lesser are 245, 366, 392. see 423. **T W Y**

124. Colle gelatin ('gluten'). Vellis vaccini is cowhide as a source. see 204. **W H**

124a. Colchicum crocus. see 141, 219. **Y**

Colcothar vitriol. see 490. **T**

125. Colocynth "bitter apple' or bitter cucumber, cucurbite, citrullus. see 280, et al. *Cucumis colocynthis.* **W L H Y**

126. Colophony pitch. see 352. **R B T W L H Y**

127. Columbine culver-wort, sparagus, geranium molle, pigeon foot. *Geranium columbinum.* **B T**.

Comfrey consolida. see 128.

127a. Condisicale condes. Not identified, perhaps an ointment based on rye flour. see 395a. **T**

128. Consolida comfrey, consoude, greinure. *Symphytum officinalis (large) or Brunella vulgare (small).* **R B T W L H Y**

Convolvulus scammony. see 416. **Y**

129. Cooked meats beef, lamb, pork, veal, snake, frog and various domestic and wild fowls, and their organs. Sometimes the specifiied source was a cas-

	trated male animal. Drippings from roasts. **T W L Y**	
130.	Copper	calchanthum, malachite, salts see 106, 482, etc. **T W L H Y**
131.	Corail	coral polyps(red and white), sponge stone. see 162. **W L H Y**
132.	Coriander	herb belsegensima. *Coriander sativum*. **T W H Y**
	Corigiola	see 361
	Cornel	the dogwood berry. see 63b
133.	Cornu	powdered horns of deer and goats, etc. see 62. **L W H**
134.	Cortex	pini bark of pine tree. see 350. *Pinus sylvestris*. **T L H**
135.	Costus	costmary. roots and oils. See 49, 454 *Costus arabicus*. **T W H Y**
	Cotonia	and cotonea malum. quince. see 372.
136a.	Coudrier.	hazel. see 215a. **Y**
136.	Cotyledon	umbilicus venus, wall pennyroyal. see 420. **L H**
136a.	Couperose	see 106, 482, 490. **L H Y**
137.	Courges	zucchini, watermelon et al. Juices are elacterina. Watermelon is cocomero see 144a, 280. *Cucurbita maxima*. **R W H Y**
	Cowslip	primrose. see 368a.
138.	Crab (river)	cancer fluvialis, granchia titrata, crab-meat and shells. **B W L Y**
138a.	Crayfish	flesh, juice and ashes. **H Y**
139.	Crassula	major and minor, sedum, stonecrop, orpine, andrachne, mamilla muris, tegularia, vermicularis. *Sedum purpurascens*. **R L H**
	Cress	plantain. see 353
	Creta marina	chalk. see 251.
140.	Crisomel	oil from orange seeds. **W**
140a	Crithimum	samphire, St. Peter's herb, cretani. *Crithimum maritimum*. **T**
141.	Crocus	saffron. see 124a, 219, 398. **W L H**

142. Crows' feet   pes corvus, pes milvi. see 33, 120, 376. *Ranunculus sceleratus.* **T W L H**

143. Cubebs   a pepper. *Piper cubeba..* **W L Y**

144. Cucumber   cultivated or wild, momordique, cucumiscelle. *Cucumis var. Ecballium elaterium.* **R W L H Y**

144a Cucurbite   melon. see 137, 144. see 280. Many species. **R W L Y**

145. Cumin   comin, the herb *Cumin cyminum.* **R W Y**

146. Curcuma   turmeric. see 503. *Curcuma longa.* **T L H Y**

147. Currants   red, fresh or dried.see 210a, 393. *Rubis rubrum.* **W H**

148 Cuscuta   dodder; see 148, 169. **T W**

Cuttle-fish   bone squid. see 62

Cylotrum   an arsenical and lime corrosive. see 327. **Y**

148a. Cynoglossus   cinoglossus, hound's-tongue herb, leaves and roots. *Cynoglossus officianale.* **H**

148b. Cyperes succus.   sedge, papyrus. see 422. berries are from *Cyperus longus, C. rotundus .* **B W L H Y**

149. Cyprés   the tree. nuts (seeds), bark, leaves. see 396, 479. The nuts are from *Cupressus sempervirem.* **B W L H Y**

150. Dactylus   dates of palm *Phoenix dactilifera .* Diaphoenicon is a laxative electuary of dates. see 155c. **R T W H Y**

Daffodil   roots and flowers. see 301. **T**

151. Damascus plums   see 355 **W**

Dates   see 150

152. Daucus   carrot, baucia. see 52. *Daucius carota.* **T H Y**

Delphinium   larkspur. see 445.

152a Dentale   entale, lead-wort. *Plumbago europaea.* **T**

153. Diachylon   Mesüe's (one of several versions, see 284a.) ointment made of: 18, 26, 76, 124, 181, 185, 206, 228, 252, 253, 311, 379, 443, 459, 493. **T W H Y**

153a Diadragon   an electuary. see 8, 466. **H Y**

153b Diagridum   an electuary. see 416 **W**

154. Diamargaritum   rubis troscicata, troche based on 342 and 393.
W H Y

155. Diamoron   a syrup of 294. see 317a. **W H Y**

155a. Dianthus   a betony (56) and an electuary based on 387.
T Y

155b Diapenidon   a potion based on barley sugar. see 323. **H**

155c. Diaphoenicon   Diapalma. see 150

156. Diarhodon   an astringent powder from 2, 27, 59, 116, 407(3kinds),460.**W**

156a. Diateron   piperion see 341 **Y**

156b. Diatesseron   see 462. **T H**

157. Diazinziber   a purgative made from 79, 86, 93, 201, 276, 295. **W**

158. Dill   leaves and seeds. see 26. **B**

159. Dipsaccus   teazle thistle, carduus, cardo. see 100, 458, 487. *Cardo fullonum and Dipsaccus sylvestris.* **L H Y**

Dock   sorrel. see 395.

Dodder   cuscuta, Hell weed, (lesser dodder). see 148, 169

160. Dogwood   box-wood, stink-weed, punaise. The oil the berry is cornel. see 63b. **T H**

160a. Dove's Dung   star of Bethlehem. *Ornothogalum umbellatum.* **T**

160b. Dove's Foot   sparagi, *Geranium Molle.* **R Y**

161. Dragantum   iron peroxide, calcantum, colcothar chalcidis. see 490. sometimes confused with 466. **T L H Y**

161a. Dragon-weed   tarragon. *Dracunculus vulgaris.* **T**

161b. Dwarf elder   goat-weed, hieble. see 205. **H**

Earthworms   see 258 and 499.

161c. Ebulus   elder tree. see 165 and 406. **H Y**

162. Écume de Mer   meerschaum, spuma maris, at least 5 varieties, including sponges, algae and corals, halcyon. see 131. **R W H L Y**

163. Eggs   ova. whites (album), yolks (moel), shells, whole. **B R T W L H Y**

163a. Eglantiere   see 389. **H**

164. (H)Ellebore — eleborum, ellebre, Christmas rose. *Helleborus album and nigrum, Veratrum album.* **R T W H Y**

165. Elder — sureau, sambucus, ebulus. juice and a tube of bark slipped off a twig to serve as a cannula. see 161c, 406. **B T W H Y**

165a. Elm — slippery elm tree bark. *Ulmus fulva.* **R T**

166. Emeralds — aluminum silicate gemstones, smaragdus, praze, prassium . **W H**

167. Emperor's herb — an umbellifer similar to angelica. see 26a. *Angelica archangelica.* **W H**

167a. Encaustrum — caustic red ink, or vernis. see 479, 490. *Terminalis vernis.* **T W**

168. Encens — see 188, 316, 463. **R Y**

Endive — pig-snout, groin du porc, chicory. see 113, 392. **T**

Entale — dentale. see 152a

168a. Enula — inula, elecampani. see 437. **W H Y**

169. Epithyme — like cuscuta. see 160. *Cuscuta major and minor.* **W H**

170. Equisetum — asperella, cauda equina, queue equina, horsetail reed, shave grass. *Equisetum arvense.* **T W H**

Ers — vetch. see 325, 483.

171. Eruca — mustard weed, charlock, rocket-root, sinapus. see 297, 426. *Sinapus avensis.* **R T W Y**

171a Esula — a spurge. see 173, 442. **T W H Y**

172. Eupatorium — agrimony. see 13. **T W Y**

173. Euphorbia — amblete, custos hortis, marsilium, manne, solsequium, esula, titimalle, cataputia. anabulle is the sap. see all named here. *Many varieties of spurges, Euphorbeacea.* **R B T W L H Y**

174. Fabaria — lovage, water parsnip. see 247, 256, 430. **T H**

175. Faex — precipitate at bottom of oil jugs, faex olei. **T W H Y**

176. Faex cerae — beeswax, faex alvearum, eryngium. see 293, 329a.368aa, 397. **H**

177. Farina de Moulin — amidon, far, amylum, farina volatica, mill-dust

		(fine wheaten flour) also found at bake-ovens, see 21,187,494. **R T W L H Y**
178.	Fava	feve, fabba, beans or their stalks, especially *Vicia faba*. **W L H**
179.	Feces	stercus, tordus; sheep, goat, deer, birds, horses, human etc. see 184. **R T W L Y**
180.	Fennel	fenoil, marathon. leaves. see 307. *Foeniculum dolce et vulgare, and Nigella sativa*. **R T W L H Y**
181.	Fenugrec	aegoceros, buceros, telis. seeds, Greek fennel, ferrugine. seeds usually powdered. see 180. *Trigonella foenum-graecum*. **R B T W L H Y**
	Fermentum	see 502. **W H**
181a.	Ferns	filix, beech fern, royal fern etc. see 7,362 363. var. *Osmundia* **H Y**
182.	Fesire	white bryony. see 67. **W**
	Fever-few	tansy. see 454.
	Ficus fig.	see 185.
183.	Fiel	bile, fel, felles, (dog, cow, bull, ox, felles avium, colre, choler etc.). see 57. **W L H Y**
184.	Fiente	fimus columbinus or equus. pigeon or horse droppings. see 179. **R T W L H**
185.	Figs	alos, coctana, citonia. caprificus is a wild fig. see 84, 122b, 260. *Ficus arboris*. **B T W L H**
185a.	Figwort	pigamon, quadrangula. see 56.
186.	Filipendula	spirea, dropwort, meadow-sweet. *Spirea filipendula*. **H**
186a	Fish	many varieties by name.All authors
	Fisticus	pistachio. see 351.
	Flammula	clematis. see 120.
	Flaura	an herb of various sorts: a clover, a fumitory, etc. see 122a, 191.**R**
	Flax	linen. see 252.
	Flies	house flies. **H**
186b.	Flos	'flower', battitura aeris, aloxan. various films (usually metallic salts) deposited on metals and fluids. see 481, 482, etc. **W L H Y**

187. Flour   farina, furfur, samich, froment, pigle (coarse-ground). see 21, 177, 395a, 436, 494. **R T W L H Y**

188. Frankincense   gum resin. see 168, 316, 463. *Boswellia cartorii* . **R B T W L H Y**

189. Fraxinus   bark of ash tree, fiêne, stone-mint, manna. see 264, 389, 453. *Fraxinus excelsior.* **T W H Y**

Frog   see 375. **B T**

190. Fuchsia   the flower. see 334. *Parietaria officianalis.*

191. Fumitory   fumiterre, gingidium, perhaps flama, lady's mantle, hen's foot. *Fumaria officinalis or Gingidium.* **R T W L H Y**

192. Fusco   unguentum fuscum, Brown ointment of Nicolas see 306. **R H**

193. Galanga   galingale, melingalata, China root. see 276. *Alpinia galanga.* **R T W H Y**

194. Galbanum   a ferula resin. *Ferula galbaniflua.* **R B T W L H Y**

194a. Galen's Ointment   72, 105, 206, 253, 312, 388, 439, 493. **T L H**

Galigan   rue. see 394. **Y**

195. Galls   oak galls. **B T W L H Y**

196. Gallitricum   salvia, centrum galli, crista galli, oculi christis, sclaria. see 400, 405. **H Y**

197. Garance   madder root, rubeau, spargula. see 392a et al., 434a, 474, 497. *Galium molugo, G. aparime and Rubia tinctorum.* **Y**

198. Garlic   affodil, ailes, aulx, allium. see 16a, 43. **R T W**

Garyophyla   see 93

199. Gentian   genista. bitter roots of *Gentiana lutea* . **T W L H Y**

Geranium   see 6, 209.

200. Germander   scordium, polium, chalmedrys, camedrios, yva. see 346, 418. *Teucrium polium and montanum.* **R T W L H Y**

Geum   Eugenia. see 93

201. Ginger   zingiber, genevrier, abel. see 24. *Amomum*

zingiber. **R B T W L H Y**

202. Girofle   cloves, caryophyllus. see 93 et al. **R Y**

     Git   coriander. see 307

202a. Gladiolus   sword-grass, yellow flag, see 228. *Iris pseudoacoris.* **H**

203. Glans   acorns (quercus). see 309a. **H Y**

     Glue   see 368aa. **W L**

204. Gluten   colle, gelatin from fish or domestic animals, mucilage, animal collagen (not from grains). see 124, 242a, 430bb. **R B T W L H**

     Glycyrrhyza   licorice. see 246, 381.

     Goat's beard   salsify. see 49a.

205. Goatweed   gout-weed, another umbellifer, sometimes Bishops-wort, Agnus caste. see 11a, 22. *Ammi majus, Aegropodium podagraria* .**T W H**

     Gold   incinerated or decocted. see 43b, 121.

     Goudron navire   ship-tar. see 304 et al., 352, 359, 360. **Y**

206. Graisse   animal fat—chicken, geese, pork, turtle, etc., pinguedo, sepum, ysopus, bovis, gras, sui, adeps. see 225, 235, 311. Grassede are the drippings from roasts. **R B T W L H Y**

207. Gramen   sedges, couch grass. see 422 et al. *Agropyrum repens.* **L H**

     Grana paradisi   cardamon. see 86, 332

208. Grape   uva. leaves and fruit, and skins. raisins, sapa michum (with honey), saramitum, capreoli are the tendrils. see 12. **R T W**

208a. Grasses and Reeds see 378a, and 386. **R T W H**

209. Gratia dei   geranium. see 6 *Gratiola officianalis.* **H Y**

210. Green Oint.   basically 14 and 273, with supplements by various authors including 188, 256, 272, 329, 360, 424, 459. **R T W L H Y**

210a. Groseille   currants or gooseberries. see 147 or *Ribes grossularia.* **W H Y**

211. Gui.   mistletoe. leaves, berries, twigs. *Viscum album.* **T W**

Guimauve	malva. see 18, 273 **Y**
212. Gum Arabic	from acacias. **R T W L H Y**
213. Gummi	sap of cherry, plum, other gums as gumme d'eve, gum evry, Persian gum. see 466. **T W L H**
214. Gypsum	cockel, selenite, alabaster, plaster of Paris, calcium sulfate. **T W L Y**
Hair	see 111
215. Handacote	septemnerviée. see 428. **W**
Hare's Beard	see 395
Hare's foot	pes leporis, see 344a
Hawkweed	mouse-ear. see 219a, 347
215a. Hawthorne	spina, hazel. fruits and flowers. *Crategus oxyacantha.* **B**
215b. Hedera	clematis, funis pauperum. see 120. **R H Y**
216. Hematite	rust, emathitis, pierre sanguinis, lapis sanguinis, red ochre. see 227, 228a. **T W L Y**
Hemlock	see 116. **T Y**
Hemp	see 78. **T Y**
217. Henbane	jusquiame, hyoscyamus, solathrum, nightshade, belladonna, cassilago, chenille, fabe lupini. see 232, 290a, 431. **R T W H Y**
Henna	alkanna. see 15.
Hen's foot	pes gallinacia, fumitory. see 191
Hepatica	liver-wort, marchantia. see 268.
218. Hericium	sea urchin bristles. ericium, herisson, hircis, lupis iudaici. see 249. **W H**
219. Hermodactyl	digitus hermetis, colchicum and other related tubers. see124a. *Hermodactylus tuberosus.* **R T W L H Y**
219a. Hieracium	hawkweed. see 347.
219b. Hieralogodon	Galen's laxative. see 344c. **H**
219c. Hierapicra	picra. see 344c. **W H**
Hieromandrea	mandrake. see 263
219d. Hierarufinum	a laxative of colocynth, germander, asafoetida, wild parsley, aristolochia, pepper, cinnamon,

saffron, polium, myrrh and honey. see cochia, and 125. **H Y**

220. Honey   miel, various kinds. hydromel is a mixture with water. beehive honey contained some wax. see 330. **R B T W L H Y**

Honeysuckle   also oculum. see 84. **R**

Hordeum   barley. see 323.

Horehound   marrubium. see 271.

Horse's tail   equisetum. see 170.

221. Houx bruscus.   holly. see 226a. *Riscus aculeatus..* **T W**

222. Hyacinth   squill, blue-bell, jacinth. see 443. *Hyacinthus nonscriptus.* **T W H**

Hydromel   see honey, 220.

Hyoscyamus   see 217, 232, 431.

223. Hypericon   St. John's Wort. see 287, 501. *Hypericium perforatum.* **R H**

224. Hypocystus   hypoquistidos. fungus on roots of *Cistinus hypocystus.* **T W L H Y**

225. Hysop   humidus arabic for lanolin. see 206, 235. **T W**

226. Hyssop   herb hasca. *Hyssopus officinalis.* **W H**

226a. Ilex holly.   berries, leaves, bark. see 221. *Ilex aquafolium.* **T**

Ink   vitriol. see 167a, 479, 490

Inula   enula. see 168a, 437 et al. **W H**

227. Irundinum   iron. see 228a, et al.

228. Iris   yreos, powdered orris root, eris ustis is burnt iris flowers, oil. see 202a. *Iris germanica, illyrica, florentinma, etc.* **T W L H Y**

228a Iron   fer. yellow ochre. see 227, 249a, 267, 289, 419. **R T L H Y**

Isis   ysis. see 502a. **T**

Ivy   various. see 120

228b. Jacea   scabious.dijaciton is a laxative. see 414. **H Y**

Jacinth   hyacinth. see 222, 443.

John Saint.   see 372a, 401a et al.

229. Joubarbes   Jove's beard. house leeks, stonecrop, tettesuriz,

	poireaux, sticado. see 101, 229, 243, 319, 425. *Sempervivum tectorum.* **R T W H Y**
230. Jujubes	fruit of the trees. *Zizyphus vulgaris and Z. saturna.* **T W Y**
231. Juniper	savine, sabine. needles, cones, oil. see 479. *Juniperus sabina.* **R H Y**
232. Jusquiaime	henbane, aconite, marsilium, faba luparia, luparis, chenille, morel, caniculata, dens caballinus, symphoniaca. see 217, 290a, 431. *Hyoscyamus albus and niger.* **R T W H Y**
Kabiteji	lupin. see 259. **R**
233. Kekenji	winter cherry. *Physalis alkekenji.* **H**
Knot grass	polygonum. see 361.
234. Labdanum	sometimes ladanum or laudanum. resin of cistus trees, especially *Cystus creticus.* **B T L H Y**
Labrusca	bryony. see 67.
Lac	milk. see 286. **H**
234a. Lacca	lactea. a red resin from litmus. see 325. *Roccella tinctoria* .
Lacertus	lizard. see 257, 446
Lactucca	lettuce. see 245. **H**
Lana succida	wool-fat. see 235, et al. **H**
Lanceola	plantain. see 353. **H**
235. Lanolin	suint, lana succida, hysop, ysopus, oesype. see 206, 311, 498. **W L**
236. Lapathum	sorrel, rumex, burdock paradella, lappa, lapazio. see 49b, 395. *Lappatum acutum.* **R T W L H Y**
236a. Lapis lazuli	powdered blue gem, ferrous sulfate. **T W**
Lappa	sorrel, burdock, lapathum. see 236 and 395. **H Y**
Larkspur	delphinium. see 445.
237. Laterinum	oil of the small fish. **T**
Laudanum	labdanum. see 234. **L**
238. Lauriers	lorier, baccis lauri. berries, leaves of bay trees.

Laurin is oil of bay leaves. *Laurus nobilis.* **R T W L H Y**

239. Laureole   de-barked daphne twig, spurge laurel, medulla milici. *Daphne laureola.* **R W L H**

240. Lavender   *Lavandula stoechas and L. officinalis.* **T W Y**

241. Lead,   filings limailles, minium. See 249a. **R W L**

242. Lead,   white lead sulfate is galena. see 105, 253. **R T W L**

242a. Leather   especially shoe-soles. See 124, 204, 431a **H Y**

243. Leeks   see 229, 319. Prassium (emerald) because of its green. see 166. **W H**

Lemon   the peel. see 250. **H**

243a. Lentigo   water-moss, probably sphagnum. *Sphagnum cymbifolium.* **T H Y**

244. Lentils lens, lentes. **R W L H Y**

244a. Lessive   a strong soap, a weak lye. see 254, 412, 430c. **H Y**

245. Lettuce   laitues, lactuca, lettue. *Lactuca sativa; Lactuca agresta* i is wild lettuce (escarolle, endive). **R T W L**

245a. Levain   leaven. Bakers' yeast. **H**

Levisticus   lovage. see 247. **R**

246. Licorice   liquoritia, herb reglisse. see 381. *Glycyrrhiza glabra* . **T W L H**

247. Ligusticum   levisticus, lovage. see 174, 256, 430. *Ligusticum levisticum.* **L H**

248. Lily   lis, arcus daemoniacus, crinon. usually oil of bulbs and leaves. *Lilium candidum et al.* Lily often included iris, narcissus and gladiolus. **R B T W L H Y**

248a. Lily of the Valley mayblossom (? May butter). *Convallaria majalis.* **T**

249. Limacons   limax, limazun. snails with shells. **R T W H Y**

249a Limailles   metal filings including bronze, iron, lead. see 241, 289, 419. **R T H Y**

250. Limes   limo. limes, lemons. see 119. *Citrus limonum.* **H**

W Y

251. Lime (stone)   quick lime, chaux vive, calx, creta, chauz. fresh lime, powdered, used in cylotrum. See 74a. **R B T W L H Y**

252. Lin   linois, semence, semen lini, flax seeds and oil or meal. *Linum usitatissimum.*. **R B T W L H Y**

Linaria   penny-wort. see 420. **R H Y**

253. Litharge   litargerie, yellow lead oxide, scum of melted lead or silver. see 121, 242. for litharge nutritum (spumie argentum) see 441. **R T W L H Y**

253a Liver wort   hepatica, marchantia *Peltigera canina or Marchantia polymorphi.* **H**

254. Lixivium   aqua cineris, lessive, lye, also very strong soap. see 83, 240a et al. **B T W L H Y**

Lizard   see 257, 446. **R B T**

254a. Lodestone   magnetite, ainant, black iron oxide. **H**

255. Lolium   panicium, zizania. darnel grass. *Lolium temulentum and perenne.* **R T H**

256. Lovage   "Alexander's Medicine". see 174, 247. Black lovage is *Smyrnum dusatrum,* **T W L Y**

257. Lucertoli lacertus. lizard. see 446. **B L**

257a. Lucius magna   the pike fish, Esox lucius. **W**

258. Lumbrici   ges entera. earthworms (or maggots). see 499. **R L H Y**

258a. Lungwort   water lentil, palma Marina, muscus aquae. *Lemna minor .* **R H**

259. Lupin   kabitegi, flowers of faba lupina, usually powdered. *Lupinus album.* **R T W H**

260. Lycium   licium. made from 84. see 185. **W H**

Lye   aqua cineris. see 83, 244, 254. **H**

261. Mace   myristica. *Myristica fragrans.* **W H Y**

Madder   garance. see 197, 392a, 474.

Magnet   see 254a.

Maiden hair   venus hair. see 7, 363.

Malum   punicum pomegranate. see 364. **H**

262. Malum   terrae cyclamen, malot, earth-nut, etc. see 114.

R L H Y

Malva	mauve. see 18, 273. **B H**
263. Mandragora	mandrake, belladonna. Hieromandrea is a potion based on mandragora. *Mandragora officinarium.* **R T W L H Y**
264. Manna	tamarix, ash-tree. see 189, 453. **T H Y**
265. Manne	euphorbia, esula resin. see 173 et al. **W Y**
266. Manuchriston	like diamargariton, with added honey. **W**
Marathrum	saxifrage. See 349, 413
266a. Marble	powdered. **L**
267. Marcassita	iron pyrites (sulfites). **T H**
268. Marchantia	liver wort, hepatica. *Marchantia polymorphia and M. conica.* **T L**
269. Margarita	pearls or daisies. see 342. **R H**
269a. Marigolds	various. *Calendula officinalis.* **H**
269b. Marine pumace	a coral fish. **T**
270. Marjoram	marjolaine, oregano, hortensa, amoracus, maiorama. sweet marjoram. see 324. *Origanum marjorana and O.vulgare.* **T W H Y**
Marrow	bone. see 275. **R T W**
271. Marrubium	maruil neir, samsucus, linoscrofon. horehound. *Marrubium vulgare.* **B T W H**
Marsilium	wolf-bean. **H**
271a. Martiaton	soldier's ointment. 1, 51, 72, 238, 270, 312, 394, 400, 493, 496. **T L**
Mary	Saint. See 361, 401a.
272. Mastic	resin and oil. *Pistachia lentiscus .* **R W L H Y**
273. Mauve	guimauve, mallow (various), althea, sanaticula, malve, ebiscus malaviscum, cubes, dialthea, diante, mallachee. see 18. *Althea officianalis.* **R B T W L H Y**
Meadow-sweet	see filipendula, see186
273a. Meats	carnes, including snakes and moles. see 88, 129, 375. 451. **T L H Y**
274. Medlar	nespole, mespilus, the fruit. *Mespilus germanica.* **L H Y**

275. Medulla   moelle, meule, midolle, bone marrow, specific animals and bones are named. see 61. **B T W L H**

     Meerschaum   spuma maris. see 162.

     Mel   also miel. honey. see 220, 330

276. Meligalata   galanga. see 193. **W**

277. Melilot   corona regia. sweet clover. *Melilotus leucothea and arvensis.* **T W L H**

278. Melissa   sweet balm, calamint. see 72. *Melissa officinalis.* **T W H Y**

279. Mellicrate   pomegranate fruit, or a sweet honey-water beverage. See 364 **R**

280. Melon   barecha, citrullus, pumpkin, melo, citri, pepo, squash. See 50, 144a, 492. **R T W H Y**

280a. Memitte   yellow-horn poppy (confused with 109) *Glaucum flavum.* **R T H**

281. Menthastrum   wild mint, aquatic mint, horse mint, sysimbro. See 288a. *Menthastrum sylvestris.* **R T H**

282. Mercuriale   linozostis, mercurelle. common weed. *Mercurialis annua.* **T W H**

283. Mercury   argentum vivum. quick-silver. see 186b. **T W H Y**

284. Mesûe's Fetid Pills   a laxative containing 11, 19, 79, 125, 220, 228, 271, 272, 299, 398, 410, 469. **W Y**

284a. Mesûe's Oint.   19, 65 (old white), 253, 278, 299, 321, 388 (or 300), 411, 496. see153. several were attributed to Mesúe. **R B T L H**

285. Mie a pain   mica panis. bread crumbs. see 65. **W L Y**

286. Milk   mother's is lactus muliebris. cow's milk is lait de scroppha, albugasse is donkey's milk, also goat-milk-whey and cheese-water. **T W L H Y**

     Mill Dust   see 177

287. Millefuilles   yarrow, St. John's herb. see 501. *Achillea millefolium, Hypericum perforatum et al.* **B T H**

288. Millet   milium, granum. *Panicum miliaceum.* **T W Y**

     Minium   lead filings. see 241. **Y**

288a. Mint   menthe. see 72, 281, 367. **R T H Y**

Mistletoe   gui. see 211.

288b. Mithradates   penny cress. the Mithradaticon was a theriac *Thrapsus arvense.* **T H Y**

Moles   see 273a. **H**

Moly rue.   see 394

289. Molo   molendini stercus irundini, cimolia, molybdenum. bits of iron or powder from mill grindstones, limailles. see 116a, 228a, 249a. **R T L H Y**

290. Money wart   wood pimpernel, serpentaria, nummularia. see 292, 348. *Lysimachus nummularia.* **Y**

290a Morel   (not the mushroom) henbane. see 232, 431. *Morel officianalis* **H Y**

291. Moschus   deer musk. see 96,446. *Moschus moschifer.* **H Y**

291a. Moss   muscus, musceline, muscus aquae, sphagnum, etc. see 258a, 296. *Sphagnum cymbifolium and Usnea barbata. etc.* **T H**

291b. Moss Ointment   27, 29, 35, 51, 72, 128, 180, 201, 226, 238, 270, 271a, 290a, 309 (oil), 367, 396, 411. **T**

292. Mourons   scarlet pimpernel, anagallis. See 290, 348.

293. Mu   beeswax. see 176, 329a, 397. **W H**

294. Mulberries   mûres, mora, omorusia. see 155, 317a. *Morus nigra.* **W L H Y**

294a Mullein   see 395, etc. **H Y**

295. Mummy   momie, mumie, flecks of desiccated cadavers collected from tombs and catacombs. **R B W L Y**

Muriate   of soda salt. see 404.

Musa   plantain. see 353.

295a. Muscade   nutmeg, muscat. see 308. **W H Y**

296. Muscus   arboris tree-moss, lichen. see 291a. *Usnea barbata.*

Mushrooms   various. see 11.

Musk   deer, beaver. see 96,291, 446. **T W Y**

297. Mustard   see 171,426. *Synapus alba.* **R B T W L H Y**

297a. Mustard Garlic *Sysimbrium allaria.* **R**

298. Myrobalans Indian, or yellow. unripe are chebules. emblicus, belliricus. see 108 *Myrobalans indica.* **T W L H Y**

299. Myrrh mirre, musa, smyrna, resins of commiphora plants. *Balsamodendron myrra.* **R B T W L H Y**

300. Myrtle seeds, leaves, berries, oil, wood, water. *Myrtis communis.* **R B T W L H Y**

301. Narcissus daffodils, affodil, asphodel. *Narcissus pseudo-narcissus.* **R B T L H**

302. Nard spikenard, spic, and oil. see 437, 475. *Valeriana jatamansi and Nardostachys jatamansi.* **R B T W L H Y**

303. Nasturtium cresson, water-cress, senationes, garden crew. *Nasturtium officinalis.* **B T W H**

304. Navale goudron de navire, ship tar. see 352, 455. **B T W**

304a Nenufar water-lily, farfar. see 491. **L H Y**

Nespole medlar. see 274. **H**

305. Nettles ortie, califex ignita, castrangula, millemorbia. seeds. Quadrangular, ficaria see 326. *Urtica urens.* **T L H Y**

306. Nicolas' Ointment see 365. Ung.Fuscum (Brown Ointment), see 192. **T W H**

307. Nigella Roman coriander, ciminum, nielle, gith. see 180. *Nigella sativa.* **B T W H Y**

Nightshade henbane. see 217. **T**

Nitre nitrum. see 402. **R H**

Nummulare money-wort. see 290, 292, 348 **Y**

308. Nutmeg muscade, nux muscata, noiz muscate, centrum galle. See 295a *Myristica fragrans.* **R W L H Y**

309. Nux meats shells and oils of nuts. chestnuts are castana, hazel nuts are avellanum, nual is walnut, brou is walnut shells. See17, 110, 309a **R T W L H Y**

Oak fern see 362

309a Oak tree   quercus, robur, chene, glans. tan bark is cortex stypticus. See 203 **W L H Y**

310. Oats   avoine, aegilope. *Avena sativa.* **T W L H**

311. Oesypus   Ysopus, lanolin. see 206, 235. **T W L H**

312. Oil   usually from mature olives, whereas onfacium (318) was made from the thin juice of green olives and was not classed as a real oil. see 248, 313, 317, 344b, 389, 394, 486. **R B T W L H Y**

313. Oil of Deben   see 53b. from seeds of *Moringa aptera.* **W**

314. Ointments   Apostles', Basilicon, Black, Brown, Diachylon Galen's, Green, Martiaton, Mesües, Moss, Mummy Nicolas', Palm, Populeum, Rhaze's White, Saracenic,William Somer's, Aurgheons, Yellow (citrin). **R B T W L H Y**

315. Oleander   shrub. *Nerium oleander.* **T H**

316. Olibanum   thus, frankincense, cortex olibanum. (thus masculinum from Lebanon). See 188, 463. **R B T W L H Y**

317. Olives   oil of green or ripe fruits. wood of tree. *Olea sativa.* **R B T W H**

317a. Omorusia   mulberry. see 294. *Morus nigra.* **T**

318. Onfacium   omphacus, infantium. thin oil of green olives. see 312. **W H Y**

319. Onions   cepa, as distinct from leeks, allium, poirium. see 101, 415. **R T W H**

Opirus   bread. see 65

320. Opium   pavot, philonium. seeds and pods of poppy. see 337. *Papaver somniferum.* **R B T W L H Y**

321. Opoponax   epoponac, panax. like myrrh a commiphora resin. *Opoponax chironem.* **R T W L H Y**

Orache   blite. see 24a, 42.

322. Oranges   fruit or peel, arantium. see 31b, 119. **T W**

323. Orges   barley, hordeum. penidium is barley-sugar cake, ptisan and vitis alba are barley broth. see 155. *Hordeum vulgare .* **T W L H Y**

324. Origanum   oregano, wild marjoram. see 270. **T W H**

325. Orobe   horobus, bitter vetch, ers, vicia, lacca is the gum.
                      see 234a. *Ervium ervilia and E. lens.* **W L H**
326. Ortie   nettles. see 305. *Urtie pilulifera et al. including
                      Scrophularium nodosum.* **T W H Y**
327. Orpiment   orphimentum, auripigmentum. yellow ars-
                      enious oxide, used in cylotrum. see 34, 43c. **R
                      T W H Y**
     Ossa   combusta bone-ash. see 62
     Ossisacara   and ozzizacara, see 330. **B T Y**
     Ova   eggs. see 163. **H**
328. Ova formicarum   ant eggs. **T L H**
329. Oxalis   rumex, lapathum, wood-sorrel, alleluia, trefoil,
                      oseille. see 395 et al., and 433. **T L H**
329a. Oxycroceum   beeswax. see mu, 176, 293. **H Y**
330. Oxymel oxysaccharum. a honey-vinegar laxative mixture,
                      ozzizacara, osisatum, oxylaxativum. **R T W L H
                      Y**
     Oyster   shells incinerated and powdered. see 117.
330a. Palm Ointment   made with red clay (32), 105, 121 (silver), 253,
                      289, 419, 441, 460. **W L H**
330b. Palma marina   lungwort. see 258a. **R H**
331. Palme vert   heart of palm or date palm. see 150. **W L H**
     Panada   bread soup. see 65.
     Panax   opopanax. see 321.
     Panicium   darnel grass, see 255.
     Papaver   opium. see 320. **H**
332. Paprika   cardamon. see 86.
333. Papyrus   paper, usually burnt. see 107. **T L**
334. Parietoria   pellitory, lichwort, paritarie. see 190 *Parietoria
                      erecta and P. diffusa.* **R L H**
334a. Parsnip   wild. *Pastinacia sativa.* **T H**
335. Passula   agresta. see 12, 478. **W L**
336. Patience   wild dock, rumex, oxalis. see 395.
337. Pavot   white and black papaver, poppy (seeds). see
                      320. **W Y**
338. Peach   persica. fruit, seeds or leaves. *Persica vulgaris or*

	Prunus persica. **R T W H Y**
339. Pear	fruit, flowers, leaves, wine. *Pirus communis.* **T W L H**
340. Peas	pisum, any type, or beans. see 358.
340a. Peganum	piganum, wild rue (not a rue) probably a scrofularia. **H**
Penidium	barley sugar. see 323. **H**
Pennyroyal	see 367
340b. Peony	flower of *Nus paionia.* **R**
341. Peppers	piper, serpyllum, various regions. Diateron piperion was made of three kinds of peppers. see 156a. *Polygonum hydropiper.* **W L H Y**
342. Perles	pearls or marguerite flowers. leaves or oyster-pearls. see 269. **R T W**
343. Persicaria	water-pepper, smart weed, cul-rag. *Polygonum varieties and Persicaria hydropiper.* **R H**
344. Persil	parsley, selinum is the seed of apium. *Carum petroselinum.* **R T W H Y**
Pes corvinus	crow's foot. see 142. **W**
344a. Pes leporis	Haresfoot clover, sanamunda. see 122a. *Trifolium arvensis.* **T H** 344b.Petroleum oil of. Benite, Holy Oil. **R**
Petroselinium	see 29, 247. **L H**
Philonium	opium. see 320
Pierre de lanternes	unidentified. probably crumbled sandstone. **Y**
Pigle	wheat. see 494.
344c. Pigra	picra, hierapicra and Galen's hierologodon. a laxative pill. see, 199, 79, 125, used with or as alternative to cochia. Contains 19, 58, 79, 220, 272, 398, 437. **T W H Y**
Pig-snout	endive , groin du porc. see 113, 392
Pigweed	dog-foot. see 109a **H**
345. Pili leporis	mullein. see 356. **B T L Y**
346. Pilium	a germander. see 200, 418. **W**
347. Piloselle	hieracium, hawkweed. see 219a. *Hieracium*

pilosella. **T L H Y**

348. Pimpernels — anagallis, scarlet pimpernel, ipia, wood pimpernel is moneywort, a lysimachia. see 290, 292. *Anagallis arvensis or Stellaria media.* **R T W H Y**

349. Pimpinelle — pimprinelle, saxifrage, lesser burnet, anise. see27, 413. *Sanguisorbe officinalis.* **R T H Y**

350. Pine — stone pine and others. tree bark, seeds etc. *Pinus pinus.* see 134. **H**

Pinguedo — pork lard. see 206.

Piper — pepper, serpyllum. see 341.

Pira — and pyra. see 339.

351. Pistachia — fisticus. see 459 *Pistacia vera.* **L H**

Pisum — peas. see 340, 358. **H**

352. Pix — peize, pix alba and nigra, poix, pissa, resin, turbentyne, colophony. see 126, 304, 359, 360, 379, 469a. **R B T W L H Y**

353. Plantain — plantago, many varieties including water-cress, psyllium, rib-wort, lanceola, lancelette, policaria, quinque nervicium, arnoglossa, waybread, yva. see 428. *Plantago psyllium, P. cynops, etc.* **R T W L H Y**

354. Plomb — brûle alanauch, plumbum ustum, yellow oxide of lead. see 242, 253. **W L H Y**

355. Plum — prune, prunella, plums, tree sap (see gummi), seneste, sebeste Damascus, etc. Diaprunum is an electuary of plums. *Prunus domestica,* also *P.spinosum,* the blackthorn, sloe. **T W L H Y**

356. Poil de lievre — pili leporis, hare's-beard (Great Mullein). see 395, 433, 457. *Verbascum thapsus.* **R T W H Y**

357. Poireux — garlic. see 43. *Allium porrum .* **W**

358. Pois — pisum, peas of all kinds. *Pisum sativum.* **H**

359. Poix greque — probably hemlock tree resin, see pix. **W**

360. Poix (noir) — shoe-makers' pitch or wax. **W Y**

360a. Polycaria — pulicaria. inula. see 168a. **T Y**

361. Polygonum — knot grass, corrigiola, cesune, geniculata, St.

Mary's Herb, Solomon's seal. see 49, 361, 454, *Polygonum aviculare.* **T L H Y**

362. Polypode   oak fern, beech fern. ee 181a. *Polypodium vulgare or Gymnocorpium dryopteria.* **R T W L H Y**

363. Polytric   beech fern, hair-cap moss, golden maiden hair fern. *Polytrichium juniperium.* **R T W**

363a Poma   Apples, sour apples pears, etc. fruit, wood, leaves, bark. **T L H**

364. Pomegranate   malum punicum, pomme gernette, fruit, leaves, flowers or bark (ecorce, cortica), mellicrate, psidia (the fruit peel), wine, water.

    Punica   *granatum.* see 47, 279. **R B T W L H Y**

    Pome de terre   cyclamen. see 114

364a. Poplar   aspen. leaves. buds are oculi populi and bourgeons, bacca, aigeros. see 364a et al. *Populus tremuloides.* **T L H Y**

    Poppy   opium. see 320. **R B T W L H Y**

365. Populeum Oint.   also populeon (contained poplar tree-buds— bourgeone de peuplier) also called Nicolas' Ointment, one of several recipes included. 44, 49, 217, 263, 336, 348. **R T W L H Y**

365a. Porrum   garlic, ptasion. see 43. **R Y**

366. Portulaca   wild and domestic. purslane, chicken-feet, olus fatuum, Herb Robert. see 368. *Lepidum campestre and L.ruderale.* **T L H Y**

    Potentilla   tormentilla. see 465

367. Pouliot   pulegium, pennyroyal, polial roial, Dragon-tea used mint. *Menthe pulegium..* see 288a. **R T W Y**

368. Pourpier   purslane. see 366. *Portulaca oleracea.* **H**

    Prassium   emeralds or leeks. see166, 243. **W H**

368a. Primavera   primrose, primula, cowslip. see 25a. *Primula vera.* **H**

368aa. Propolis   bee glue and wax. see 293, 329a. **T H**

368b. Prunella   self-heal, fruit of blackthorn sloe, sanicula *Prunella vulgaris.* see 424a. **T H Y**

    Prunum   plums. see 355

	Psidia	pomegranate peel. see 364. **T H**
368bb.	Psyllium	plantain. see 353. **T L H Y**
	Pulegium	penny-royal. see 367.
368c.	Pumice	spuma maris. see 162. **T H**
369.	Pumpkin	citrouille, zucca see 50, 280. **R W H**
	Purslane	portulaca. see 368.
370.	Pyrecanthum	lycium. **T H**
371.	Pyrethrum	peretrum, pellitory. flowers of fever-few, chry-santhemum. *Anthrum pyrethrum.* **B T W H Y**
	Quercus	oak. see 309a.
	Quicklime	see 251
372.	Quince	coing, cotonia, cydonium malum, citonium malum. pulp and seeds. see 123. *Pyrus cydonia.* **T W L H**
	Radish	see 373
372a	Ragweed	St. John's wort. *Senecio jacobea.* **T**
373.	Raifort	radish, raiz, horse-radish, rapistrum, raphanus, rave. *Cochlearia armoracia, Raphanus sativus and other Raphani.* **R T W L H Y**
	Raisins	uva passa. see 473. **T H**
374.	Ramich	an Arabian compound 19, 30 (berries), 93, 195, 299, 308, 318, 264, 407, 433. **H**
375.	Rana scortica	frog-meat. see 273a. **B T**
376.	Ranunculus	clematis, pes corvus, crow's feet. See 33, 120, 142. *Flammula jovis.* **H**
377.	Rape	a mustard. *Brassica rapa and napus.* see 64a. **W L H Y**
377a.	Rave	turnip or radish. see 373 and 377.
377b.	Red Powder	Roger's suture powder. 59, 126, 128, 272, 316, 408. **R Y**
378a.	Reeds	canes, marsh grass, canne, panicium, darnel etc. see 386. **R T W L H**
379.	Resin	gumma pini. pine pitch rosin. see 15a, 352. **R T W L H Y**
380.	Realgar	red arsenic ore. see 34 and 327. **B W L H Y.**
381.	Reglisse	licorice. see 246. **W**

381a Rhazes' Oint.   Ung. album, contained 17, 77, 105, 163(whites), 253, 388,493 **Y**

382. Rhubarb   *Rhababarum of many species.* **W Y**

    Rib-wort   plantain. see 353.

    Robert's Herb   portulaca. see 366. **Y**

383. Roche   alum. see 20.

    Rocket-root   eruca. see 171. **T W**

384. Rognons   (oil from) castrated testes,—calves, sheep, etc. **T**

    Ronces   rubis,blackberry. see 393.

385. Rosat   roset, rosamel, honey with crushed rose petals. see 390. **R W Y**

386. Roseau   marsh reeds, canne. see 378a. *Arundo donax.* **W.**

387. Rosemary   herb. see 155a. *Rosemarinus officinalis.* **W Y**

388. Rose-oil   oleum rosarum, oil of petals. **R W L H Y**

389. Rose   powder of petals or whole flowers including the anthers. Eglantiers are wild roses. see 53c. *Rosacea, var. species.* **T W H Y**

390. Rose-syrup   rosamel, rosat syrup of petals with honey or sugar, see 385. **W H Y** 391. Rose-water water of petals, eau rosat. **W H Y**

392. Rostrum   porcinum endive, groin du porc. see 113. *Cichorium endivia.* **W H Y**

392a. Rubia   madder. see 197, 434a, 474, 497 *Rubia tinctoris.* **T H Y**

393. Rubis   blackberry, bramble, framboisier moron. ronces rouge are unripe. see 154. *Ronces nemorosus et al.* **R T W H Y**

394. Rue herb   ruta, moly, galigan. oil. *Ruta angustifolia and R. graveolans. A. montana.* **R T W H Y**

395. Rumex   patience, sorrel, oxalis, lappa, burdoch, dock, acedula, great mullein, shepherd's crook, bouillon, hare's-beard. see 16, 49b, 236, 294a, 329, 356, 433, 457. *Rumex acetosa et al.* **T W H Y**

395a. Rye   flour. siligo. *Secale cereale.* **T**

396. Sabina   cypress, or juniper. the resin is sandarac. see 149, 479. **T**

397. Saccharum   beeswax. see 220, 293.

397a. Safflower   carthamus.(not saffron). see 91. *Catrhamus tinctorius.* **R W**

398. Saffron   safron, colchicum, zafranatis, crocus. see 91, 141, 219. *Crocus sativus.* **R T W L H Y**

399. Sagapenum   another ferula plant resin. see 37, 429 *Ferula persica.* **R B T Y**

400. Sage   many varieties. herb salvia, sange, lungwort, palma marina, pulmonaria, gallitricum. see 196, 258a, 405. **R T W L H Y**

401. Sagimen   aphroniton, spuma nitri. precipitate of potassium nitrate. **H Y**

401a Saints' Herbs   Saint Bennett's, see 116. **T.** Saint John's, see 13, 35, 287, 287a, 372a,**T,** Saint Mary's, see 49, 361, 454 Saint Peter's, see 140a.

Sal armoniac   see 424. **W L H Y**

Sal baurachi   borax. see 63, 402. **R W L H Y**

402 Sal de nitre   nitrum, borax, saltpeter. see 63,402. **R W L H Y**

402a Salex   salix. see 495. **H Y**

403. Saliva   spittle. **R T W L**

403a. Salsola   samphire, glass-wort, sal alkali. see 140a, 406a. *Salsola kali.* **H**

404. Salt   sal. common or rock, sel gemma, brine, aloxan (brine 'flower'), muriate of soda. **R B T W L H Y**

405. Salvia   sage (many varieties), centrum galli, also darnel, cockle, clary, ieble, salge-damasche, salge-savage. see 196, 400. *Salvia officinalis.* **R H Y**

406. Sambucus   elder tree, sureau, seu, ebulus. see 165. *Sambucus nigra.* **R L H Y**

406a. Samphire   saphira, glass-wort, marine crest. see 140a, 403a, 487, 501.**T H**

407. Sandalwood   sandalus. *Santalum album and rubium.* **R T W L H**

	Sanamunda	hare's foot, caryophylla. see, 93 et al. **H**
	Sandarac	the resin. see 396. **H**
408.	Sang dragon	sang de dragunt, sedge. resin of *Calamus draco.* **R B T W H Y**
	Sanguinaria	see 140a, 406a, 487, 501. **H**
409.	Sanguis	blood: goat, sheep, deer, tortoise, bat, frog, snake, ox, dove hare, menstrual etc. **B T H**
	Sapa	grape syrup. see 208, and sappa michum, a syrup with honey.
409a.	Saracenic ointment	102, 105, 173, 206, 242, 242, 286, 368c. **R T**
410.	Sarcocolla	argemone. resin of *Pinea mucronata or Astragalus fasciculoformis.* **R B T W L H Y**
411.	Saturieia	herb savory. *Satureia hortensis.* **T H**
411a.	Satyrion	an aphrodysiac orchid. see 472. *Satyrion hircinum.* **W**
412.	Savon	French soap, sapo, soapwort, saponaria, burith. soap. see 244a, 430c **R T W L H**
412a.	Savory	many varieties. *Satureia hortensis.* **H**
413.	Saxifrage	marathrum. flowers or leaves. see 27, 349. **T W H Y**
414.	Scabious	devil's bit, jacea, knautia arvensis, morsus diabole. see 228b. *Centurea scabiosa.* **R T W L H Y**
415.	Scalllions	bulbus, onions. see 101, 319. **W**
416.	Scammony	bindweed, convolvulus, anabula, diagridum. see 152b. *Scammonaciae, several varieties.* **T W L H Y**
	Scariola	chicory. see 113. **T H**
416a.	Schoenanthum	palea camelorum, juncus. see 444. **H**
417.	Scoloprendre	ceterach, hart's-tongue fern, cow-tongue, bugloss, blue weed. see 69. **W H**
418.	Scordium	wood sage, a germander. see 200, 346. *Eucrium scordium.* **W**
418a.	Scorpion	incinerated. **L H**
419.	Scoria	ferrugo, iron filings and rust, merda ferri and

	cimolea, limailles. the dross of melted iron. see 216.**W H Y**
420. Scrophularia	pennywort, centumcellie, toad-flax, umbilicus venus, linaria, cymbalaire, quadrangular, many varieties of *Scrophularaciae nodosum, aquativca, etc. Linaria vulgaris.* **R T L H Y**
421. Sebestes	sebesten plums, cordia myxa. see 355. **T Y**
422. Sedge	cyperes. see 74, 148b, 207, 434, 444. **W L**
422a. Sedum	stonecrop. see 446b. **R Y**
423. Seeds	common seeds, including lettuce, endive, purslain, chicory, melons. see 123a. **R T W**
424. Sel armoniac	sal ammoniac, ammonium chlorhydrate, (not from 23) (commonly called"arsenic"). **B W L Y**
424a Self-heal	sanicula, prunella. see 368 et al. **H Y**
Selinum	apium seeds. see 29, 344. **L**
425. Sempervivum	crassula minor, house leek, leeks, joubarbe, sticado. see 229 et al. **R T W L**
426. Senape	synapus, senevé, mustard. see 171, 297. **R B T W L Y**
Senecio	also senacio. groundsel see 102. **T Y**
427. Senna	many cassia varieties.Diasunna is a potent laxative. see 94. *Cassia fistula* **T W Y**
428. Septemnervée	handacotte, septfoil centinervia, ribwort, quinquenervia, tormentila see 215, 353. *Plantago* **R T W**
429. Serapinas	serapias, sarapinas, sagapenum. see 37, 399. *Ferula persica.* **R W L H Y**
430. Sesali	lovage, white gentian. See 174, 247, 256. *Laerpitum siler.* **W**
Shepherd's Crook	rumex. see 395.
Sicadis	white bryony. see 67. **H**
Sifula	sider, aneth, sweet absinthe see 26. **H**
430a. Silex	flint. **Y**
Siligo	rye. see 187 (white), 395a. **T**
430b. Silver	argentum. flos, ashes. **L**

Sisymbro	horse-mint, menthastrum. see 281. **R**
430bb. Skin	cow and sheep, for making collagen, parchment, pellis. see 204. **W**
Snails	see 249. **T H Y**
Snake-root	serpentaria. see 33.
Snakes	various. see 273a. **H**
430c. Soap	usually a strong soap, lessive, perhaps French soap, Saracenic soap etc. see 244a, 412. **T W L H Y**
Soapwort	see 412. **R**
Socotrin	aloes, succatrensis. see 19.
431. Solathrum	nightshade, henbane, solanum, morele, camel, mors canis, egg-plant see 217, 232, 290a. *Solanum nigrum et al.* **R T W L H Y**
431a Solea	leather, soglia. see 124, 204, 242a, 430bb. **R H**
431b. Soot	from ovens, chimneys etc. see 38, etc. **H**
432. Sorba	cormes. fruits of the mountain ash. *Sorbus domestica, and Sorbus ancuparia.* **T L H**
433. Sorrel	oxalis, oseille, rumex, lapathum, burdock see 329, 395. **T W Y**
434. Souchet	a sedge, see 5, 74, 75, 422, 444.
434a. Spergula	spargula, madder. see 392a. **H**
435. Spathula	foetida stinking iris. *Iris foetidissima.* **R T H**
436. Spelt	epeautre, hard wheat. see 21, etc. **W**
436a. Sperm	goat. **T**
437. Spic	spikenard, nard. See 43a, 168a, 302, 475. *Valeriana officinalis, Inula conyza et al* . **B T W L H Y**
438. Spider web	toile d'araignée, tela aranea. cobweb. see 31. **B W H**
438a. Spig	any lichen, especially *Lichen gyratis.* **W**
Spina	hawthorn. see 215a. **B**
438b. Spinach	*Spinacea oleracia.* **H**
438c. Spleen-wort	a scaly fern. *Asplenum ceterach.* **T**
439. Spode	zinc oxide, tuthie, pompholyx, cathimia, calamine see 121. **W L Y**

440. Spodium   calcined arrowroot. *Maranta arundinacia*. **L H**
     Sponge   whole or ashes. see 117. **T H**
441. Spuma d'argent écume d'argent, flower of silver, litharge. see
                    121, 253. **R T W**
441a Spuma maris   magnesium silicate, meerschaum. see 162. **W
                    L H**
442. Spurge   resin of a euphorbium. See 171, 173. *Euphorbia lathyris*. **R T L**
442a. Squid   os sepiae, seiche, sepia. burnt bone. see 62. **T
                    H**
443. Squill   wild hyacinth. See 222. *Scilla maritima*. **R T W L
                    H Y**
444. Squinanthus   sinancie, another calamus, schoenanthum. see
                    5, 74, 75, 416a 422, 434. *Andropogon schoenanthus.*
                    R T W L H
444a. Stag's horn   any fern of genus *Platycerum*. **T**
445. Staphisagre   larkspur, delphinium, cheif d'espurge,
                    polycaria, pes alauda, jonquarola. *Delphinium
                    staphisagre or inula policaria*. **R T W H Y**
445a. Stellaria   chick-weed. morsus gallinae. *Stellaria media*. **H**
446. Stellion   gaulus, a musk-like excrement of lizards. see
                    257.**W**
     Stercus   feces. see 179.
     Sticado   joubarbs. see 229, 446a. also *Stoechas citrinus
                    and Graphalum stoechas.*
446a Stoechas   many varieties. see sticado and 240. also *Stoechas
                    arabica*. **W H Y**
446b. Stonecrop   vermicularis. see 422a. *Sedum acre*. **R Y**
446c Straw   reeds, grasses, etc. see 378a, 386. **H**
446d. Strawberry   *Fragaria vesca*. **Y**
447. Styrax (storax) assefan, liquid amber, benzoin. calamite is inferior grade storax. see 36, 41, 73. *Liquidambar
                    orientale (a tree)*. **R B T W L H**
447a. Sudor   sweat, animal or human. **R**
448. Sugar   alun de sucre, zuccharum, nabete (powdered)

sugar candy, penedis is a droplet of sugar, sugar of violets etc. **R B T W L H Y**

Sureau   elder. see 165. **H Y**

449. Sumach   the poisonous toxicodendron. *Rhus coriaria* as well as non—poisonous *R. aromaticum*. **B T L Y**

450. Sulfur   often stated as 'live', being fresh from the mine. **R T W L H**

450a. Swallow-wort   milk-weed. *Cynanthum vincitoxicum*. **T**

450b. Sycomore   sap of *Ficus sycomorus*. sometimes the Egyptian mulberry. **Y**

451. Talpa   the mole. see 273a. **H**

452. Tamarind   tamarind fruit. *Tamarindus indica*. **T W L Y**

453. Tamariscus   sap of manna, ash tree. see 189, 264. *Fraxinus ornus, Mysicaria germanica*. **R T W H**

454. Tansy   athanasia, St. Mary's Herb, fever-few. *Tanacetum vulgare*. **T H Y**

455. Tar   naval, piotch, pix, Greek. see 304, 352, 359, 360. **R B T H Y**

Tarragon   dracunculus. see 161a.

456. Tartar   potassium bitartrate from wine lees. **R T W L H Y**

457. Tassus   Barbatus tassebarbatus. great mullein (bouillon). see 356. *Verbascum thapsus*. **R T W H Y**

458. Teazle   chardun thistle, dipsacus, cardo. see 100, 102, 159, 487. **T Y**

Tenacetum   tansy. see 454

459. Terebinth   also olibanum, xylobalsamum. closely related to mastic. alkitron is a distillate. see 272, 351. also *Pistacia terebinthus*. **R W L H Y**

Terpentine   pitch. see 352.

460. Terra sigillata   an astringent trochee of baobab fruit, *Adansonia digitata*, or a reddish clay of Lemnos, fashioned like an Egyptian seal. chimolia or cymolea. **R T W L H Y**

461. Thapsus   tapsie, another scrofularia umbellifer. see 36. *Thapsia villosa and Th. garganilla*. **R T H**

462. Theriac — many formulas through the centuries, Galen's Greater Treacle. The diatesseron variety contained 58, 199, 220 and 238(berries). Recently called treacle. see 156b. **T W L H Y**

Thistle — teazle. see 458 et al.

463. Thus — tus, cortex thuris. a thick frankincense, see 168, 188, 316. *Boswellia thurifera.* **B W L H**

464. Thyme — calamint. *Thymus capitatus.* **T W H**

Titimalle — euphorbia. see 173. **R T H Y**

Toad flax — scrophularia. see 420.

Tongue — see 69

464a. Tonnina — Mediterranean tuna. **T**

465. Tormentilla — sarsaparilla, quinquefolum, cinqfoil, potentilli, geranium maculatum, cranesbill or doves-foot, pie de colomb, pseudoselinon, callipetalon. *Potentilla reptans.* **T H Y**

466. Tragacanth — dragacanth, adracanth. see 8, 153a, 213 *Astragalus gummifer.* **B T W L Y**

Tremula — poplar. see 364a (quaking aspen). **T**

467. Tribulus — water thistle, water chestnut or Burra Gukaroo. *Tribulus terrestris or T. aqautica.* **H**

Triticum — wheat. see 494.

468. Tryphére — an electuary containing truffles and various sweets. **W**

469. Turbith — turpeth, diatesseron laxative, roots of *Operculum turpathum.* **B T L Y**

Turmeric — curcuma. see 146 and 503.

469a Turpentine — pitch. see 352.**T W L**

470. Tussilage — colt's foot. *Ungula caballina.* **H Y**

471. Tuthie (tutty) — see spode. see 121, 439. **T W L H Y**

Umbilicus — venus cymbalaria. see 136, 420. **R L H**

472. Unguis caprae — goat slipper. see 411a. **H**

472a Urine — animal and human. **B T H Y**

Urtica — nettles. see 305, 326.

Uva — grapes. see 208.

473. Uva passa — raisins. **T W H**

474. Valania   madder. see 197, 392a. *Rubia tinctorium.* **W**

475. Valerian   phu, amatilla, fistra. spikenard. see 302, 437. **T H Y**

476. Venus hair   maidens-hair fern, capillus venus, bed-straw. see 7, 36, 181a. *Adiantum capillus veneris.* **T H Y**

Venus ointment apostolicon. see 30

Verbascum   tassus barbatus, see 457. **Y**

477. Verbena   vervaine, hiera botane, verminacula. *Verbena officinalis.* **R T W L H Y**

478. Verjus   agresta, vinum acerbum, a potion from sour grapes or other sour fruits. see 12, 335, 485.

478a. Vermicularis   stonecrop, sedum. see 446b

Vermis   worms. see 258, 499. **H**

479. Vernis   juniper tree sap, encaustrum. see 167a *Thuia articulata* . **T W H Y**

480. Vespa   wasp. **H**

481. Vert d'Airain   vert d'araim, ziniar, fleur d'arain, flos aeris, viride aes, bronze flower, similar to 482. **R T L H Y**

482. Vert de Gris   ziniar, copper 'flower', copper acetate, chloride or sulfate. See 10, 65a, 106, 130, 481. **R T W L H Y**

483. Vetch   ers, orobe. see 325. **L**

484. Vinegar   acetum, aisil. **R B T W L H Y**

485. Vinum goretum raw styptic wine. see 12, 478. **W**

486. Violets   oil of or water of many varieties of *Violaria.* **R B T W L H Y**

487. Virgo pastoris   shepherd's purse, another dipsacus, sanguinary, centinodium, passerinus, proserpinaia. see 501 et al. *D. sylvestris.* **T W L H**

488. Virgo cervi   deer's penis. **H**

489. Viticella   white bryony, vitis. see 67, 120 etc. *Clematis flammula.* **R L H**

490. Vitriol rosa   red iron sulfate, couperose, atrament, chalcantum, colcothar, ink, Roman vitriol. **R T W L H Y**

490a. Water chestnut — *Trapa natans.* **T**

490b. Water cress — plantain. see 353. *Nasturtium officianale, Lepidium sativum* . **R Y**

491. Water lilies — nenuphar, dardana, fafara. see 304a. *Nymphea alba.* **T W L H Y**

492. Watermelon — fruit, wild and cultivated. see 280.**Y**

492a Water mint — *Mentha aquatica.* **T**

492b. Waters — sea, rain, spring, containing drownings etc. see 286, 300, 364, 391.

493. Wax — white and red (cera alba and rossa), cere, sire, oxycroceum. see 329a. **R B T W L H Y**

494. Wheat — froment, triticum. pigle is coarsely ground. see 21 et al. **T W L Y**

494a. Wm. Somer's Oint. 379 and 485. **T L**

Whey — serum. especially goat's. see 286. **Y**

495. Willow — salex. withe. tree bark, and flowers *Salix alba and nigra.* **W L**

496. Wines — many varieties, named by color, region, potency, acidity, thickness. see 485. **R B T W L H Y**

Winter seeds — the four cool-weather seeds. 137,144, 280, 492. see 123a. **T**

497. Woad — pastel, the dye. See 197, 392a. *Isatis tinctoria.* **Y**

497a. Wood — various kinds, including Brazil-wood. see 11a, etc **H**

498. Wool — laine muste, lana succida, unwashed fleece. see 235. **R B W Y**

499. Worms — lumbrici, ver, verm, maggots. see 258. **T L Y**

Wormwood — absinthe. see 1.

Xylobalsamum — terebinth. see 459 **W**

500. Yari — cuckoopint arum, se. see 35a. *Arum maculata.*

501. Yarrow — mille feuille, sanguinary. see 223, 287. **B W**

502. Yeast — fermentum. leaven. **W H**

Yellow Oint. — citrin. contains 181, 188, 312, 379, 493. **H Y**

502a Yerasimum — erysimus, ? Saint Simon's herb, or simissome. Yperman used it as a mild laxative for children. see 458. *Erysimum cheiranthoides* Y

	Yreos	iris. see 228.
	Ysopus	see 206, 311.
502b.	Ysis	isis. any lichen of genus *Isidium*. **T**
	Yva	gum eve, iva arthretica, a germander. see 353. *Teucrium chamaedrys*. **T**
503.	Zedoaria	turmeric. see 146. *Curcuma longa et al.* **H Y**
503a.	Zegi	ink, vitriol. **W**
	Ziniar verdigris. see 482.	
	Zinziber	ginger. see 24, 201. **H**
	Zizania	lolium. see 255
	Zucca	pumpkin. see 369 **R**
	Zuccharum	sugar. see 448.

Appendix II Persons Cited in the Text

The list includes the names cited by Yperman, by DeMets and by the English translator

ACTOR Probably Actuarius. Physician in the Byzantine Court Fl. 1250-80

AGRIPPA Fl. 100 AD, Rome

ALBERT THE GREAT The 13th C schoar and polymath 1193-1280

ALBUCASIS Fl. 1000 AD, Cordova
In Arabic he was Abul Kasim Chalaf Ben Alban el Zaroam. His *Surgery and Instruments* , Translated by MS Spink and GL
Lewis,University of
California Press, Berkeley, 1973. His work drew much from Paul of Aegina.

AVICENNA 980–1037, Persia
In Arabic he was Abou ali el Ossein, Ibn Abdallah. Shortened by the Europeans to Ibn Sinna. Author of *The Canon*. Cited eleven times by Yperman, more than any other.

BE(N)VENOUD (Bevenutus Grapheus) Fl. 1300, Palestine
A contemporary of Yperman. Author of a book on Ocular Disease. See fn.98 inBook II.

BERNARD OF GORDON French physician, author of The Lily of
Medicine
Montpellier Fl.1300
BRUNO DA LONGOBURGO (in Calabria) Fl. 1250, Padua
Un Chirurgo Italiano (contains an Italian translation of much of
Bruno's *Chirurgia*), M. Tabanelli, Leo S. Olschki, Florence,
1970. English transl. by LD Rosenman. Pittsburgh, Dorrance
Publishing Co.2002.

CONSTANTINUS AFRICANUS 1020-1087, Salerno, Monte
Cassino
A great translator in the early Salernitan Era.

DIOSCORIDES Great Greek Author of the classic Pharmcopeia
Fl. 50 AD

FOUR SALERNITAN MASTERS Fl. 1250
One or more unknowns who wrote *The Gloss on Roger and Roland*. A
description and discussion by C. Daremberg is in Vol. III of
the *Collectio Salernitana*, of S. de Renzi, 1852, pp. 205-254.
Engl. translation by LD Rosenman, 2002. See **Roland**

EXPERIMENTATOR The name of a lost treatise, cited by a
Flemish cleric.Probably
Written during the 13thC. Yperman's citations suggests the name
of a person. Sarton says no.

GALEN 120-310. Rome (Greek origin)
The dominant figure in the medical world before the Renaissance.

GILBERTUS ANGLICUS Fl. 1180-90, Salerno
One of the three leading physicians in England of that era.
Accompanied Richard I on his crusade. Claimed 'The Royal
Touch' as a cure for scrofula began with Edward the Confes-

sor (d.1066). The origin was debated; French authors claimed that it began with Clovis.

GILLES OF CORBEIL Fl. 1200, Salerno
Royal Physician at Paris. Author of a book on Urine.

.

GUY DE CHAULIAC Fl. 1360, Paris
Le Grande Chirurgie (1363), Modern French Edition by E.Nicaise; Germer, Balliere, et Cie, Paris, 1890.

HENRI DE MONDEVILLE 1260-1320, Montpellier and Paris
Chirurgie, (1306-1320), Modern French Edition by E. Nicaise;Germer, Balliere et Cie, Paris, 1893. Engl. transl. by LD Rosenman. Awaiting publication.

HIPPOCRATES 460-?370, Greece
Called the Father of Medicine.

HUGH OF LUCCA (see Theodoric) 1160-1250, Bologna

ISAAC JUDAEUS THE ELDER Egypt. Physician and philosopher Fl. 900

LANFRANCHI Fl. 1180-1205, Milan-Paris
Left Milan as a political refugee, came to Paris @ 1295. A pupil of William of Saliceto. Taught Yperman and Mondeville, et. al. A Middle-English edition was published in 1380. Edited as '*Science of Surgery'* by R.von Fleischhacker, 1894. London, Early English Text Society. English transl. by LD Rosenman. Awaiting publication.

MACER Udo von Meudon, d. 1161, Germany
The name 'Macer' was the familiar title of his book "*Macer Floridus*" rather than an author's name.

NICOLAUS Fl. 1250, Alexandria and Nicaea
Nicholas Myrepsos, Author of the great Antidotary of that era.

PETER LUCRATOR Probably Peter of Abano. Called "The Lucidator" 1250-1320

PITARD 1228-1325, Paris
Surgeon to Louis IX; founder of College of Saints Cosmos and Damien (St. Comê)
Dominant figure in guiding French surgery out of the low level of early 13th C.

PLATEARIUS Fl. 1150, Salerno
Probably Matthew, son of John. The last of a famous family of physicians and herbalists, dating from the 11thC

PLINY THE ELDER Encyclopedist. Rome 23-79 AD

RHAZES Fl. 900, Persia
In Arabic Abou Bekr Mohammed ibn Zakarias. Wrote the *Book of Almansor* and the *Continens.*

ROGER FRUGARD Fl. 1170, Salerno—Padua
The first author of a surgical text in Europe. His *Chirurgia* was transl. in Italian by L.Stroppiana and D.Spallone in 1957. Rome. Istituto di Storia della Medicina della Universita di Roma. English translation by LD Rosenman. Philadelphia. Xlibris Co., 2002.

ROLAND OF PARMA Fl. 1200, Italy
Copied, editedand revised Roger's work. Roland.s *Chirurgia* is in de Renzi's *Collectio Salkernitana*, Vol. II. An Italian edition by M. Tabanelli is in *La Chirurgia Italiana Nell'Alto Medioevo*, 1965, Florence, Leo S. Olschki, English translation by LD Rosenman,includes Daremberg's Essay on the Four Salernitan Masters (v.i.). Philadelphia. Xlibris Co., 2002

SERAPION Fl. 850 Damascus
In Arabic Ibn Seraphioun. Better known as Serapion the Elder.

DeMets confused him with an Alexandrene of the 2ndC BC.

THEODORIC 1206-1298, Bologna-Cervia
SURGERY, translated by E Campbell and J Colton, Appleton-Century-Crofts, New York, 1960. He was the follower and possibly the real son of Hugh of Lucca. His text describes his Master's methods.

WILLIAM OF CONGENIS Fl. 1250, Montpellier
Physician known for a surgical text largely copied from Roger's.

WILLIAM OF MOERBEKE **cited as Medicke. A Flemish Monk 1215-1286**

WILLIAM OF SALICETO 1210-1280, Italy
The Master Surgeon of the latter 13th C. Taught Lanfranchi. His *Chirurgia* was translated into French by P. Pifteau. 1898. Toulouse, Imprim. Saint Cyprien. English translation by LD Rosenman. Awaiting publication.